This book is to be returned on or before
the last date stamped below.

H. Löffler · J. Rastetter

Atlas of Clinical Hematology

Springer

Berlin
Heidelberg
New York
Barcelona
Hong Kong
London
Milan
Paris
Singapore
Tokyo

H. Löffler · J. Rastetter

Atlas of Clinical Hematology

Initiated by L. Heilmeyer
and H. Begemann

Fifth Revised Edition

With 199 Figures, in 1032 separate Illustrations,
Mostly in Color, and 18 Tables

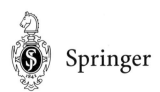 Springer

Professor Dr. med. Helmut Löffler
Ehem. Direktor der II. Medizinischen Klinik und Poliklinik
der Universität Kiel im Städtischen Krankenhaus
Seelgutweg 7, 79271 St. Peter, Germany

Professor Dr. med. Johann Rastetter
Ehem. Leiter der Abteilung für Hämatologie und Onkologie
1. Medizinische Klinik und Poliklinik
Klinikum rechts der Isar der Technischen Universität München
Westpreußenstraße 71, 81927 München, Germany

English editions

© Springer-Verlag Berlin Heidelberg
1st ed. 1955
2nd ed. 1972
3rd ed. 1979
4th ed. 1989

German editions

Atlas der klinischen Hämatologie
© Springer-Verlag Berlin Heidelberg
1st ed. 1955
2nd ed. 1972
3rd ed. 1978
4th ed. 1987
5th ed. 1999

Japanese edition

Rinsho Ketsuekigaku Atlas
© Springer-Verlag Tokyo, 1989

Editions published under license

Spanish edition
published by
Editorial Cientifico-Médica
Barcelona, 1973

Italien edition
published by
PICCIN Editore S.A.S.
Padova, 1973, 1980

Japanese edition
published by
Igaku Shoin Ltd.
Tokyo, 1975

Translated by: Terry C. Telger, Fort Worth, Texas, USA

ISBN 3-540-65085-7 Springer-Verlag Berlin Heidelberg New York

ISBN 3-540-50851-1 4th Edition Springer-Verlag Berlin Heidelberg New York

Library of Congress Cataloging-in-Publication Data applied for

Die Deutsche Bibliothek – CIP-Einheitsaufnahme

Atlas of clinical hematology / H. Löffler ; J. Rastetter. Initiated by L. Heilmeyer and H. Begemann. – 5., rev. ed. – Berlin ;
Heidelberg ; New York ; Barcelona ; Hongkong ; London ; Milan ; Paris ; Singapore ; Tokyo : Springer, 1999
   Dt. Ausg. u.d.T.: Atlas der klinischen Hämatologie. – 4. Aufl. u.d.T.:
   Begemann, Herbert: Atlas of clinical hematology
   ISBN 3-540-65085-7

Production: PRO EDIT GmbH, 69126 Heidelberg, Germany
Coverdesign: Frido Steinen-Broo, eStudio Calamar, Spain
Typesetting: Mitterweger & Partner Kommunikationsgesellschaft mbH, 68723 Plankstadt, Germany
Computer-to-film: Triltsch, 97070 Würzburg, Germany

SPIN: 10673669   24/3134 – 5 4 3 2 1 0 – Printed on acid-free paper

Preface to the Fifth Edition

The first edition of the *Atlas of Clinical Hematology* was published over 40 years ago. The first four editions were coauthored by Herbert Begemann, who died unexpectedly in April of 1994. We wish to dedicate the fifth edition as a memorial to this dedicated physician and hematologist.

Since the fourth edition was published in 1987, hematology has undergone profound changes. New methods such as cytochemistry and immunophenotyping have been joined by cytogenetics and, more recently, molecular genetic techniques, which have assumed a major role in routine diagnostic procedures. This has been due in part to significant advances in methodology and new tools in molecular biology. When used in standardized protocols, these tools can furnish swift results that are relevant to patient care. Since the advent of cytogenetics and molecular genetics, we have formulated new definitions for clinical and biological entities. An example is promyelocytic leukemia with its two variants (M3 and M3v), the (15;17) translocation, and the PML/RARA fusion gene, which has been successfully treated for the first time with differentiation therapy. Another example is acute myelomonocytic leukemia with abnormal eosinophiles (M4Eo), inversion 16, and the MYH/11/CBFB fusion gene, which has a very good prognosis. The transmission of morphologic findings by electronic data transfer is also gaining importance in hematology, as it permits the immediate review of difficult findings by specialists. Several colleagues seated at their own desks and microscopes can communicate with one another instantaneously by computer monitor. These advances do not alter the fact that hematologists must still have a sound grasp of morphologic principles. Diagnostic problems often arise when modern counting devices and cell sorters, with their impressive capabilities, are used without regard for cellular morphology. There is no question that classical morphology has gained much from its competition and comparison with the new techniques, leading to significant diagnostic and prognostic advances.

While retaining the basic concept of the previous editions, we found it necessary to eliminate several chapters. Now that many hematologic centers and laboratories are equipped with fluorescence-activated cell sorters (FACS) for immunotyping, and given the availability of reliable commercial kits and precise staining instructions for immunocytochemistry, the chapter by B. R. Kranz has been omitted from the present edition. We have also dropped the methodology section and most of the electron micrographs supplied by Prof. D. Huhn. Both colleagues merit our sincere thanks. Ever since the first edition, Prof. W. Mohr of Hamburg has authored the chapter on blood parasites as the principal causative agents of tropical diseases, and we gratefully acknowledge his contribution. Following the death of Prof. Mohr, we have chosen to include this chapter owing to the special importance of tropical diseases in the modern world. We are grateful to Prof. R. Disko of Munich, who agreed to revise and update the chapter.

The chapters on chronic myeloproliferative diseases, and especially those dealing with myelodysplasias, acute leukemias, malignant lymphomas, and malignant mastocytoses, had to be extensively revised or rewritten. We have added new sections and illustrations on therapy-induced bone marrow changes, cytologic changes in the cerebrospinal fluid due to leukemic or lymphomatous meningeal involvement, and NK cell neoplasias. We have also endeavored to give due attention to issues in pediatric hematology.

In compiling this revised fifth edition, in which over 90 % of the illustrations are new, we benefited greatly from our two decades of central morphological diagnostics for the ALL and AML studies in adults and the morphological consulting of the BFM treatment study on AML in children (H. L.). We thank the directors of these studies, Professors D. Hoelzer, T. Büchner, U. Creutzig, and J. Ritter, for their consistently fine cooperation. We also thank the Institute of Pathology of the University of Kiel, headed by Prof. Karl Lennert, and the current head of the Department of Hematologic Pathology, Prof. Reza Parwaresch, for preparing histologic sections of the tissue cores that we submitted.

Acknowledgements

We are indebted to Prof. Brigitte Schlegelberger, Prof. Werner Grote (director of the Institute of Human Genetics, University of Kiel), Dr. Harder, and Mr. Blohm for providing the cytogenetic findings and schematic drawings. We limited our attention to important findings that have bearing on the diagnosis or confirmation of a particular entity.

A work of this magnitude cannot be completed without assistance. My secretary of many years, Mrs. Ute Rosburg, often freed me from distracting tasks so that I could gain essential time. Mrs. Margot Ulrich efficiently organized the processing of the photographic materials, while Mrs. Ramm-Petersen, Mrs. Meder, and Mrs. Tetzlaff were meticulous in their performance of cytologic, cytochemical, and immunocytochemical methodologies. My senior staff members in Kiel, Prof. Winfried Gassmann and Dr. Torsten Haferlach, helped with the examination and evaluation of many of the specimens pictured in the Atlas. My colleague Dr. Haferlach collaborated with the study group of Prof. Schlegelberger to introduce the FISH technique into routine clinical use. Finally, we thank Mrs. Monika Schrimpf and the entire staff at Springer-Verlag in Heidelberg as well as Ms. Judith Diemer at PRO EDIT GmbH for their thoughtful and effective support.

St. Peter and Munich   Helmut Löffler · Johann Rastetter
Summer 1999

Preface to the Fourth Edition

Hematology, the study of the blood and its disorders, has existed as a science for approximately one hundred years. During that period it has remained true to its goals. Despite many advances in the submicroscopic and biochemical realm, hematology has clung to its basic postulate that the majority of blood disorders are expressed in morphologically distinct cellular changes. Even modern hematology relies largely on the morphologic examination of cells, and the microscope continues to be its main diagnostic tool. Today we may describe hematology as the only morphologically oriented clinical science. It owes its existence chiefly to the development of staining methods that make it possible to assign morphologic structures to specific cellular functions and thus to specific pathologic states. The first step in this direction was the brilliant discovery of panoptic stains in the early part of this century by Pappenheim, Wright, and others. This was followed in the 1950 s and 1960 s by the development of numerous cytochemical procedures for the differentiation of diverse biochemical reactions and cell types. In the last decade, immunologic methods have been employed to identify cell type-specific antigens as a means of classifying lymphatic and other cells more precisely and more objectively. This has aided in the differentiation of many important hematologic disorders.

In this fourth edition of the *Atlas of Clinical Hematology,* we have attempted to update the text and bring it in line with recent developments. As before, the book is subdivided into a theoretical part and a pictorial part which illustrates the morphologic features of specific disorders using a combination of photomicrographs and watercolor paintings created by Hans and Thea Dettelbacher. The paintings convey a sense of depth to the microscopic image that will help the student appreciate and differentiate morphologic details. We have retained the chapter on electron microscopy, which we regard as a kind of connecting link between cell structures that are visible by light microscopy and the functional significance of those structures. Tropical medicine has become a subject of growing interest to hematologists and internists in our increasingly mobile population, and therefore the section on tropical medicine has been revised and expanded. Also, we have added new photomicrographs and have replaced a number of old ones with photographs of greater clarity.

The present edition features a new, comprehensive chapter on the light-microscopic demonstration of immunologic cell markers. It is divided into a methodologic and a cytologic section and deals extensively with the subtyping of normal and malignant lymphoid cells. This new and difficult chapter was authored by Bernd R. Kranz, who proved to be not only a leading expert in his field but also a cooperative, constructive coworker who offered many helpful suggestions going beyond his area of specialization. We express our sincere thanks for his contributions. We are also indebted to our co-authors Dieter Huhn and Werner Mohr, who worked with us on earlier editions and extensively revised and updated their chapters.

We thank our colleagues Heimpel of Ulm, Kaiserling of Tübingen, Lopes-Cardozo of Leiden, Müller-Hermelink of Würzburg, and Sepp of Munich for supplying specimens and photomicrographs of rare disorders or special cell forms. We are grateful to Mr. Jorg Kuhn, who mastered the difficult task of supplementing the watercolor illustrations done for the first edition by Hans and Thea Dettelbacher. Mr. Kuhn proved to be a talented and sensitive artist, and his contribution is gratefully acknowledged.

Despite her other professional obligations, Dr. Gudula Wernekke-Rastetter has again provided an outstanding subject index. We thank her for turning our atlas into a useful reference work.

If this book recaptures the visual impact of the earlier editions, the credit belongs to Springer-Verlag and its staff as well as to the Dreher Reproduction Service in Stuttgart and Stürtz Printers in Würzburg. All contributed to the success of our book, and all demonstrated great technical expertise and understanding. Everyone with whom we worked took pains to implement our wishes as regards the finished appearance of the volume. Working with them was always a pleasant and satisfying experience. We express our sincere thanks to Dr. H. Götze, Mrs. T. Deigmöller, Mrs. U. Pfaff, Dr. J. Wieczorek, and Mr. K. Söll, to name but a few of the many persons who contributed to the success of this book. Finally we would like to express our sincere thanks to our translator, T. C. Telger.

It is the hope of the editors and authors that this fourth edition of our atlas will enjoy the same enthusiastic critical and consumer response that greeted the first three editions.

Munich, Summer 1989　　　　Herbert Begemann · Johann Rastetter

Preface to the First Edition

So far the diagnostic advances of smear cytology have found only limited applications in medical practice. This is due largely to the fact that available illustrative materials have been too stylized to give the novice a realistic introduction to the field. In the present atlas we attempt to correct this situation by portraying the great morphologic variety that can exist in individual cells and in pathologic conditions. In so doing, we rely mainly on artist's depictions rather than photographs. On the one hand the "objectivity" of color photos, though much praised, is inherently questionable and is further degraded by the process of chemographic reproduction. An even greater drawback of photomicrographs is their inability to depict more than one plane of section in sharp detail. By contrast, a person looking through a microscope will tend to make continual fine adjustments to focus through multiple planes and thus gain an impression of depth. A drawing can recreate this impression much better than a photograph and so more closely approximates the subjective observation. We have avoided depicting cells in black and white; while there is merit in the recommendation of histologists that students' attention be directed toward structure rather than color, this is rarely practicable in the cytologic examination of smears. The staining methods adopted from hematology still form the basis for staining in smear cytology. For this reason most of the preparations shown in this atlas were stained with Pappenheim's panoptic stain. Where necessary, various special stains were additionally used. For clarity we have placed positional drawings alongside plates that illustrate many different cell types, and we have used arrows to point out particular cells in films that are more cytologically uniform.

We were most fortunate to have our color plates drawn by an artist, Hans Dettelbacher, in whom the faculties of scientific observation, technical precision, and artistic grasp are combined in brilliant fashion. We express our thanks to him and to his equally talented daughter Thea, who assisted her father in his work. Without their contribution it is doubtful that the atlas could have been created.

We are also grateful to a number of researchers for providing scientific help and specimens, especially Prof. Dr. Henning and Dr. Witte of Erlangen, Dr. Langreder of Mainz, Prof. Dr. Mohr of the Tropical Institute of Hamburg, Dr. Moeschlin of Zurich, Dr. Undritz of Basel, and Dr. Kuhn of our Freiburg Clinic. We also thank our translators, specifically Dr. Henry Wilde of our Freiburg Clinic for the English text, Dr. Rene Prevot of Mulhouse for the French text, and Dr. Eva Felner-Kraus of Santiago de Chile for the Spanish text. We must not fail to acknowledge the help provided by the scientific and technical colleagues at our hematology laboratory, especially Mrs. Hildegard Trappe and Mrs. Waltraud Wolf-Loffler. Finally, we express our appreciation to Springer Verlag, who first proposed that this atlas be created and took the steps necessary to ensure its technical excellence.

Freiburg, Spring 1955   Ludwig Heilmayer · Herbert Begemann

Contents

Methodology

List of Diseases

Methodology

A. Techniques of Specimen Collection and Preparation

Blood Smear

Differentiation of the peripheral blood is still an important procedure in the diagnosis of hematologic disorders. The requisite blood smears are usually prepared from venous blood anticoagulated with EDTA (several brands of collecting tube containing EDTA are available commercially). However, many special tests require that the blood be drawn from the fingertip or earlobe and smeared directly onto a glass slide with no chemicals added. The slide must be absolutely clean to avoid introducing artifacts. Slides are cleaned most effectively by degreasing in alcohol for 24 h, drying with a lint-free cloth, and final wiping with a chamois cloth (as a shortcut, the slide may be scrubbed with 96 % alcohol and wiped dry).

Preparation of the Smear. The first drop of blood is wiped away, and the next drop is picked up on one end of a clean glass slide, which is held by the edges. (When EDTA-anticoagulated venous blood is used, a drop of the specimen is transferred to the slide with a small glass rod.) Next the slide is placed on a flat surface, and a clean coverslip with smooth edges held at about a 45° tilt is used to spread out the drop to create a uniform film. We do this by drawing the coverslip slowly to the right to make contact with the blood drop and allowing the blood to spread along the edge of the coverslip. Then the spreader, held at the same angle, is moved over the specimen slide from right to left (or from left to right if the operator is left-handed), taking care that no portion of the smear touches the edge of the slide. The larger the angle between the coverslip and slide, the thicker the smear; a smaller angle results in a thinner smear.

Once prepared, the blood smear should be dried as quickly as possible. This is done most simply by waving the slide briefly in the air (holding it by the edges and avoiding artificial warming). The predried slide may be set down in a slanted position on its narrow edge with the film side down. For storage, we slant the slide with the film side up, placing it inside a drawer to protect it from dust and insects.

The best staining results are achieved when the smear is completely air-dried before the stain is applied (usually 4–5 h or preferably 12–24 h after preparation of the smear). In urgent cases the smear may be stained immediately after air drying.

Bone Marrow

Percutaneous aspiration of the posterior iliac spine is the current method of choice for obtaining a bone marrow sample. It is a relatively safe procedure, and with some practice it can be done more easily and with less pain than sternal aspiration. Marrow aspirate and a core sample can be obtained in one sitting with a single biopsy needle (e.g., a Yamshidi needle). When proper technique is used, the procedure is not contraindicated by weakened host defenses or thrombocytopenia. However, there is a significant risk of postprocedural hemorrhage in patients with severe plasmatic coagulation disorders (e.g., hemophilia), in patients on platelet aggregation inhibitors, and in some pronounced cases of thrombocytosis. In all cases the biopsy site should be compressed immediately after the needle is withdrawn, and the patient should be observed. The procedure should be taught by "hands-on" training in the clinical setting.

Aspiration is usually performed after a core biopsy has been obtained. The needle is introduced through the same skin incision and should enter the bone approximately 1 cm from the biopsy site. A sternal aspiration needle may be used with the guard removed, or a Yamshidi needle can be used after removal of the stylet.

The operator rechecks the position of the spine and positions the middle and index fingers of the left hand on either side of the spine. The sternal aspiration needle, with adjustable guard removed, is then inserted until bony resistance is felt and the needle tip has entered the periosteum. This is confirmed by noting that the tip can no longer be moved from side to side. The needle should be positioned at the center of the spine and should be perpendicular to the plane of the bone surface. At this point a steady, gradually increasing pressure is applied to the needle, perhaps combined with a slight rotary motion, to advance the needle through the bone cortex. This may require considerable pressure in some patients. A definite give will be felt as the needle penetrates the cortex and enters the marrow cavity. The needle is attached to a 20-mL glass syringe, the aspiration is performed, and specimens are prepared from the aspirated material.

After the needle is withdrawn, the site is covered with an adhesive bandage and the patient instructed to avoid tub bathing for 24 h.

The usual practice in infants is to aspirate bone marrow from the *tibia*, which is still active hematopoietically.

We prefer to use the needle described by Klima and Rosegger, although various other designs are suitable (Rohr, Henning, Korte, etc.). Basically it does not matter what type of needle is used, as long as it has a bore diameter no greater than 2–3 mm, a well-fitting stylet, and an adjustable depth guard. All bone marrow aspirations can be performed in the ambulatory setting.

Sternal aspiration is reserved for special indications (prior radiation to the pelvic region, severe obesity). It should be practiced only by experienced hematologists. It is usually performed on the sternal midline at approximately the level of the second or third intercostal space. The skin around the puncture site is aseptically prepared, and the skin and underlying periosteum are desensitized with several milliliters of 1 % mepivacaine or other anesthetic solution. After the anesthetic has taken effect, a marrow aspiration needle with stylet and guard is inserted vertically at the designated site. When the needle is in contact with the periosteum, the guard is set to a depth of about 4–5 mm, and the needle is pushed through the cortex with a slight rotating motion. A definite "give" or "pop" will be felt as the needle enters the marrow cavity. Considerable force may have to be exerted if the cortex is thick or hard. When the needle has entered the marrow cavity, the stylet is removed, and a 10- or 20-mL syringe is attached. The connection must be airtight so that an effective aspiration can be performed. The plunger is withdrawn until 0.5 to 1 mL of marrow is obtained. Most patients will experience pain when the suction is applied; this is unavoidable but fortunately is of very brief duration. If no marrow is obtained, a small amount of physiologic saline may be injected into the marrow cavity and the aspiration reattempted. If necessary, the needle may be advanced slightly deeper into the marrow cavity. The procedure is safe when performed carefully and with proper technique. Complications are rare and result mainly from the use of needles without guards or from careless technique. The procedure should be used with caution in patients with plasmacytoma, osteoporosis, or other processes that are associated with bone destruction (e.g., metastases, thalassemia major). Bone marrow aspirations can be performed in the outpatient setting.

For preparation of the smears, we expel a small drop of the aspirated marrow onto each of several glass slides (previously cleaned as described on p. 3) and spread it out with a coverslip as described for the peripheral blood. We also place some of the aspirate into a watch glass and mix it with several drops of 3.6 % sodium citrate. This enables us to obtain marrow particles and prepare smears in a leisurely fashion following the aspiration. If the aspirate is not left in the citrate solution for too long, the anticoagulant will not introduce cell changes that could interfere with standard investigations. We vary our smear preparation technique according to the nature of the inquiry and the desired tests. Spreading the marrow particles onto the slide in a meandering pattern will cause individual cells to separate from the marrow while leaving the more firmly adherent cells, especially stromal cells, at the end of the track. In every bone marrow aspiration an attempt should be made to incorporate solid marrow particles into the smear in addition to marrow fluid in order to avoid errors caused by the admixture of peripheral blood. We see no advantage in the two-coverslip method of smear preparation that some authors recommend. We find that simple "squeeze" preparations often yield excellent results: Several marrow particles or a drop of marrow fluid are expelled from the syringe directly onto a clean glass slide. A second slide is placed over the sample, the slides are pressed gently together, and then they are pulled apart in opposite directions. This technique permits a quantitative estimation of cell content. All marrow smears are air dried and stained as in the procedure for blood smears. Thicker smears will require a somewhat longer staining time with Giemsa solution. Various special stains may also be used, depending on the nature of the study.

If cytologic examination does not provide sufficient information, the *histologic examination of a marrow biopsy specimen* may be indicated. This is especially useful for the differentiation of processes that obliterate the bone marrow, including osteomyelosclerosis or -fibrosis in neoplastic diseases and abnormalities of osteogenesis, the blood vessels, and the marrow reticulum. In recent years the Yamshidi needle has become increasingly popular for bone marrow biopsies.

Fine-Needle Aspiration of Lymph Nodes and Tumors

The fine-needle aspiration of lymph nodes and tumors is easily performed in the outpatient setting. The diagnostic value of the aspirate varies in different pathologic conditions. An accurate histologic classification is usually essential for sound treatment planning and prognostic evaluation, and so the histologic examination has become a standard tool in primary diagnosis. The unquestioned value of the cytologic examination of aspirates is based on the capacity for rapid orientation and frequent follow-ups, adding an extra dimension to the static impression furnished by histologic sections.

The technique of lymph node aspiration is very simple: Using a 1 or 2 gauge (or smaller) hypodermic needle with a 10- or 20-mL syringe attached, we fixate the lymph node between two fingers of the free hand, insert the needle into the node, and apply forceful suction to aspirate a small amount of material. A thinner needle should be used for tissues that contain much blood, and some authors routinely use needles of gauge 12, 14, or 16 (outer diameter 0.6–0.9 mm). Special equipment is available that permits one-handed aspiration (e.g., the Cameco pistol grip syringe holder) and even the use of one-way syringes.

The tissue fragments on the needle tip and inside the needle are carefully expelled onto a glass slide, and a smear is prepared. It is rare for tissue to be drawn into the syringe, but if this material is present it may be utilized for bacteriologic study. The smears are stained like a blood film, and special stains may be used as needed. The aspiration is almost painless and does not require anesthesia. If the lymph node is hard or if histologic examination of the aspirate is desired, we use a somewhat larger gauge needle (approximately 1–2 mm in diameter) that has a stylet and a sharp front edge. The stylet is withdrawn before the node is punctured. Of course, the use of a larger needle requires preliminary anesthesia of the skin and lymph node capsule. All *tumors* that are accessible to a percutaneous needle can be aspirated in similar fashion.

Splenic Aspiration

Splenic aspiration is rarely practiced nowadays and is always performed under some form of radiologic guidance. Today it is indicated only in certain forms of hypersplenism or unexplained splenic enlargement. We consider the Moeschlin technique to be the safest. Splenic aspiration is contraindicated in patients with hemorrhagic diathesis, septic splenomegaly, splenic cysts, or painful splenomegaly due to excessive capsular tension or infarction. The procedure should be used with caution in patients with hypertension of the portal or splenic vein (Banti syndrome, splenic vein thrombosis, splenomegalic cirrhosis). It should be withheld from dazed patients who are unable to cooperate. Moeschlin recommends that splenic aspiration be performed only when definite splenic enlargement is noted and only under stringent aseptic conditions. The procedure is safest when performed under ultrasound guidance, as this will demonstrate not only the size and position of the spleen but also any pathologic changes (e.g., splenic cysts) that would contraindicate the procedure.

Concentrating Leukocytes from Peripheral Blood in Leukocytopenia

Principle. White blood cells are centrifuged after sedimentation of the erythrocytes to concentrate the nucleated cells and make it easier to detect abnormal cell forms.

Reagents

1. Gelatin, 3 %, in 0.9 % NaCl (or plasma gel infusion solution; B. Braun, Melsungen)
2. Heparin (cresol-free)

Method. Place 3–5 mL of venous blood or EDTA-treated blood into a narrow tube, add 1/4 volume gel to the sample and carefully mix by tilting. Let stand at 37 °C for 14 min, 7 min at a 45° slant, and 7 min upright. Pipet off the leukocyte-rich layer and centrifuge lightly at 2000 rpm. Decant the supernatant, gently shake out the sediment, and prepare the smears.

Demonstration of Sickle Cells

Method. Place 1 drop of blood onto a slide and cover with a coverslip.

Place 1 drop of 2 % sodium thiosulfate ($Na_2S_2O_4$) along one edge of the coverslip and hold a blotter against the opposite edge, the object being to draw the Na thiosulfate beneath the coverslip so that it mixes with the blood. (If this is unsuccessful, it may be necessary to raise the coverslip slightly or even add the Na thiosulfate directly to the blood before covering. However, it is best to mix the thiosulfate and blood in the absence of air, as described above!)

Create an airtight seal around the coverslip with paraffin, and let stand for 30 min at room temperature. Examine the unstained slide under the microscope.

B. Light Microscopic Procedures

1. Staining Methods for the Morphologic and Cytochemical Differentiation of Cells

Pappenheim's Stain (Panoptic Stain)

The hematologic stain that we use most frequently, and which was used in most of the plates pictured in this atlas, is Pappenheim's panoptic stain. It is based on a combination of the Jenner-May-Grünwald stain and Giemsa stain.

Method. Place the air-dried slide with the film side up in prepared May-Grünwald eosin-methylene blue solution for 3 min. Dilute with water or buffer solution (phosphate buffer pH 7.3, see below) for an additional 3 min. Pour off this solution and apply Giemsa stain immediately, without intermediate rinsing. The stock Giemsa stain is diluted with neutral distilled water by adding 10 mL water per 10 drops of Giemsa solution. Stain the specimen for 15 to 20 min. The dilution ratio and Giemsa staining time should be individually adjusted to allow for inevitable variations in the composition of the solution. After Giemsa staining, wash the slide with neutral water and tilt to air-dry. Fixation is effected by the methyl alcohol already contained in the May-Grünwald solution. The quality of the stain depends greatly on the pH of the water that is used. The smear will be too red if the water is too acidic and too blue if the water is too alkaline. Standard pH strips can be used to test the water for proper acidity. Water left standing in the laboratory can easily become too acidic through exposure to acid fumes, especially from carbon dioxide. The latter problem is solved by preboiling. A more accurate way to ensure correct acidity for staining is to use a pH 7.3 buffer solution (22.3 mL of 1/15 mol/L KH_2PO_4 + 77.7 mL of 1/15 mol/L Na_2HPO_4) instead of water.

Undritz Toluidine Blue Stain for Basophils

Reagent. Saturated toluidine blue-methanol: dissolve 1 g toluidine blue in 100 mL methanol. The solution will keep indefinitely.

Method. Fix and stain the air-dried smears on the staining rack by covering with the toluidine blue-methanol for 5 min. Wash in tap water, air dry.

Interpretation. The granulations in basophils and mast cells stain a red-violet color owing to the strong metachromatic effect of the sulfate present in the heparin. As a result, these cells are easily identified even at moderate magnification. By contrast, azurophilic granules (even in severe "toxic" granulation) and the coarse granules in leukocytes affected by Adler anomaly show very little violet transformation of their blue color.

Mayer's Acid Hemalum Nuclear Stain

This is used for the blue contrast staining of nuclei in assays of cytoplasmic cell constituents (glycogen, enzymes; pp. 10 ff.) and in immunocytochemistry.

Reagents. Dissolve 1 g hematoxylin (Merck) in 1 L distilled water and add 0.2 g sodium iodate ($NaIO_3$) and 50 g aluminum potassium sulfate ($KAl(SO_4)_2 \cdot 12H_2O$). After these salts are dissolved, add 50 g chloral hydrate and 1 g crystallized citric acid. The hemalum will keep for at least 6 months at 20 °C with no change in staining properties. The solution can also be purchased in ready-to-use form.

Method. The necessary staining time in the hemalum bath varies with the method of specimen preparation and must be determined by progressive staining. After staining, wash the slide for at least 15 min in several changes of *tap* water (acid residues may reduce the intensity of the stain).

Heilmeyer's Reticulocyte Stain

Draw a 1 % brilliant cresyl blue solution in physiologic saline to the 0.5 mark of a white cell counting pipet, and draw up the blood to the 1.0 mark. Expel the mixture carefully, without forming air bubbles, into a paraffinated watchglass dish, mix carefully with a paraffinated glass rod, and place in a moist chamber for 15–20 min. Then remix carefully with a paraffinated glass rod. With the rod, transfer 1 or 2 drops of the mixture to a microscope slide and smear in standard fashion using a ground coverslip. Examine the air-dried slides under oil-immersion magnification, and count the number of reticulocytes per 1000 red cells at multiple sites in the smear. Very high-quality films can be obtained by Giemsa counterstaining.

Heinz Body Test of Beutler[1]

This test is used to detect defects of red cell metabolism that do not allow glutathione to be maintained in a reduced state. The defect may result from a glucose-6-phosphate dehydrogenase deficiency, a glutathione reductase deficiency, diseases with "unstable hemoglobin," or an "idiopathic" Heinz body anemia. The test involves the oxidative denaturation of hemoglobin to intraerythrocytic "Heinz bodies" following incubation of the red cells with acetylphenylhydrazine.

Reagents

1. Sörensen phosphate buffer, pH 7.6, 0.67 M:
   $1/15$ M KH_2PO_4 13 parts.
   $1/15$ M Na_2HPO_4 87 parts.
2. Glucose phosphate buffer: dissolve 0.2 g glucose in 100 mL phosphate buffer. The solution may be stored frozen or at $4\,^{\circ}C$ (watch for clouding!).
3. Acetylphenylhydrazine solution: dissolve 20 mg acetylphenylhydrazine in 20 mL glucose phosphate buffer at room temperature. This solution is prepared fresh and should be used within 1 h.
4. (a) Dissolve saturated alcohol solution of brilliant cresyl blue; or (b) 0.5 g methyl violet in 100 mL of 0.9 % NaCl, and filter; blood: heparinized, defibrinated, or treated with EDTA.

Method. Centrifuge the blood lightly for 5 min. Pipet 0.05 mL of test erythrocytes into 2 mL of the acetylphenylhydrazine solution. Suspend normal erythrocytes in an identical solution to serve as a control. Aerate the suspensions by drawing them up into the pipet and carefully blowing them out with a small quantity of air; repeat several times. Incubate for 2 h at $37\,^{\circ}C$, aerate again, and incubate 2 h more.

To stain with brilliant cresyl blue: spread a small drop of stain solution 4(a) onto a clean, degreased slide and dry the thin stain film rapidly in air. Place a small drop of the incubated erythrocyte suspension on a coverglass and invert the glass onto the stain; examine with the microscope.

To stain with methyl violet: mix a small drop of the erythrocyte suspension with 2 or 3 drops of stain solution 4b on the slide and cover with a coverslip. Let the mixture stand for 5–10 min and examine with the microscope.

Interpretation. The percentage of erythrocytes that contain more than four Heinz bodies is determined. Normal values range from 0 % to 30 %. The number of Heinz bodies is elevated in the diseases listed above.

Nile Blue Sulfate Stain

This stain is used for the visualization of Heinz inclusion bodies. A 0.5 % Nile blue sulfate solution in absolute alcohol is transferred to the end of a slide with a glass rod until about 1/3 of the slide is covered. The slide is dried by blowing on it, and the stain film is spread out evenly with a cotton swab. Slides prepared in this way are placed face-to-face and wrapped in paper for storage. Staining is performed by dropping 2 or 3 large drops of blood onto the prepared part of the slide and covering with the prepared part of the second slide. The slides, held by their unstained outer ends, are separated and placed back together several times to thoroughly mix the blood with the stain. Finally the slides are left together for 3 to 5 min, separated, and a ground coverslip is used to collect the blood from each slide and smear it onto another slide, which is allowed to dry. The Heinz bodies appear as small, dark blue bodies situated at the margin of the yellow to bluish erythrocytes.

---

[1] After Huber H, Löffler H, Faber V (1994) Methoden der diagnostischen Hämatologie. Springer, Berlin Heidelberg New York.

Kleihauer-Betke Stain for Demonstrating Fetal Hemoglobin in Red Blood Cells

Principle. Normal adult hemoglobin (HbA) is dissolved out of the red cells by incubating air-dried and fixed blood smears in citric acid phosphate buffer (of McIlvain), pH 3.3, at 37 °C. Fetal hemoglobin (HbF) is left undissolved in the red cells and can be made visible by staining.

Reagents

- Ethyl alcohol, 80 %
- McIlvaine citric acid-phosphate buffer, pH 3.3
- Stock solution A:
  Sörensen citric acid, 21.008 g in 1 L water = 0.1 M
- Stock solution B:
  Disodium hydrogen phosphate Na_2HPO_4 $2H_2O$, 27.602 g in 1 L water = 0.2 M
- For pH 3.3:
  266 mL of solution B + 734 mL of solution A, Ehrlich hematoxylin, 0.1 % erythrosin solution

Method. Prepare thin blood smears, air dry, and fix in 80 % ethyl alcohol for 5 min. Wash in water and dry. If further processing is delayed, the slides may be stored in a refrigerator for 4–5 days. For elution, place the slides upright in a beaker containing the buffer in a 37 °C water bath for 3 min, moving the slides up and down after 1 and 2 min to keep the buffer mixed. Then wash in running water.

Staining. Stain in Ehrlich hematoxylin for 3 min, then poststain in 0.1 % aqueous erythrosin solution for 3 min. Examine at 40× using dry or oil-immersion magnification.

Interpretation. Erythrocytes that contain HbA appear as unstained "shadows," while cells that contain HbF will stain a bright red color.

The method can be used for the diagnosis of thalassemia major and for the detection of fetal erythrocytes that have entered the maternal circulation.

Kleihauer-Betke Stain for Demonstrating Methemoglobin-Containing Cells in Blood Smears

Principle. Methemoglobin combines with KCN to form cyanmethemoglobin, while oxyhemoglobin does not react with cyanides. Oxyhemoglobin functions as a peroxidase, whereas cyanmethemoglobin has very low perixodase activity.

Method. Add 1/50 vol of a 0.4 M KCN solution to blood anticoagulated with heparin or sodium citrate. Prepare thin smears from this mixture, dry, and immerse in the following mixture at room temperature: 80 mL of 96 % ethyl alcohol + 16 mL of 0.2 M citric acid + 5 mL of 30 % H_2O_2. Move the smears rapidly in the solution for about 1 min, then leave them in the solution for 2 min. Wash the smears first in methyl alcohol, then in distilled water, and stain with hematoxylin and erythrosin (see stain for HbF). Examine at 40× using dry or oil-immersion magnification.

Interpretation. Oxy-Hb-containing cells stain a bright red. Cells that contain met-Hb (converted to cyanmet-Hb) are eluted and appear as shadows.

The same staining procedure can be used to differentiate erythrocytes with a glucose-6-phosphate dehydrogenase (G-6-PDH) deficiency by combining it with the Brewer test (method of Betke, Kleihauer and Knotek). This test is based on the principle that hemoglobin converted to met-Hb by the addition of nitrite reduces to oxy-Hb in the presence of methylene blue and glucose. Red blood cells with a G-6-PDH deficit cannot undergo this reduction. Even after several hours, when all the methemoglobin in normal erythrocytes has converted back to oxy-Hb, cells with a G-6-PDH deficiency retain all or most of their met-Hb. This causes the deficient cells to appear "blank" with appropriate staining (see above: stain for demonstrating methemoglobin).

Berlin Blue Iron Stain

Principle

The Berlin blue reaction is used for the histochemical demonstration of trivalent iron. Iron in protein compounds can also be demonstrated by the addition of dilute hydrochloric acid. Iron in hemoglobin is not detected.

Reagents

- Methanol
- Potassium ferrocyanide (potassium hexacyanoferrate), 2 %
- HCl, 37 %
- Pararosaniline solution in methanol, 1 % (alternative: nuclear red stain)

Method

- Fix the air-dried smears in formalin vapor for 30 min (alternative: fix in methanol for 10–15 min).

- Wash in distilled water for 2 min and air dry.
- Place the specimens in a cuvet that contains equal parts of a 2 % solution of potassium ferrocyanide and a dilute HCl solution (1 part 37 % HCl mixed with 50 parts distilled water) for 1 h.
- Wash in distilled water.
- Nuclear stain in pararosaniline solution: 300 µL of 1 % pararosaniline solution in methanol diluted with 50 mL distilled water.
  Alternative. Stain nuclei with nuclear true red solution (which yields a fainter nuclear stain).

All materials should be iron-free, and metal forceps should not be introduced into the solution. Pappenheim- or Giemsa-stained smears can subsequently be used for iron staining. They are first prepared by destaining them for 12–24 h in pure methanol. These smears do not need to be fixed prior to staining.

Interpretation

Iron is stained blue, appearing either as diffusely scattered granules or as clumps in the cytoplasm. There are two applications for iron staining in hematology:
(a) demonstrating sideroblasts and siderocytes, and
(b) demonstrating iron stored in macrophages and endothelial cells.

Regarding (a): sideroblasts and siderocytes are, respectively, erythroblasts and erythrocytes that contain cytochemically detectable iron. This iron can be demonstrated in the form of small granules that may be irregularly scattered throughout the cytoplasm or may encircle the nucleus of erythroblasts like a ring. Normally the granules are very fine and can be identified in erythroblasts only by closely examining the smears with oil-immersion microscopy in a darkened room. Generally 1 to 4 fine granules will be seen, rarely more. When iron deficiency is present, the percentage of sideroblasts is reduced to less than 15 %. Sideroblasts containing coarse iron granules that form a partial or complete ring around the nucleus (ringed sideroblasts) are definitely abnormal. The detection of siderocytes has little practical relevance: they are increased in the same diseases as sideroblasts, and they are elevated in the peripheral blood following splenectomy, as the spleen normally removes iron from intact red blood cells.

Regarding (b): the content of stored iron is assessed by examining bone marrow fragments in smears or sections. Iron stored in macrophages

may occur in a diffusely scattered form, a finely granular form, or in the form of larger granules or clumps that may cover part of the nucleus. Iron can also be demonstrated in plasma cells as a result of alcohol poisoning or sideroblastic anemia and hemochromatosis.

The differential diagnosis afforded by iron stain is summarized in **Table 1**.

Cytochemical Determination of Glycogen in Blood Cells by the Periodic Acid Schiff Reaction and Diastase Test (PAS Reaction)

Principle

This method is based on the oxidation of α-glycols in carbohydrates and carbohydrate-containing compounds. The resulting polyaldehydes are demonstrated with the Schiff reagent (leukofuchsin).

Reagents

- Formalin.
- Periodic acid solution, 1 %, in distilled water.
- Sulfite water: add tap water to 10 mL of a 10 % sodium metabilsulfite solution ($Na_2S_2O_5$) and 10 mL of 1 mol/L HCL to make a volume of 200 mL. The stock solutions can be stored in the refrigerator; the mixture should always be freshly prepared.
- Prepare Schiff reagent (commercially available) as follows: completely dissolve 0.5 g pararosaniline in 15 mL of 1 mol/L HCl by shaking (no heating) and add a solution of 0.5 g potassium metabisulfite ($K_2S_2O_5$) in 85 mL distilled water. The clear, bright red solution will gradually lighten to a yellowish color. After 24 h, shake with 300 mg activated charcoal (powdered) for 2 min and then filter. The colorless filtrate is ready to use and, when stored in a dark stoppered bottle in a cool place, will keep for several months. Schiff reagent that has turned red should no longer be used!

Method

- Fix the smears for 10 min in a mixture of 10 mL 40 % formalin and 90 mL ethanol (alternative: fix for 5 min in formalin vapor).
- Wash for 5 min in several changes of tap water.
- Place the smears in 1 % periodic acid for 10 min (prepared fresh for each use).
- Wash in at least two changes of distilled water and dry.
- Place in Schiff reagent for 30 min (in the dark at room temperature).

Table 1. Differential diagnosis by iron stain in the bone marrow

	Sideroblasts	Iron-storing reticulum cells, sideromacrophages	Special features
Normal bone marrow	$\sim$ 20 – 60 % finely granular, 1 – 4 granules	Isolated, mostly finely granular deposits	Siderocytes in peripheral blood 0 – 0.3 ‰
Hypochromic anemias			
– Iron deficiency	< 15 % finely granular	None	Serum Fe ↓
– Infection, tumor	< 15 % finely granular	Increased finely granular or (rarely) coarsely granular deposits	Serum Fe ↓
– Sideroachrestic anemias (RARS)	> 90 % coarsely granular; ringed sideroblasts (> 30 %)	Greatly increased, many diffuse or coarsely granular deposits	Serum Fe ↑, siderocytes may be increased
– Lead poisoning	> 90 % coarsely granular; ringed sidero-blasts	Greatly increased, many diffuse or coarsely granular deposits	Serum Fe ↑, siderocytes may be increased
– Thalassemia	> 90 % coarsely granular; ringed sidero-blasts	Greatly increased, many diffuse or coarsely granular deposits	Serum Fe ↑, siderocytes may be increased
Hemolytic anemias	≤ 80 % finely granular	Increased finely granular or (rarely) coarsely granular deposits	
Secondary sideroachrestic anemias	≤ 80 % finely granular	Increased finely granular or (rarely) coarsely granular deposits	
Vitamin B_6 deficiency	≤ 80 % finely granular	Increased finely granular or (rarely) coarsely granular deposits	
Megaloblastic anemias	≤ 80 % finely granular	Increased finely granular or (rarely) coarsely granular deposits	
Aplastic anemias	≤ 80 % finely granular	Increased finely granular or (rarely) coarsely granular deposits	
Myeloproliferative disorders	≤ 80 % finely granular	Increased finely granular or (rarely) coarsely granular deposits	
Hemochromatosis	≤ 80 % finely granular	Increased	Bone marrow is not useful for diagnosis except positive plasma cells
Postsplenectomy state	≤ 80 % finely granular	Somewhat increased	Siderocytes greatly increased

- Rinse in sulfite water (changed once) for 2–3 min.
- Wash in several changes of distilled water for 5 min.
- Nuclear stain with hemalum for approx. 10 min, then blue in tap water for approx. 15–20 min, and air dry.

Even older slides that have been stained with Giemsa or Pappenheim can be reused for the PAS reaction. Specimens that have been treated several times with oil or xylene should not be used for PAS staining. The smears can be placed unfixed in periodic acid after washing in distilled water (Step 3) to remove the color.

Interpretation

PAS-positive material in the cytoplasm may produce a diffuse red stain or may appear as pink to burgundy-red granules, flakes, or clumps of varying size that may occupy large areas of the cytoplasm. The distribution of PAS-positive material in normal leukocytes is summarized in the **Table 2.** Some plasma cells, macrophages, and osteoblasts may also show a positive PAS reaction, and megakaryocytes are strongly positive.

Table 2. PAS reaction in normal leukocytes

Cell type	PAS reaction
Myeloblast	$\varnothing$
Promyelocyte	(+)
Myelocyte	+
Metamyelocyte	++
Band and segmented cells	+++
Eosinophils	+ (intergranular reaction)
Basophils	+ (granular!)
Monocytes	(+) to +
Lymphocytes	$\varnothing$ to + (granular)

Reaction: $\varnothing$ = negative; (+) = weakly positive; + = positive; ++ = markedly positive; +++ = strongly positive

Sudan Black B Stain

Principle

Sudan black B is a fat-soluble dye that becomes highly concentrated in lipids. The sudanophilia, which occurs even after degreasing, is based on an oxidative coupling of Sudan black derivatives with phenols. It is peroxidase-dependent and thus corresponds to the peroxidase reaction.

Reagents

- Formaldehyde solution
- Staining solution A: mix well 0.3 g Sudan black B and 100 mL absolute ethanol and filter (can be stored).
- Staining solution B: buffer solution: a) dissolve 16 g phenol crystals in 30 mL absolute ethanol; b) dissolve 0.3 g of $Na_2HPO_4 \cdot 12H_2O$ in 100 mL dw (store at 4 °C); mix 15 mL of solution a) + 50 mL of solution b).
- Staining solution C (working solution): mix 60 mL of solution A (dye) and 40 mL of solution B (buffer) and filter; will keep for 2–3 months.

Method

- Fix the air-dried smears in formalin vapor for 10 min.
- Wash in tap water (running or several changes) for 10 min.
- Immerse in staining solution C for 60 min.
- Wash in at least 3 changes of 70 % ethanol to remove the excess dye.
- Wash in tap water for 2 min.
- Nuclear stain with dilute Giemsa solution or hemalum.

Interpretation

Black or grayish-black staining in the cytoplasm constitutes a positive reaction. The result is very similar to that of the peroxidase reaction.

Cytochemical Determination of Peroxidase

Principle

Benzidine or diaminobenzidine (more often used) is converted, in the presence of peroxide, from the leuko form into a high-polymer form that is detectable by cytochemical staining.

Reagents.

- Fixative: methanol + 37 % formalin (10:1).
- DAB solution: 5 mg diaminobenzidine tetrahydrochloride in 20 mL of 0.05 mol/L tris-HCl buffer (pH 7.6) with 50 µL of 1 % H_2O_2 added
- Tris-HCl: 50 mL of solution A (121.14 g trishydroxymethylaminomethane dissolved in 1 L distilled water) + 40 mL of solution B (1 mol/L HCl) + 960 mL distilled water
- Mayer's hemalum:

Method

- Fix the air-dried smears for 15 s at 4 °C (30 s for thicker bone marrow smears).

- Wash 3 times in tap water.
- Air dry.
- Incubate in DAB solution for 10 min.
- Wash briefly in tap water.
- Incubate in Mayer's hemalum for 3 min.
- Wash in tap water for 3 min.
- Air dry.

Interpretation

From the promyelocytic stage on, neutrophils and eosinophilic granulocytes show a yellowish green to brownish granular stain. Monocytes may show a positive reaction, which is weaker than that of granulocytes.

Hydrolases

Principle

The principle is the same for all hydrolases and may be summarized as follows: Today only the azo dye method is still in routine clinical use. It is based on the hydrolytic splitting of an aryl ester by the enzyme and the immediate coupling of the liberated phenol derivative to a dye substance, usually a diazonium salt or hexazotized pararosaniline.

Cytochemical Determination of Leukocyte Alkaline Phosphatase (LAP) in Blood Smears

Reagents

- Fixative: 10 % formalin in absolute methanol (one part 37 % formalin, 9 parts 100 % methanol)
- Staining solution: dissolve 35 mg sodium-α-naphthyl phosphate in 70 mL of 2 % veronal sodium solution, pH 9.4; add 70 mg concentrated variamine blue salt B, and stir. Immediate filter the solution and use.
- Mayer's hemalum.

Method

- Fix the air-dried smears at 4 °C for 30 s.
- Wash 3 times thoroughly in tap water.
- Incubate in refrigerator at 4 – 7 °C for 2 h.
- Wash thoroughly in tap water.
- Nuclear stain in Mayer's hemalum for 5 – 8 min.
- Air dry the smears and mount in glycerine gelatin or Aquatex.

Interpretation

Neutrophilic granulocytes (a few band cells, mostly segmented forms) are the only types of blood cell that show enzymatic activity. The intensity of the phosphatase reaction is usually scored on a four-point scale. The activity score, or index, is based on groups of 100 cells and is calculated from the sum of the cells assigned to the different reaction grades, which is multiplied by a corresponding factor (1 – 4). The index ranges from 0 to 400. Cells in the bone marrow that have phosphatase activity are neutrophilic granulocytes, vascular endothelial cells, and osteoblasts. The location of structures in bone marrow smears, lymph node touch preparations, and sections can be determined more accurately by using methods that employ the substrates naphthol-AS-BI phosphate or -MX phosphate.

Cytochemical Determination of Acid Phosphatase

Reagents

- Fixative: see Appendix
- Staining solution: mix together 0.8 mL hexazotized pararosaniline (mix equal parts 4 % sodium nitrite and 4 % pararosaniline in HCl, see Appendix) + 30 mL Michaelis buffer pH 7.4 (58 mL of 0.1 mol/L sodium barbital + 41.9 mL of 0.1 mol/L HCl) + 10 mg naphthol-AS-BI phosphate, dissolved in 1 mL dimethylformamide. Adjust the solution to pH 4.9 – 5.1 and filter before use.
- Mayer's hemalum

Method

- Fix the air-dried smears at 4 °C for 30 s.
- Wash 3 times in tap water.
- Air dry.
- Incubate in stain solution for 3 h at room temperature.
- Wash briefly in tap water.
- Place in Mayer's hemalum for 3 min.
- Blue in tap water for 3 min.
- Air dry.

Interpretation

A bright red homogeneous or granular precipitate forms in the cytoplasm of cells with acid phosphatase activity. In the case of plasmacytomas, the abnormal plasma cells tend to show stronger activity than normal plasma cells or plasma cells affected by reactive changes. A dotlike staining pattern is seen in T-lymphocytes, while the blasts of T-ALL usually show a circumscribed (focal) paranuclear acid phosphatase reaction.

Acid Phosphatase Reaction with Inhibition by Tartrate

Method

Add 60 mg of L-tartaric acid to 30 mL of the staining solution, then analyze as described for acid phosphatase. Fast garnet GBC can be used as a coupling salt instead of the pararosaniline solution. This requires the following modifications in the staining solution: Dissolve 10 mg naphthol-AS-BI phosphate in 0.5 mL dimethylformamide, and add 0.1 mol/L acetate buffer pH 5.0 to make 10 mL. Dissolve 10–15 mg of fast garnet GBC in 20 mL of 0.1 mol/L acetate buffer solution. Mix both solutions well. Filtering is not required. Incubate the smears at 37 °C for 60–90 min.

Interpretation

Most of the cells of hairy cell leukemia are positive even after tartrate inhibition, and macrophages and osteoclasts do not show significant inhibition.

Detection of Esterases with Naphthyl Acetate or Naphthyl Butyrate ("Neutral Esterases")

Reagents

- Solution a: mix 1 drop (0.05 mL) sodium nitrite solution (4 %) + 1 drop (0.05 mL) pararosaniline solution (4 % in 2 mol/L HCl) for about 1 min (yields a pale yellow solution), then dissolve in 5 mL of 0.2 mol/L phosphate buffer, pH 7.0–7.1 (250 mL Na_2HPO_4+130 mL NaH_2PO_4).
- Solution b: dissolve 10 mg α-naphthyl acetate in 0.2–0.3 mL chemically pure acetone; add 20 mL of 0.2 mol/L phosphate buffer pH 7.0–7.1 while stirring vigorously.
- Mix solutions a and b and filter into small cuvets.

Method

- Fix the thin, air-dried smears (will keep up to 3 days when sheltered from dust, longer at 4–8 °C) in formalin vapor for 4 min or in the fixative solution for 30 s (see Appendix).
- Wash in tap water.
- Incubate for 60 min.
- Wash in tap water.
- Stain in Mayer's hemalum for approx. 8 min.
- Blue in tap water for approx. 15 min.
- Mount smears with glycerine gelatin or Aquatex (Merck).
- Air-dried smears may be mounted with Eukitt.

Interpretation

Positive cells stain with a brown to reddish-brown diffuse or granular pattern. The α-naphthyl butyrate stain yields a dark red color. The result is very similar to the α-naphthyl acetate stain, so the slightly different method used with α-naphthyl butyrate will not be described in detail.

Monocytes in the peripheral blood are strongly positive for α-naphthyl acetate stain, while neutrophilic and eosinophilic granulocytes are negative. Some lymphocytes stain with a circumscribed, dotlike pattern. The strongest activity in bone marrow cells is found in monocytes, macrophages, and megakaryocytes.

Acid α-Naphthyl Acetate Esterase (ANAE)

Reagents

- Fixative: see Appendix.
- Staining solution: dissolve 50 mg α-naphthyl acetate in 2.5 mL ethyleneglycolmonomethyl ether + 44.5 mL of 0.1 mol/L phosphate buffer pH 7.6 + 3.0 mL hexazotized pararosaniline (1.5 mL 4 % pararosaniline in 2 mol/L HCl + 1.5 mL 4 % sodium nitrite solution). Adjust the solution to pH 6.1–6.3 with 1 mol/L HCl and filter before use. The solution must be clear.
- Mayer's hemalum.

Method

- Fix air-dried smears in fixative solution at 4 °C for 30 s.
- Wash 3 times in tap water.
- Air dry for 10–30 min.
- Incubate in staining solution at room temperature for 45 min.
- Rinse briefly in tap water.
- Place in Mayer's hemalum for 3 min.
- Blue in tap water for 3 min.
- Air dry.

Interpretation

The reaction product appears as a reddish-brown homogeneous or granular precipitate. Acid esterase is used to identify T-lymphocytes. The method is reliable only for more mature forms, however, and inconsistent results are obtained in acute lymphocytic leukemias with T characteristics.

Naphthol AS-D Chloroacetate Esterase (CE)

Reagents

- Methanol-formalin solution, 9 : 1 (v/v).
- 0.1 mmol/L Michaelis buffer, pH 7.0.
- Naphthol AS-D chloroacetate.
- Dimethylformamide.
- Sodium nitrite solution, 4 %.
- Pararosaniline solution, 4 %, in 2 mol/L HCl.
- Staining solution A: mix 0.1 mL sodium nitrite solution and 0.1 mL pararosaniline solution with 30 mL Michaelis buffer.
- Staining solution B: dissolve 10 mg naphthol AS-D chloroacetate in 1 mL dimethylformamide.
- Staining solution C: mix solutions A) and B), adjust to pH 6.3 with 2 mol/L HCl, and filter into a cuvet. Use immediately.

Method

- Fix smears in methanol-formalin for 30 s at room temperature, wash thoroughly in tap water without delay.
- Place smears in staining solution for 60 min, then wash thoroughly in tap water.
- Nuclear stain with hemalum for 5–10 min, wash thoroughly with tap water, and blue for approx. 10 min.
- After air drying, the smears may be directly examined or mounted with Eukitt.

Interpretation

A bright red reaction product forms at sites of enzymatic activity in the cytoplasm. Neutrophilic granulocytes normally display a positive reaction from the promyelocytic stage on, the late promyelocyte to myelocyte stages showing the strongest reaction. A slightly weaker reaction is seen in band and segmented forms. Monocytes may also show a weak chloroacetate esterase reaction. Besides neutrophils, tissue mast cells display very strong activity. In acute myelomonocytic leukemia, which is associated with an anomaly of chromosome 16, some of the abnormal eosinophils show a positive chloroacetate esterase reaction. Normal eosinophils are negative.

Dipeptidylaminopeptidase IV (DAP IV)

Reagents

- Fast blue B (Sigma, Munich)
- Glycerine gelatin
- Glycyl-proline-4-methoxy-β-naphthylamide (Sigma)
- Phosphate buffer, 0.2 mol/L, pH 7.0
- Solution A: 13.8 g $NaH_2PO_4 \cdot 1H_2O$ in 500 mL distilled water
- Solution B: 17.8 g $Na_2HPO_4 \cdot 2H_2O$ in 500 mL distilled water
- Solution C: mix 250 mL solution B + 130 mL solution A, pH 7.0
- Dimethylformamide

Method

- Fix in methanol-formaldehyde (9 : 1, v/v) for 4 s or in fixative solution a) (see Appendix) for 30 s, wash 3 times in tap water, dry.
- Dissolve 7.5 mg glycyl-proline-4-methoxy-β-naphthylamide in 1 mL dimethylformamide.
- Dissolve 20 mg fast blue B in 1 mL dimethylformamide.
- First add solution C to 20 mL phosphate buffer and mix, then add solution B and mix.
- Filter mixture and use right away.
- Incubate 45 min, mixing several times or using a vibrator plate, then rinse briefly in tap water.
- Nuclear stain in hemalum solution for 3 min.
- Wash in running tap water for 5–10 min.
- Mount with glycerine gelatin or Aquatex (Merck).

Interpretation

The reaction product is red. Only some of the T lymphocytes, mainly the T helper cells, show a positive reaction. Vascular endothelial cells in bone marrow smears are weakly positive.

Appendix

Fixation (Suitable for Esterase, Acid Phosphatase, DAP IV)

The fixative solution is composed of:
- 30 mL buffer solution (20 mg disodium hydrogen phosphate · 12H$_2$O and 100 mg potassium dihydrogen phosphate dissolved in 30 mL distilled water; pH should be 6.6)
- +45 mL analytical grade acetone
- +25 mL formalin (37 %)

Fix air-dried smears in this solution for 30 s at 4–10 °C, wash in three changes of distilled water, and dry at room temperature for 10–30 min.

Schaefer universal fixative. Mix 0.5 mL of 25 % glutardialdehyde solution and 60 mL analytical grade acetone in distilled water to make 100 mL. Air-dried smears are incubated in this fixative solution at room temperature: 1 min for peroxidase, 10 min for chloroacetate esterase, 5 min for detecting esterase with naphthyl acetate or naphthyl butyrate, 1 min for acid phosphatase, 1 min for alkaline phosphatase, 10 min for detecting iron, and 10 min for the PAS reaction.

Sodium Nitrite Solution 4 %

Dissolve 4 g sodium nitrite in distilled water to make 100 mL.

Pararosaniline Solution 4 %

Dissolve 2 g Graumann pararosaniline (Merck) in 50 mL of 2 mol/L HCl by gentle heating. Cool and filter the solution.

The sodium nitrite and pararosaniline solutions will keep for several months when stored in a dark bottle under refrigeration. Most of the reagents and even commercial staining kits can be ordered from pharmaceutical houses (Merck, Serva, Sigma, etc.). Before kits are used for routine tests, they should be compared against solutions prepared by the methods indicated.

The cytochemical features of blood cells and bone marrow cells are reviewed in **Table 3.**

Table 3. Cytochemistry of blood and bone marrow cells

	Per-oxidase	PAS	Esterase α-Naphthyl-acetate-, Naphthol-AS-acetate-	Esterase Naphthol-AS-D-chloracetate-	Phosphatases alkaline	Phosphatases acid	Remarks
Reticulum cells	Ø	Ø – +	++	Ø	Ø (1)	++	(1) vascular endothelia +++
Plasma cells	Ø	Ø	(+)	Ø	Ø	+	Acid phosphatasc is strongly positive in multiple myeloma
Myeloblast	Ø	Ø – (+)	Ø – (+)	Ø	Ø	Ø	
Promyelocyte	++	(+)	Ø – (+)	+++	Ø	+	
Myelocyte	++	+	Ø – (+)	+++	Ø	+	
Metamyelocyte	++	++	Ø – (+)	+++	Ø – (+)	(+)	
Band form	++	+++	Ø – (+)	+++	Ø – (+)	(+)	
Segmented form	+++	+++	Ø – (+)	+++	Ø – +++	(+)	
Eosinophils	++	+	Ø – (+)	Ø	Ø	(+) – +	
Basophils Blood	Ø – +	+	Ø – (+)	Ø	Ø	Ø	
Basophils Tissue				++		++	
Monocytes	Ø – +	(+) – +	+++	(+)	Ø	Ø	
Lymphocytes	Ø	Ø – +	+	Ø	Ø	Ø	Hair cells are acid-phosphatase positive
Erythroblasts	Ø	Ø	++	Ø	Ø	Ø	Positive PAS reaction in erythremias and erythroleukemias and some MDS
Erythrocytes	Ø	Ø	(+)	Ø	Ø	Ø	
Megakaryocytes and platelets	Ø	+	+++	Ø	Ø	++	PAS reaction may be decreased in Werlhof's disease
Osteoblasts	Ø	Ø	+	Ø	+++	+	
Osteoclasts	Ø	Ø – (+)	++	Ø	Ø	+++	

Reaction: Ø = negative; (+) = weakly positive; + = positive; ++ = markedly positive; +++ = strongly positive

2. Immunocytochemical Detection of Cell-Surface and Intracellular Antigens

Today the immunologic characterization of cells is based on the use of monoclonal antibodies. This may involve the immunocytologic staining of smears or analysis by flow cytometry, in which a number of different fluorochrome-labeled antibodies are used for studies of cell suspensions. We refer the reader to commercial kits, which come with detailed instructions, and to the information that has become available in recent textbooks on immunocytology and diagnostic hematology.

3. Staining Methods for the Detection of Blood Parasites[1]

"Thick Smear" Method

One drop of blood is placed on a slide and spread with the edge of a second slide to cover an area the size of a dime. The film should not be too thick, or it will flake off during drying or displace during staining (it should be thin enough that printed text can still be read through it). The film is air dried and may be stained after it is completely dry.

The film is *stained* without preliminary fixation. Owing to the concentrating effect of the thick smear method, a parasitic infection can be detected even when the organisms are present in small numbers. Staining without preliminary fixation induces a massive hemolysis that dislodges the parasites from the erythrocytes so that they can be identified.

The staining solution is prepared fresh for each use and consists of 1 drop of stock Giemsa stain distilled to 1.0 mL and buffered water (pH 7.2). This solution hemolyzes and stains simultaneously.

The stain is applied for 20 – 30 min, then the slide is carefully washed by dipping it in tap water. It is dried in an upright position.

Besides the thick smear preparation, a thin blood smear (fixed in methanol for 5 min) should also be prepared so that the parasites can be accurately identified if doubt exists. Often this is difficult to accomplish in thick smears.

Thick smear preparations for trypanosomes (T. *gambiense*, T. *rhodesiense*, T. *cruzi*) are stained in the same way as for malaria parasites. This method is also used to examine for *Borrelia recurrentis*.

Bartonellosis

Bartonella organisms are most readily detected by the examination of Pappenheim-, or Giemsa-stained blood smears.

Detection of Blood Parasites in Bone Marrow Smears

Blood parasites are best demonstrated in marrow smears by Giemsa staining (17 mm) after fixation in methanol (5 min) (see p. 7).

---

[1] Revised by Prof. Dr. R. Disko, Munich

Toxoplasmosis

Giemsa staining of the touch preparation or other sample is also recommended for the detection of toxoplasmosis. Direct immunofluorescence and the peroxidase reaction can detect the organism with high sensitivity.

Microfiliariasis

1. **Wet preparation (thick smear method):** Examine a drop of fresh (anticoagulated) blood under a coverslip on a microscope slide (bearing in mind the periodicity in microfilarial activity, see p. 403). The highly motile organisms are clearly visible even at low magnification (250×).

2. **Concentrating the sample:** To 3 – 5 mL of drawn venous blood, add 10 – 15 mL of a mixture of 95 mL formalin (5 %), 5 mL acetic acid, and 2 mL of an alcoholic gentian violet solution (4 g per 100 mL 96 % alcohol). Centrifuge the mixture, and examine the sediment for stained microfilariae. (Membrane filtration methods provide a particularly good yield.)

3. **Examination of a skin snip for microfilariae** (*Onchocerca volvulus*). Place a large drop of physiologic saline solution onto a slide. Immerse in the saline a pinhead-size piece of skin excised with a Walser dermatome (if that is not available, use a razor blade). Cover with a coverslip, let stand 20 min, then examine with the microscope at low power (~300×). The organisms will pass from the skin into the saline medium and will move vigorously in the fluid.

Mycobacterium Species (M. tuberculosis, M. leprae)

One or two of the following reactions are used to examine a suspicious sample. The Kinyoun and auramine stains are usually combined and have largely replaced the Ziehl-Neelsen stain. The mycobacteria stain red with both the Kinyoun and Ziehl-Neelsen stains.

a. Kinyoun cold stain (alternative to Ziehl-Neelsen):
1. Fix the specimen (with heat or methanol).
2. Immerse in Kinyoun solution for   3 min.
3. Wash with water for   30 s.
4. Place in Gabett solution for   2 min.
5. Wash and dry.

b. Auramine stain:
1. Fix the specimen with heat.
2. Stain with Auramin solution for 3 min.
3. Decolorize with acid alcohol for 1 min.
4. Wash off acid alcohol with water.
5. Restain with blue-black ink solution for 1 min.
6. Rinse off ink solution with water and dry.

c. Ziehl-Neelsen stain:
1. Fix the specimen with heat.
2. Cover with 10 % carbolfuchsin and heat to steaming 3 times; stain for 3 min.
3. Decolorize in 3 changes of acid alcohol for 3 min.
4. Wash with water.
5. Counterstain with dilute methylene blue solution for 3 min.
6. Wash with water and dry between sheets of blotting paper.

Illustrations

A. Overview of Cells in the Blood, Bone Marrow, and Lymph Nodes

Figure 1 presents an overview of the various cells of hematopoiesis. The figure does not attempt to answer unresolved questions of cell origins and is intended only as an introductory scheme to help the beginner find some order in the bewildering variety of cells. The cells of hematopoiesis develop from CD 34 – positive stem cells, which resemble large lymphocytes or small, undifferentiated blasts (**Fig. 2**). When cultured, these cells form colonies that can sometimes be identified by their intrinsic color (**Fig. 3**).

Red and white cell precursors account for most of the cells found in normal bone marrow. In addition there are variable numbers of *reticulum cells, vascular and sinus endothelial cells, megakaryocytes, tissue mast cells, lymphocytic elements, plasma cells* and, very rarely, osteoblasts and osteoclasts (more common in children). The earliest precursors of the red and white blood cells have a basophilic cytoplasm and are very similar to one another. As hemoglobin synthesis increases, the *erythroblasts* lose their basophilic cytoplasm while their nuclei undergo a characteristic structural change. After losing their nuclei, the young erythrocytes still contain remnants of their former cytoplasmic organelles as evidence of their immaturity. They are reticulocytes and are released as such into the peripheral blood. The reticulocytes can be demonstrated by supravital staining (see p. 8).

The *myeloblasts*, which are the precursors of neutrophilic granulocytes and monocytes, develop into neutrophilic promyelocytes and promonocytes. The eosinophilic and basophilic granulocytes pursue their own lines of development and therefore have their own promyelocytes with specific granules.

Platelets (thrombocytes) develop from the cytoplasm of the megakaryocytes.

The common progenitor cell from which monocytes and neutrophilic granulocytes originate might be termed the myelomonoblast (CFU-GM).

The *reticulum cells* described and counted in cytologic preparations from bone marrow, lymph nodes, and spleen form a heterogeneous group. A large portion belong to the macrophage system and are derived from blood monocytes. They also include segregated vascular and sinus endothelial cells in addition to dendritic cells belonging to the stroma. The reticulum cells of the bone marrow constitute the reticular or spongy tissue of the bone marrow in which the actual hematopoietic cells reside. Apparently they perform important tasks relating to nutrition and differentiation of the blood cell precursors.

Two different types of reticulum cell are known to occur in the lymph nodes and spleen: the "dendritic reticulum cell," which occurs exclusively in germinal centers, primary follicles, and occasionally in the peripheral zones of follicles, and the "interdigitating reticulum cell," which is specific to the thymus-dependent region of the lymph node (see **Fig. 132** for details).

The "fibroblastic reticulum cell" described by Lennert and Müller-Hermelink can occur in all regions of the lymph node as well as in bone marrow, but as yet it has not been positively identified by light microscopy. The cells formerly described as small "lymphoid reticulum cells" are probably tissue lymphocytes.

In the *lymphatic system,* a basic distinction is drawn between B lymphocytes and T lymphocytes based on the development, differentiation, and function of the cells. Unfortunately, the differentiation of these two cell types cannot be accomplished with traditional staining methods and must rely on immunocytologic or flow cytometric analysis. Both lymphatic cell lines appear to arise from a common, committed stem cell that probably resides in the bone marrow. Thereafter the primary differentiation of the T cell line takes place in the thymus, while that of the B cells (in humans) takes place in the bone marrow, which today is viewed as the equivalent of the *fabrician bursa* in birds. Further development and proliferation of both cell lines take place in the lymph nodes.

The final maturation stage of B lymphocytes is the plasma cell, whose function is to produce immunoglobulins. Plasma cells occur ubiquitously.

Apparently they can develop anywhere in the body but are most plentiful in lymph nodes, spleen, and bone marrow. A positive correlation exists between the amount of immunoglobulins present in the serum and the size of the plasma cell population.

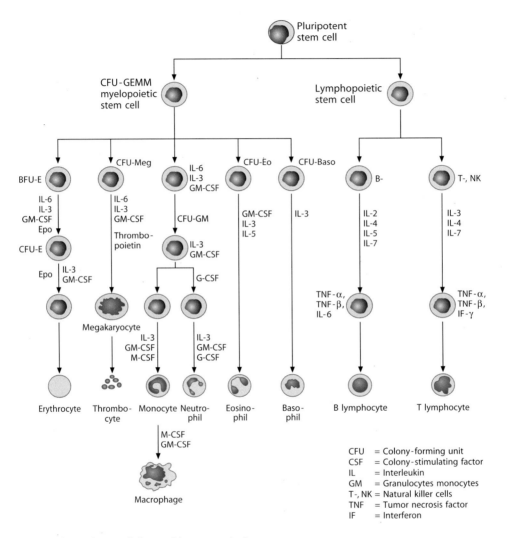

Fig. 1. The various cell lines of hematopoiesis

Fig. 2. CD 34 – positive stem cells

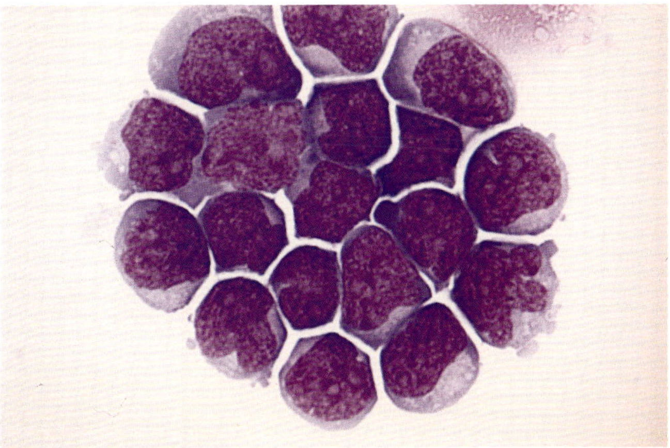

Fig. 3. Colonies of CD34-positive
stem cells in cultures

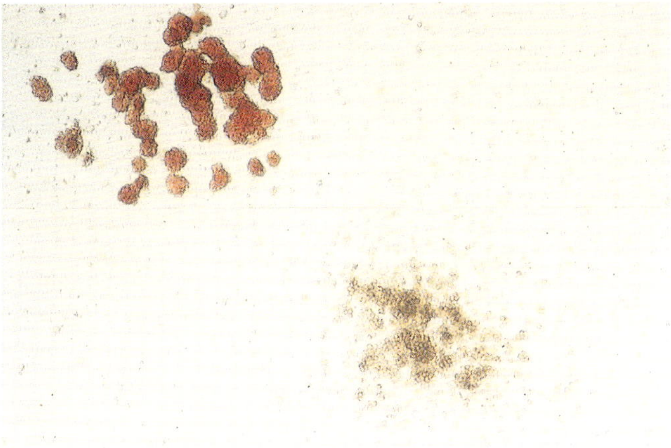

B. Blood and Bone Marrow

1. Individual Cells

Light Microscopic Morphology and Cytochemistry

Fig. 4 a–f. Cells of erythropoiesis

The **proerythroblasts,** called also **pronormoblasts** or **rubriblasts,** are the earliest precursors of erythropoiesis. They range from 15 to 22 µm in size and do not yet contain hemoglobin. They typically have a darkly basophilic, often shadowy cytoplasm that sometimes shows pseudopodia. The nucleus has a dense, finely honeycombed chromatin structure (**Fig. 4 a–c**). Most proerythroblasts have several (at most five) indistinct pale blue nucleoli, which disappear as the cell matures. Like all erythropoietic cells, proerythroblasts tend to produce multinucleated forms. Typically there is a perinuclear clear zone, which is found to contain minute granules on phase contrast examination. Hemoglobin first appears adjacent to the nucleus and produces a flaring of the perinuclear clear zone, later expanding to occupy the whole cell and heralding a transition to the polychromatic forms. Meanwhile the nucleus undergoes a characteristic structural change: the nucleoli disappear while the chromatin becomes coarser and acquires typical erythroblastic features.

A continuum exists from the basophilic proerythroblasts to the **macroblasts** (**Fig. 4d**). These cells tend to be smaller than proerythroblasts (8–15 µm in diameter). The nuclear-cytoplasmic ratio is shifted in favor of the cytoplasm, which is polychromatic due to the co-existence of basophilic material with a greater abundance of hemoglobin. The nucleus appears coarse and smudgy, and there is partial clumping of the nuclear chromatin.

As development progresses, the cell loses more of its basophilic cytoplasm and further diminishes in size (7–10 µm in diameter), gradually entering the stage of the **orthochromatic normoblast** (**Fig. 4e**). The nuclear-cytoplasmic ratio is further shifted in favor of the cytoplasm, which acquires an increasingly red tinge ultimately matching that of the mature erythrocyte. Supravital staining of the youngest erythrocytes reveals a network of strands (see p. 8) called the "substantia reticulofilamentosa" of the reticulocytes. Staining with brilliant cresyl blue causes the aggregation or precipitation of ribonucleoproteins. It takes four days for the cells to pass through the four maturation stages. The clumplike erythroblastic nucleus then condenses to a streaklike, featureless, homogeneous mass. Some authors subdivide the normoblasts into basophilic, polychromatic, and orthochromatic forms according to their degree of maturity, while others use the terms *rubricyte* (basophilic normoblast) and *metarubricyte* (orthochromatic normoblast). Such fine distinctions are unnecessary for the routine evaluation of marrow smears, however. Normoblasts are incapable of dividing. The nucleus is expelled through the cell membrane.

Particularly when erythropoiesis is increased, examination of the smear will reveal *nests or islands of erythroblasts* with central reticulum cells whose cytoplasm is in close contact (metabolic exchange) with the surrounding erythroblasts (**Fig. 4 f**).

Fig. 4 a–d

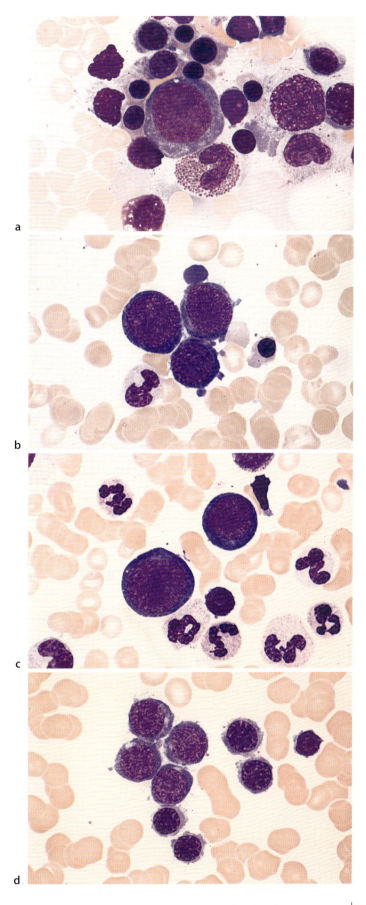

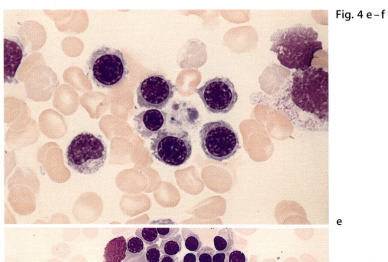

Fig. 4 e–f

e

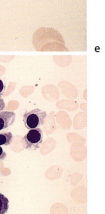

f

Fig. 5 a – f. Erythrocytes 1

The morphologic evaluation of erythrocytes is based on the following criteria:
- Size
- Shape
- Hemoglobin: concentration, distribution
- Stainability
- Distribution in the smear
- Inclusions

a. Normal erythrocytes (diam. 7 – 8 µm).

b. Hypochromic erythrocytes in iron deficiency anemia. The cells, which have normal diameters, are conspicuous for their paucity of hemoglobin, which may form only a thin peripheral rim (anulocytes).

c. Poikilocytes are dysmorphic erythrocytes of variable shape that occur in the setting of severe anemias. Their presence indicates a severe insult to the bone marrow. Teardrops and pear shapes are particularly common and are not specific for osteomyelosclerosis or -fibrosis.

d. Microspherocytes are smaller than normal erythrocytes (diam. 3 – 7 µm) but are crammed with hemoglobin and have a greater thickness, giving them an approximately spherical shape. They are typical of congenital hemolytic jaundice (spherocytic anemia) but also occur in acquired hemolytic anemias.

e. Elliptocytes (ovalocytes) result from an inherited anomaly of erythrocyte shape that is usually innocuous but may be linked to a propensity for hemolytic anemia (elliptocytic anemia).

f. Basophilic stippling of erythrocytes is a sign of increased but abnormal regeneration. It is particularly common in lead poisoning. The normal prevalence of basophilic stippling is 0 – 4 erythrocytes per 10,000

Fig. 5 g, h. Erythrocytes 2

g. Polychromatic erythrocytes (diam. 7 – 8 µm), **Cabot rings.** Polychromasia occurs when mature erythrocytes show increased staining with basic dyes (violet stain) in addition to hemoglobin staining. It is usually associated with reticulocytosis. Polychromasia occurs in red cells that still have a relatively high RNA content and in which hemoglobin synthesis is not yet complete. It is especially common in chronic hemolytic anemias.

The variable staining of the erythrocytes is also termed *anisochromia*. Cabot rings are remnants of spindle fibers and are a product of abnormal regeneration (see also **Fig. 46c**).

h. Megalocytes are very large, mostly oval erythrocytes that are packed with hemoglobin (> 8 µm in diameter). They occur predominantly in megaloblastic anemias (see p. 88)

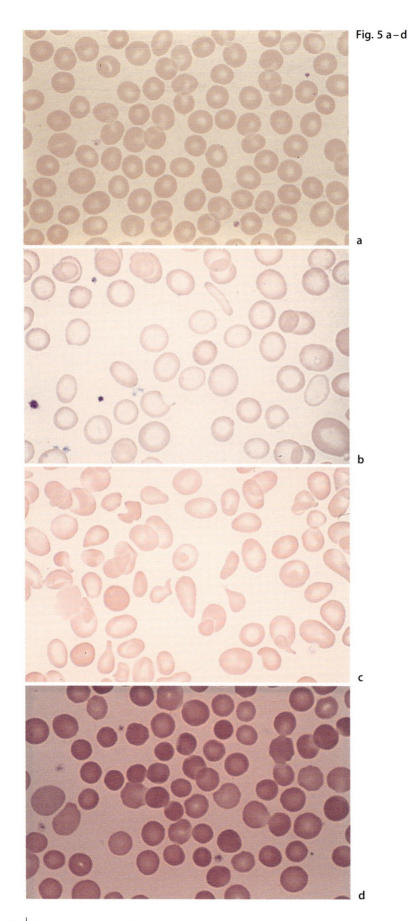

Fig. 5 a–d

Fig. 5 e–h

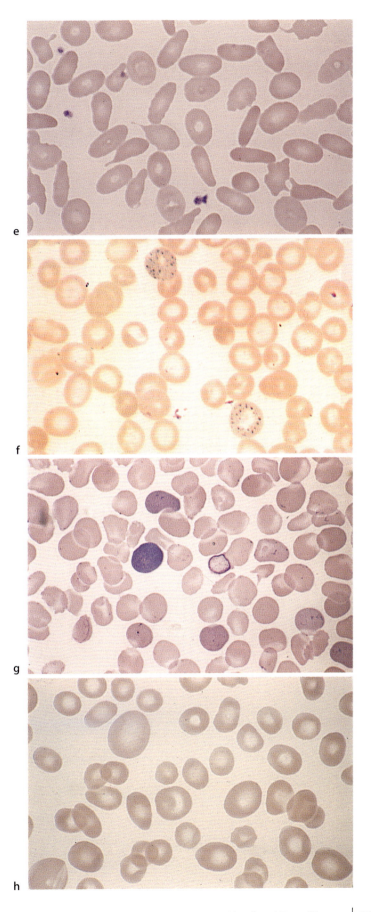

e

f

g

h

Fig. 6 a – i. Erythrocytes 3

a. Erythrocytes containing *nuclear remnants* in the form of *Howell-Jolly bodies*, which are observed after splenectomy and in cases of splenic atrophy. Chromatin dust, like the Howell-Jolly bodies, consist of nuclear remnants.

b. Target cells (Mexican hat cells) are distinguished from anulocytes by the deeper staining of their central zone and peripheral rim. They are particularly common in hemoglobin abnormalities, occurring also in other hemolytic anemias, severe iron deficiency, and after splenectomy.

c. Acanthocytes or "burr cells" are distinguished by their jagged surface, which usually is deeply clefted. Acanthocytes are seen in a rare hereditary anomaly, A-β-lipoproteinemia. They are also a feature of uremia and hepatic coma, where large numbers of these cells are considered a poor prognostic sign. Acanthocyte formation has also been linked to the use of alcohol and certain drugs.

d. Sickle cells (drepanocytes). Sickle-shaped erythrocytes occasionally form spontaneously, but sickling is consistently induced by oxygen withdrawal in the sickle cell test (see p. 5). It signifies a common hemoglobinopathy, HbS disease (sickle cell anemia), which affects blacks almost exclusively. Red cell sickling also occurs in the less common HbC disease.

e. Knizocytes (triconcave erythrocytes) occur mainly in hemolytic anemias. The affected erythrocyte appears to have a "handle."

f. Stomatocytes have a slitlike central lucency. They are found in the very rare hereditary stomatocytosis and in other anemias.

g. Schizocytes (fragmentocytes) result from the fragmentation of erythrocytes, consisting either of a fragmented red cell or a fragment detached from such a cell. They resemble bits of broken egg shell. They may be caused by increased mechanical hemolysis (turbulence from artificial heart valves) or by increased intravascular coagulation (e.g., in hemolytic uremic syndrome) as fast-flowing red cells are sliced apart by fibrin filaments.

h. Siderocytes are erythrocytes that contain iron granules detectable with iron staining. They are a common feature of severe hemolytic anemias, lead poisoning, and pernicious anemia. Siderocytes containing coarse iron granules, which may encircle the nucleus (see Fig. 60), are pathognomonic for sideroachrestic anemias. Normal blood contains 0.5–1 siderocyte per 1000 red cells.

Left: At the center is a siderocyte containing several large iron granules and two sideroblasts also containing coarse iron granules, which normally are very small and difficult to see.

Right: At the center are three erythrocytes with numerous gray-violet granules that contain iron. This is a clear-cut pathologic finding that is rarely observed.

i. Reticulocytes in various stages of maturity. The more filamentous reticula are characteristic of younger cells (brilliant cresyl blue stain, see p. 8)

Fig. 6 a–d

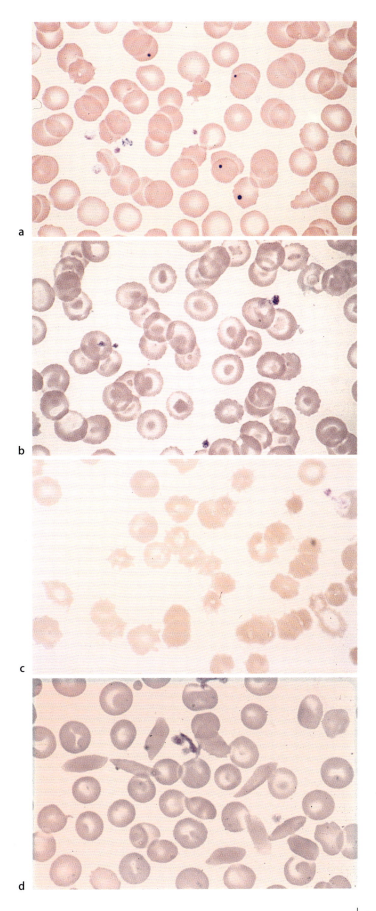

a

b

c

d

Fig. 6 e–h

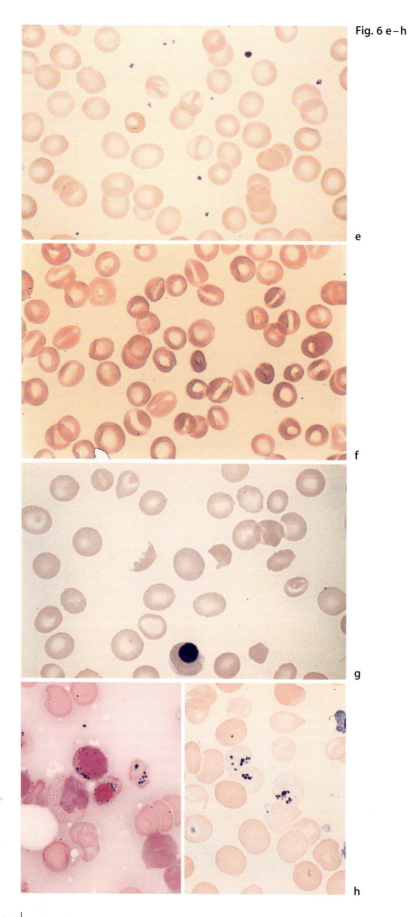

e

f

g

h

Fig. 6 i

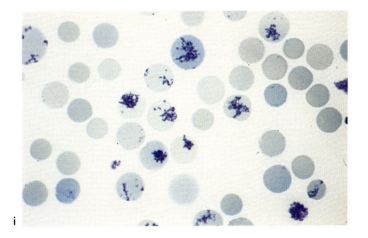

i

Fig. 7 a–h. Myeloblasts and promyelocytes

Myeloblasts are the earliest precursors of granulocytopoiesis that can be identified by light microscopy. Today it is believed that they also function as precursors of monocytes, i.e., as myelomonoblasts. They range from 12 to 20 μm in diameter (**a–c**). The cytoplasmic rim is basophilic but may show a range of hues from soft pale blue to dark blue. The cytoplasm is agranular on ordinary panoptic staining, although older cells frequently show incipient granulation signifying transition to the promyelocyte stage (**d**). The peroxidase reaction is usually negative, but there is no question that agranular, peroxidase-positive myeloblasts exist. The nucleus shows a very fine, dense chromatin structure with as many as six nucleoli, which generally are distinct and pale blue.

Promyelocytes evolve directly from the myeloblasts by incorporating azurophilic granules into their cytoplasm in a concentric pattern surrounding the clear zone in the nuclear indentation (Golgi zone), which itself is devoid of granules. Initially there are few granules, but these subsequently thicken and spread to fill the cytoplasm. At first the cytoplasm is basophilic but gradually lightens until it acquires the typical myelocytic tinge. The variable staining properties of the cytoplasm have led some authors to subdivide the promyelocytes into mature and immature forms, groups 1 and II, etc. As in myeloblasts, the promyelocyte nucleus is finely structured and contains up to six nucleoli. The cells are peroxidase-positive. First to appear are the primary or azurophilic granule, which contain peroxidase; they are joined later by the specific secondary granules (peroxidase-negative), which increase as maturation proceeds. The cells are 20–25 μm in diameter, making promyelocytes the largest cell of the granulocytopoietic and erythropoietic lines. In absolute terms, mitoses are more frequent than in the myeloblasts (**d–h**)

Fig. 7 a–d

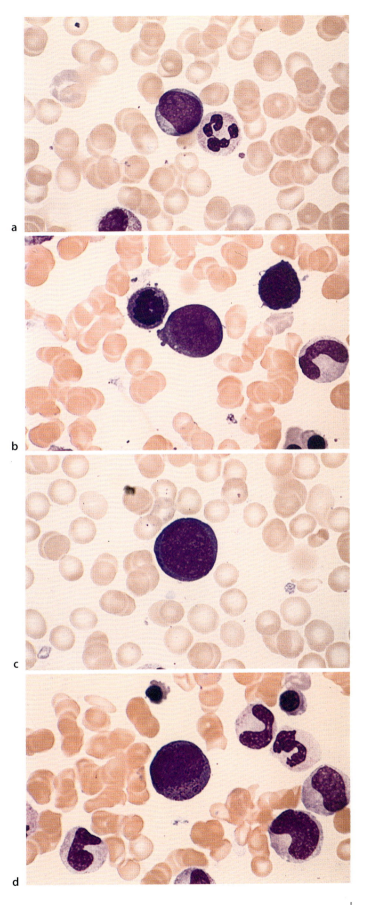

a

b

c

d

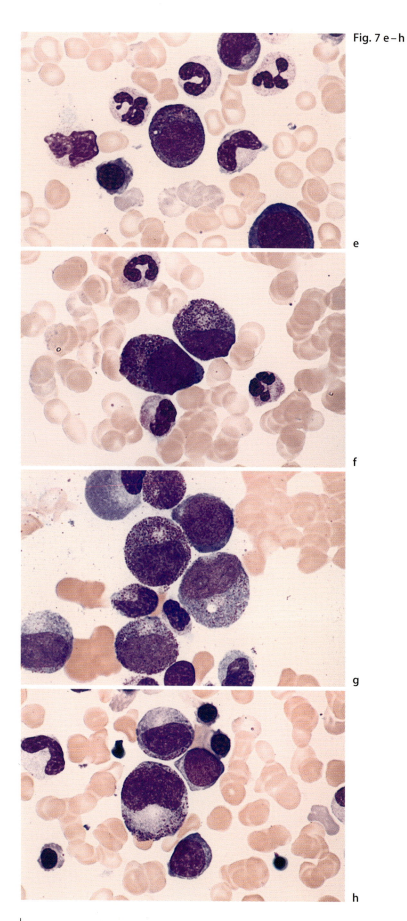

Fig. 7 e–h

e

f

g

h

Fig. 8 a – h. Neutrophilic myelocytes, metamyelocytes, band and segmented forms, also eosinophilic and basophilic granulocytes and tissue basophils

The offspring of the promyelocytes are the **myelocytes** (**a – e**). Generally these cells are somewhat smaller than their immediate precursors, with diameters ranging from 14 to 20 μm. As the coarse promyelocytic granules become more sparse, the typical fine neutrophilic granularity becomes predominant. The basophilic cytoplasm lightens from the nucleus outward, becoming acidophilic, while the nuclear chromatin acquires a coarser structure. Nucleoli are rarely visible. The myelocyte is the most plentiful granulocytopoietic cell type found in the bone marrow.

As maturation proceeds, the nuclear chromatin becomes even coarser and more dense. The nucleus becomes indented or horseshoe-shaped, while the cytoplasm and granules remain essentially the same as in mature myelocytes. The cells at this stage are called **metamyelocytes** or *juvenile forms* (**d**). A few may be found in the peripheral blood. Metamyelocytes are no longer capable of division.

The **band neutrophil** (**e**) is distinguished from the metamyelocyte by its smaller and more coarsely structured nucleus. Its cytoplasm and granules are like those of metamyelocytes. Constrictions begin to appear in the nucleus, but the cell is not classified as a *segmented form* until the bridge between two nuclear lobes is filiform or less than one-third the width of the adjacent lobes.

The nuclear lobes of the *segmented neutrophil* (**b, c, g**) present a coarse, clumped chromatin structure. Most of these cells contain 3 – 5 nuclear lobes usually joined by thin, short chromatin filaments. A cell containing more than 5 lobes is said to be hypersegmented. This is especially common in pernicious anemia but is not pathognomonic for that condition. The band and segmented forms range from 10 to 15 μm in size.

Eosinophilic granulocytes (**b, e, f**) develop in much the same way as neutrophils, but the two cell types are always distinguishable from the promyelocyte stage onward. The nuclei have structures similar to the corresponding maturation stages. The typical large eosinophilic granules almost completely obscure the cytoplasm. Conspicuously large granules, sometimes of a deep blue color, may be found among these mature eosinophilic granules in the early stages of promyelocytes and myelocytes (**b, e**) but are no longer present in the mature stages. Another typical feature of eosinophils is their nuclear segmentation, with most cells possessing two nuclear lobes and a smaller number having three. Mitoses of eosinophils are also occasionally found in bone marrow. All eosinophils are peroxidase-positive.

Basophilic granulocytes (**g**) also have a developmental pathway similar to neutrophils but usually are not distinguishable until the myelocyte stage. Typically they contain large basophilic granules that obscure the cytoplasm and even cover the nucleus. In segmented basophils the nucleus consists of multiple lobes and often presents a cloverleaf shape. The cells tend to be somewhat smaller than neutrophils and eosinophils. They are usually peroxidase-negative when standard technique is used.

Mast cells (tissue basophils, h) are classified into two types based on nuclear size and shape and granule density. *Mastoblasts* and *promastocytes* have a relatively large nucleus with an indistinct structure and sparse granules. *Mastocytes* are large cells (diam. 15 – 30 μm) with a round, compact nucleus showing structural similarities to the lymphocyte or plasma cell. Acid mucopolysaccharides are responsible for the typical *metachromasia* of the granular stain pattern and can be demonstrated cytochemically with toluidine blue stain (for method, see p. 7). A strong naphthol AS-D chloroacetate esterase reaction is also typical (**h**, *right*). Mast cells produce heparin and histamine in a ratio of 3 : 1. Isolated mast cells may be found in fragments of normal bone marrow. The mast cell population in bone marrow is increased in severe inflammatory disorders, panmyelophthisis, non-Hodgkin lymphoma, and especially in Waldenström disease (lymphoplasmocytoid immunocytoma) and hairy cell leukemia. Atypical mast cells may be found in mastocytoses (**Figs. 128, 129**).

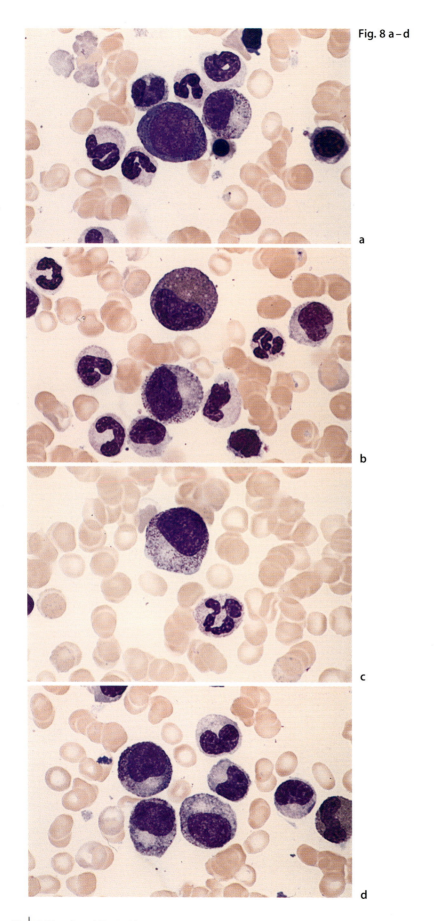

Fig. 8 a–d

a

b

c

d

Fig. 8 e–h

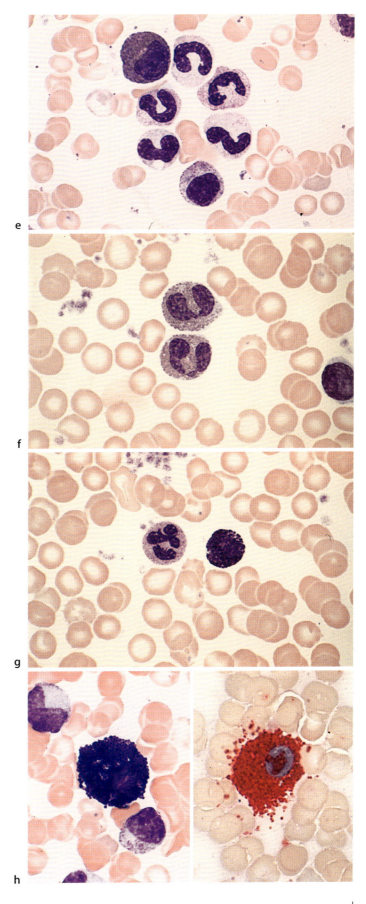

e

f

g

h

Fig. 9 a – d. Degenerate forms, toxic changes and artifacts

Rarely, **degenerate leukocyte forms (a)** may be found in the peripheral blood of patients exposed to certain irritants. They are more commonly seen in smears prepared from long-stored blood previously treated with EDTA or citrate solution. Most of these cells have the same diameter as segmented forms, but many are considerably smaller (4 – 8 μm). Usually their cytoplasm is slightly more basophilic than in segmented forms, and their granules are coarser and often smudged. Pronounced nuclear pyknosis is typical, and 3 – 5 solid, featureless nuclear remnants may be found scattered like droplets in the cytoplasm. There are few if any filaments interconnecting the nuclear remnants.

In cases of severe infection or bone marrow injury, it is common to find large purple granules in the myelocytes and in more mature stages up to the segmented forms. Often they are similar to the granules seen in promyelocytes, and many authors consider them to be identical. This **"toxic granulation" (b)** is variable in its intensity. In very pronounced cases the neutrophils may come to resemble basophilic granulocytes.

Cytoplasmic vacuoles in leukocytes, like toxic granulations, can develop in response to various *toxic insults.* They are often observed during long-term *chloramphenicol therapy, phenylketonuria, diabetes mellitus,* and in the setting of severe bacterial and viral infections. The vacuoles reflect a metabolic disturbance in the affected cells.

Heparin artifact. Adding heparin to peripheral blood or especially bone marrow before preparing smears leads to artifacts when a panoptic stain is used (Giemsa or Pappenheim): the cells show scant or atypical staining, and a purple, crumbly precipitate forms on the background, making it difficult or impossible to identify the cells **(c).**

Necrotic bone marrow. Bone marrow that has been aspirated and stained may be found to contain unstructured purple material or faint, shadowy cells with indistinct outlines. The cause is necrotic bone marrow at the aspiration site. The necrosis may be quite extensive and is occasionally seen in acute leukemias and other diseases **(d)**

Fig. 9 a–d

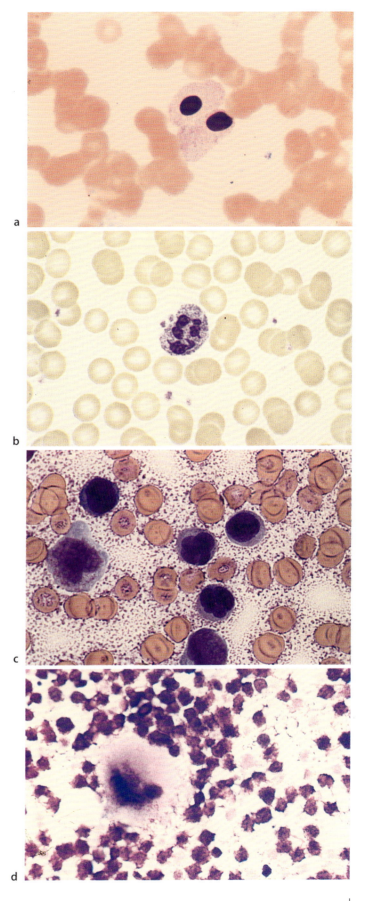

Fig. 10 a–f. Congenital anomalies of granulo-cytopoiesis

The **Pelger-Huet anomaly** (a–c) is an inherited anomaly involving the nuclei of granulocytes. The heterozygous form predominates in man while the homozygous form, characterized by small round or oval nuclei (c), is extremely rare. The nucleus of neutrophils is indented and resembles the band form, giving rise to a "pseudo-regenerative" white blood picture. When nuclear segmentation (lobulation) occurs, the neutrophils acquire two nuclear lobes and rarely three. These lobes are exceptionally short, thick, and chromatin-rich. Pelger myelocytes and band forms also have very coarse, clumped nuclei rich in chromatin. The patient is classified as a full carrier if all neutrophils are affected by the anomaly and a partial carrier if normal band and segmented forms are also present. The Pelger-Huet anomaly is harmless in its effect on leukocyte function. Severe infections and particularly myelodysplasias, acute myeloid leukemia, and advanced chronic myeloid leukemia can produce transient, qualitatively similar changes in white cell nuclei, creating what is known as "pseudo Pelger-Huet forms."

In the **Alder-Reilly anomaly** (d–f), the granulocytes contain large, bluish granules that often resemble those of promyelocytes. The abnormal granulation is especially marked in eosinophils, which appear basophilic rather than eosinophilic (e, *left*). The lymphocytes also contain particularly large azurophilic granules (f). Carriers of this anomaly frequently have associated bone and joint deformities (gargoylism). The anomaly is known to occur in mucopolysaccharidosis VI and VII

Fig. 10 a–d

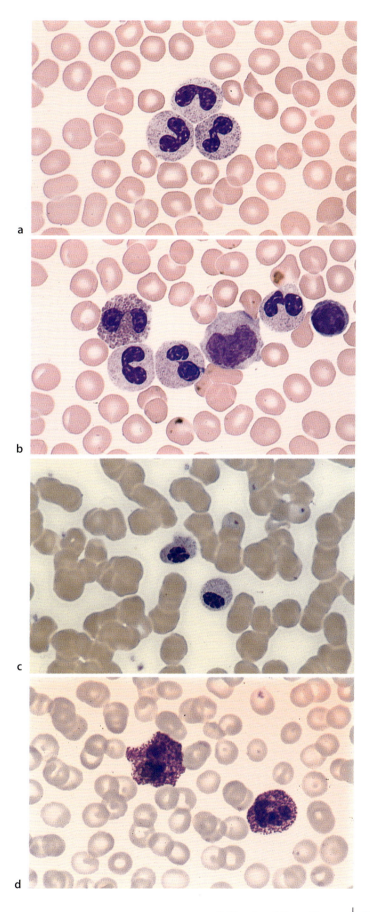

a

b

c

d

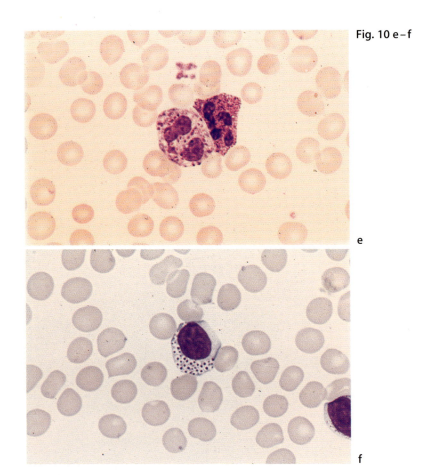

e

f

Fig. 11 a–f. Steinbrinck-Chediak-Higashi anomaly (granular gigantism of leukocytes)

This condition affects virtually *all leukocytes*. The *neutrophils* contain irregular, grayish-blue cytoplasmic inclusions 1–3 μm in diameter. These bodies are sharply demarcated and contain peroxidase and also CE in some cases, identifying them as primary granules (**a, b, e, f**). The granules of *eosinophilic leukocytes* are also enlarged to 2–3 times the size of normal eosinophilic granules. They are round to oval in shape and variable in size. Most *lymphocytes* and *monocytes* also contain intensely red-staining granules 1–2 μm in diameter. The inclusions in the monocytes are 5 μm in diameter and stain pink (**d**). In the *bone marrow*, red-violet bodies 1–3 μm in diameter can be demonstrated in semimature and mature cells starting with the promyelocytes. In addition, the myeloblasts and myelocytes frequently contain large vacuoles in which a large, round inclusion is often found (**c–f**). Phase contrast and electron microscopy reveal coarse cytoplasmic inclusions of a pleomorphic structure in neutrophils and eosinophils, lymphocytes, and even in erythroblasts. There is further evidence indicating that the disease is based on a defect in the lysosomal membrane. This pathogenic disturbance, which exerts its major biochemical effect on glycolipids, affects not only the blood cells but other organs as well and thus cannot be considered innocuous. Affected individuals usually die at an early age

Fig. 11 a – d

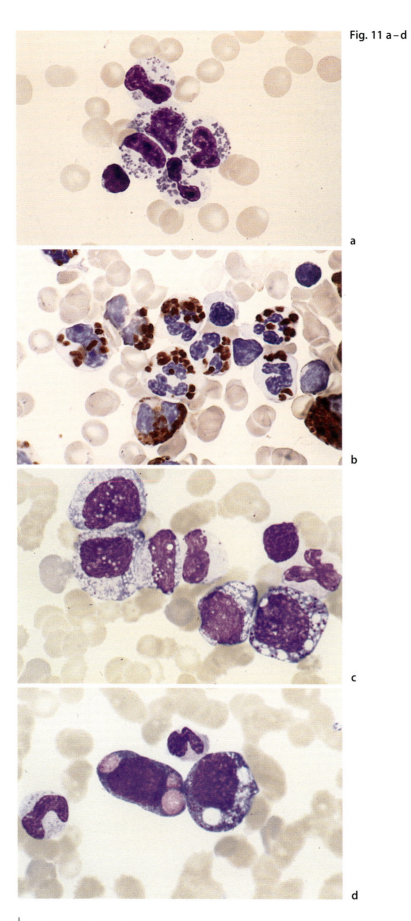

a

b

c

d

Fig. 11 e–f

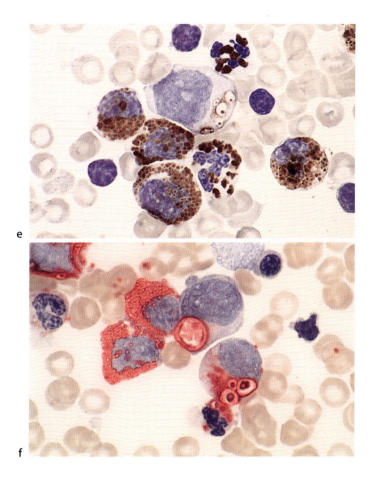

e

f

Fig. 12 a–d. May-Hegglin anomaly

This disorder has an autosomal dominant mode of inheritance and is associated with mild leukopenia and thrombocytopenia. The neutrophilic granulocytes contain predominantly rod-shaped inclusions of a pale- to dirty-blue color, approximately 2–5 µm in diameter, which are found on electron microscopy to consist of dense RNA fibrils and are distinguishable from the Döhle bodies that occur in severe infections. The inclusions also occur in monocytes and eosinophils, but they are very difficult to detect in these cells. They can be selectively demonstrated with methyl green-pyronine stain (red) (**a, b**). Giant platelets are also detected (**c**). There is one reported case (H.L.) in which bone marrow examination revealed a coarse, nonhomogeneous clumping of granules in the cytoplasm of the megakaryocytes (**d**)

Fig. 12 a–d

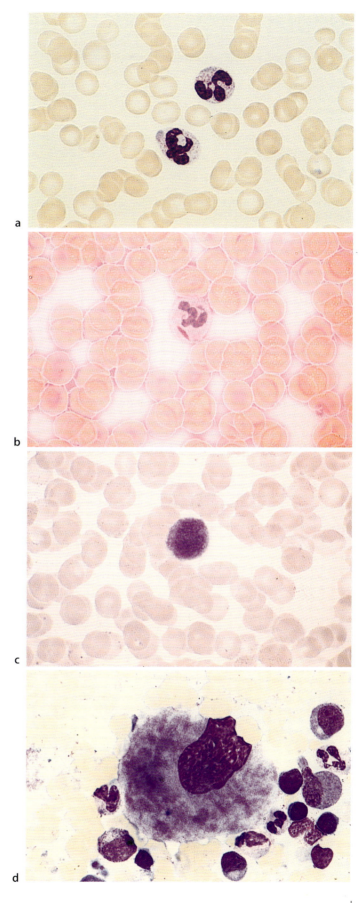

a

b

c

d

Fig. 13 a–h. Cells of the monocyte-macrophage system

a, b Typical monocytes with pleomorphic nucleus, pale blue cytoplasm, and fine, barely perceptible azurophilic granules.

c Monocyte, with a metamyelocyte at *upper left*.

d Monocyte with a small nucleus and, below it, a segmented neutrophil.

e Two promonocytes in a bone marrow smear.

f Two promonocytes with nucleoli, and a monocyte at *upper left*.

g Monocyte with phagocytized nuclear residue.

h Monocyte with phagocytized material in the cytoplasm (macrophage).

Monocytes. The monocyte is an exceptionally pleomorphic blood cell ranging from 12 to 20 μm in size. Its cytoplasm often has irregular borders and stains a characteristic grayish blue. Some monocytes contain azurophilic granules much finer than those seen in lymphocytes. The nucleus is seldom round; usually it is deeply indented and lobulated (often bean-shaped). Its loose, delicate chromatin pattern is unique among the blood cells. Clumps of chromatin may be found scattered among larger, chromatin-poor areas. Nucleoli are rarely present

Fig. 13 a–d

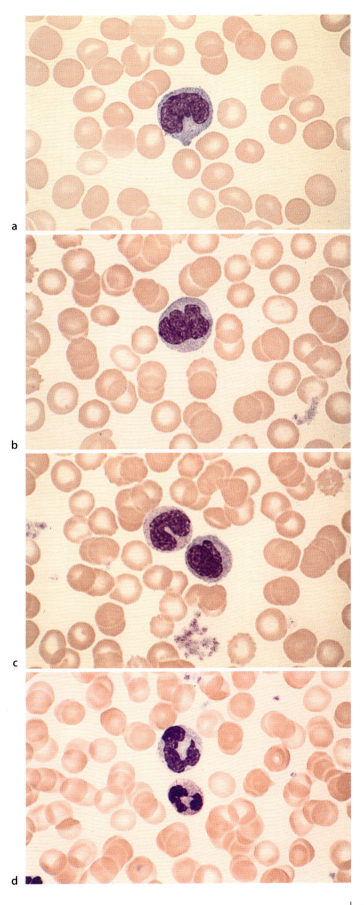

a

b

c

d

Fig. 13 e–h

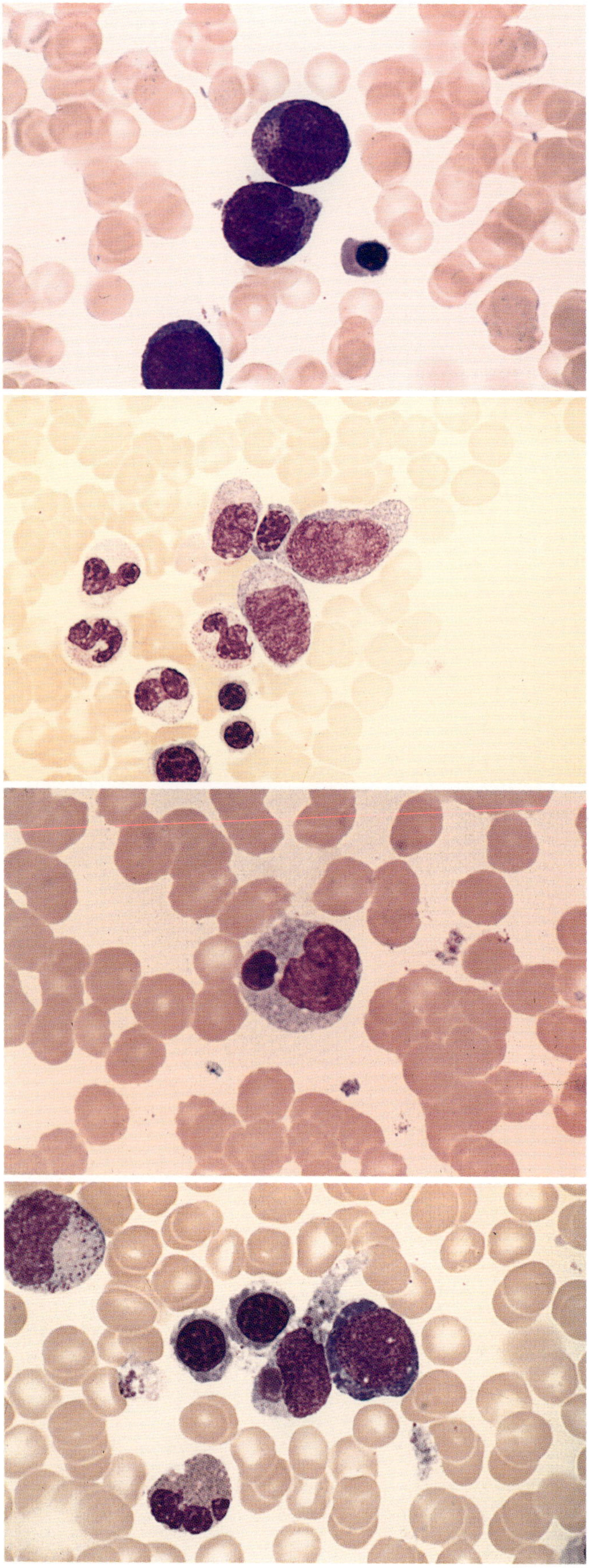

e

f

g

h

Fig. 14 a – h. Macrophages in the bone marrow

a Macrophage with nuclei, erythrocytes and platelets in the cytoplasm (nucleus at *lower right*).

b Two macrophages with cellular residues.

c Macrophage showing high acid phosphatase activity (red) and nuclear residues (bluish gray).

d Binucleated macrophage with predominantly fine-grained hemosiderin in the cytoplasm (yellow-gold).

e Abundant hemosiderin, some coarsely granular, in the cytoplasm.

f Clumped and diffusely scattered iron in the cytoplasm of macrophages (Berlin blue reaction).

g Peculiar blue pigment in the cytoplasm.

h Two lipophages containing droplets of stored fat.

The bone marrow cells formerly known as reticulum cells in cytologic practice are actually quite diverse. A great many cells that cannot be fitted into standard classification schemes have been grouped under the heading of "reticulum cells." Current concepts regarding the origin and classification of the cell forms of interest here will be discussed below. A large portion of the *"reticulum storage cells,"* but probably not all, are derived from the monocyte-macrophage system. The reticulum cells of the bone marrow in the strict sense form the reticular or spongy tissue that constitutes the matrix of all hematopoiesis. Other types are vascular endothelial cells and sinus endothelial cells, which occasionally are found in clusters. Arterial endothelial cells are distinguishable from other "reticulum cells" by their positive alkaline phosphatase reaction. When spread onto a slide, the cells lose part of their cytoplasm and present as *"naked nuclei."* The cells formerly called *small lymphoid reticulum cells* probably represent tissue-bound lymphocytes. The *shape and appearance of reticulum cells* vary greatly with the purpose and functional status of the cell. The typical nucleus presents a loose "reticular" structure with one or more small nucleoli that are fairly indistinct. Usually there is a broad rim of cytoplasm that is poorly demarcated from its surroundings. The cytoplasm usually appears clear or pale blue on staining. Vacuoles are common.

Dendritic and interdigitating reticulum cells, which carry out important immunologic functions, will be described later

Fig. 14 a–d

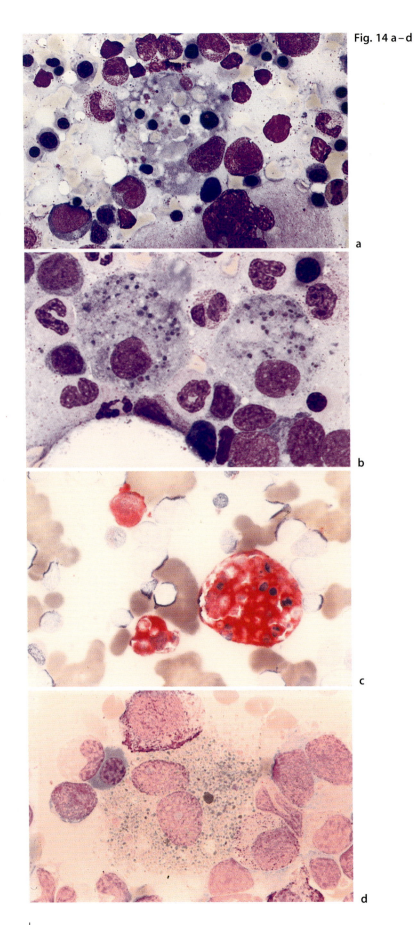

Fig. 14 e–h

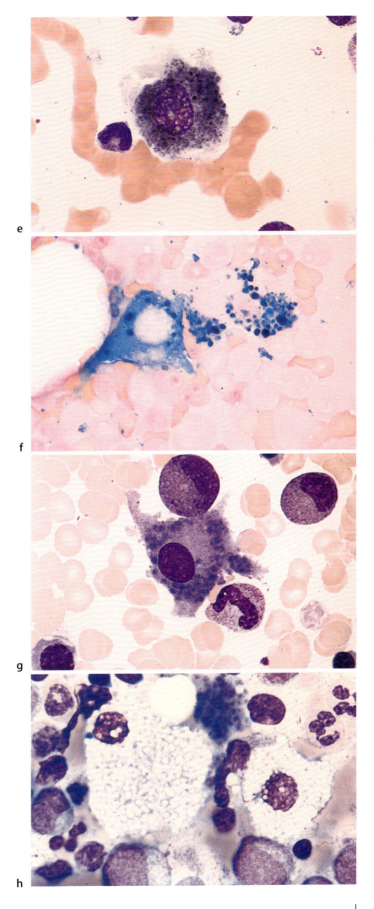

e

f

g

h

Fig. 15 a–e. Megakaryocytes

These largest of the bone marrow cells show extreme morphologic diversity. The young precursors are called *megakaryoblasts*, of which the smallest diploid forms are only slightly larger than myeloblasts, which they resemble (**a**). The diploid forms develop into polyploid forms, which have two or four small nuclei or one large nucleus depending on whether the nucleus undergoes true division or simple reduplication (endomitosis). A polyploid *promegakaryocyte* with only one nucleus is shown in panel **b**.

Cell **c** is somewhat more mature, as we see from its polychromatic cytoplasm in which acidophilic elements coexist with the basophilic ground substance.

Cell **d** is a mature megakaryocyte with an indented nucleus, blurred chromatin pattern, and a red-violet, shadowy cytoplasm.

Cell **e** conveys the impression of platelet formation at *lower left* and *upper right*.

Fig. 15 a–d

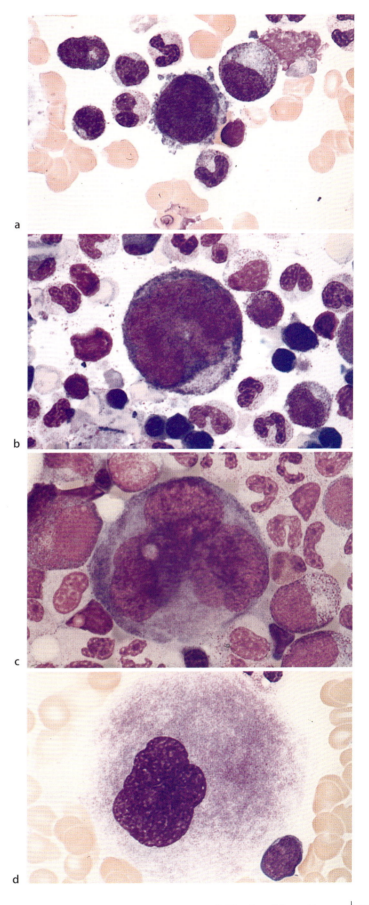

a

b

c

d

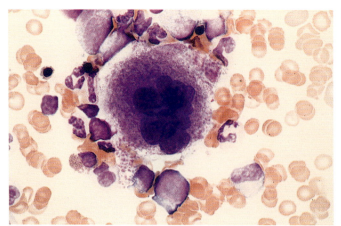

Fig. 15 e

e

Fig. 16 a – f. Osteoblasts and osteoclasts

a Group of osteoblasts in a bone marrow smear. The clear area in the cytoplasm lies distant from the nucleus (Golgi region).

b Cluster of osteoblasts at high magnification. The clear area in the cytoplasm is plainly visible and lies farther from the nucleus than in plasma cells.

c Extremely high alkaline phosphatase activity in osteoblasts. Besides mature granulocytes and vascular endothelial cells, these are the only cells in the bone marrow that display high alkaline phosphatase activity.

d Multinucleated osteoclast (separate round nuclei) in the bone marrow.

e Elongated portion of an osteoclast, showing a series of adjacent nuclei.

f Twisted osteoclast with coarse inclusions (resorbed bone).

A familiarity with **osteoblasts** is important so that they can be distinguished from plasma cells or, when clustered, from tumor cells. Most osteoblasts are oblong with a maximum diameter of approximately 30 µm. As a rule the nucleus is eccentrically placed, has a reticular chromatin pattern, and usually contains several deep-blue nucleoli. The cytoplasm is dark blue and contains a clear zone, the archoplasm, situated some distance from the nucleus. Osteoblasts have high alkaline phosphatase activity.

Osteoclasts are a special type of foreign-body giant cell derived from monocytes. They contain several or numerous round or oval nuclei, usually with one small nucleolus. They display high acid phosphatase activity. The cytoplasm is reddish-violet and finely granular. It may contain coarse inclusions believed to be remnants of resorbed bone. Exceptionally large osteoclasts with as many as 100 nuclei (*polykaryocytes*) may be found in the bone marrow of children and especially in patients with osteitis fibrosa generalisata

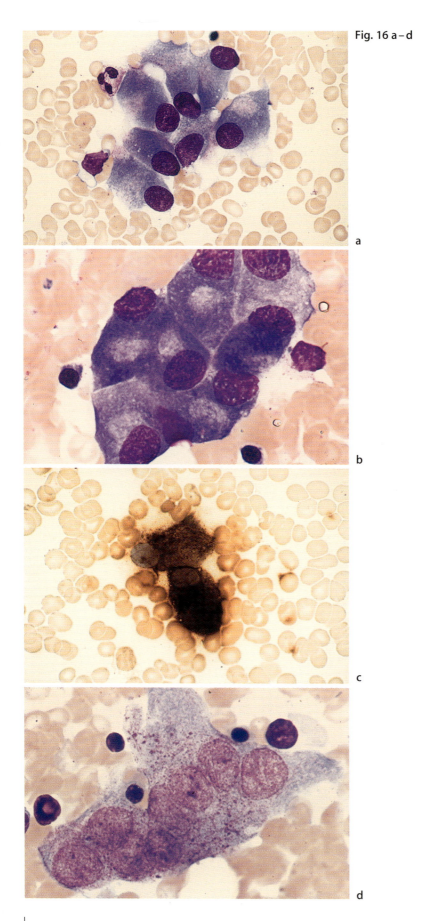

Fig. 16 a–d

a

b

c

d

Fig. 16 e–f

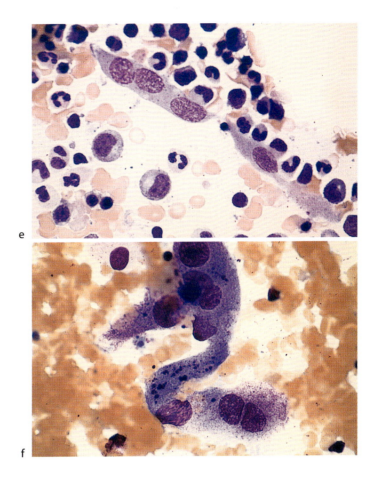

e

f

Fig. 17 a–g. Lymphocytes and plasma cells

a Small lymphocyte with narrow rim of pale to moderate blue cytoplasm.

b Small lymphocyte at *top*, compared with a monocyte *below*. Note the difference in nuclear structure.

c Coarsely granular lymphocyte with numerous, relatively coarse azurophilic granules in a broad, pale cytoplasmic rim. Cellular morphology is consistent with a T cell or NK cell.

d Plasma cell from peripheral blood ("blood plasma cell") with highly basophilic cytoplasm and a perinuclear halo.

e Typical mature plasma cell in the bone marrow with an eccentric nucleus and perinuclear halo.

f Group of mature plasma cells with a spoked-wheel nuclear structure, which usually is apparent only in tissue sections.

g Binucleated mature plasma cell (not uncommon in reactive states).

The dominant forms in healthy adults are small **lymphocytes** with a compact nucleus. Occasionally they are accompanied by larger cells that may contain *azurophilic granules* in their cytoplasm.

Plasma cells in the bone marrow are characterized by a basophilic cytoplasm and an eccentric nuclear position. The cells range from 14 to 20 µm in size. The cytoplasm of mature forms is darkly basophilic (due to a high content of ergastoplasm), often shadowy, and always agranular. Small to moderately large cytoplasmic vacuoles also are commonly seen. The nucleus of immature cells is centered, shows a delicate chromatin pattern, and contains 1–3 nucleoli. The nucleus of mature plasma cells is always eccentric and shows a coarse chromatin pattern similar to that in mature lymphocytes. Nucleoli cannot be demonstrated in the mature forms with ordinary stains. Binucleated or even multinucleated forms are not uncommon. The individual chromosomes in mitotic figures are relatively coarse

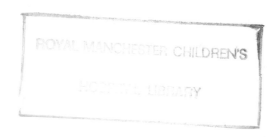

Fig. 17 a–d

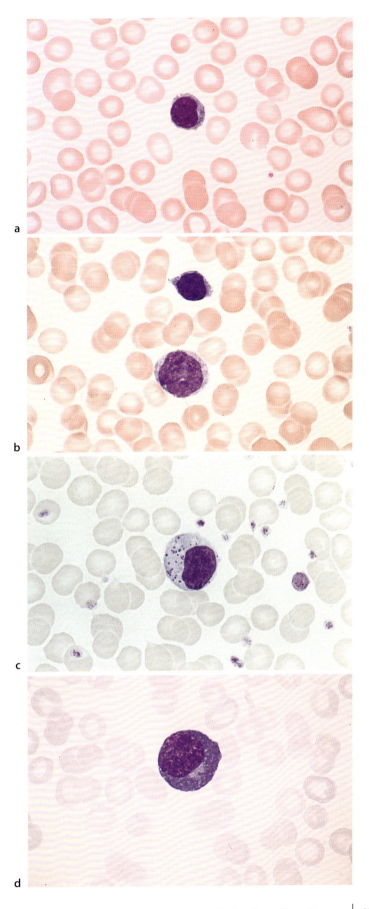

a

b

c

d

Fig. 17 e–g

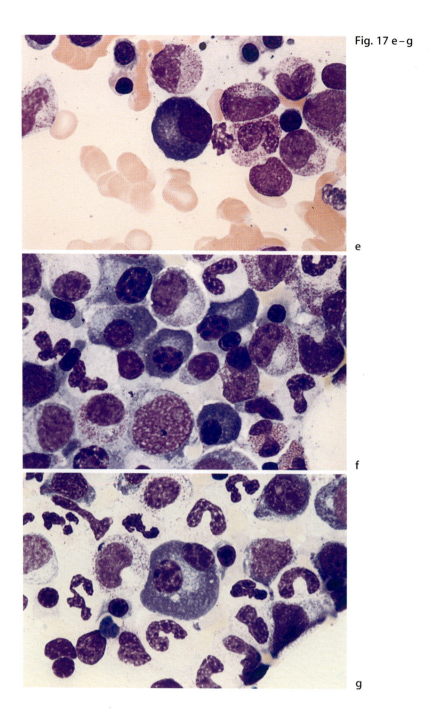

e

f

g

2. Normal and Abnormal Bone Marrow

Composition of Normal Bone Marrow

As stated on p. 23, normal bone marrow contains the precursors of erythrocytes, granulocytes, platelets, stromal cells, tissue mast cells, B lymphocytes, and occasional osteoblasts. The abundance of stromal cells varies with the smear technique that is used. Reticulum cells are sparse in pure bone marrow fluid but are more plentiful in the smear from a bone marrow fragment. Mature hematopoietic cells develop within a few days after bone marrow transplantation and even more rapidly following peripheral stem cell transplantation (**Fig. 20a – c**).

Various techniques can be used to perform a *differential cell count* in bone marrow aspirates. Formerly we determined the cell counts per 100 leukocytes and their precursors. In the counting of marrow fragments, which should be free of blood if possible, a maximum of 10 lymphocytes are found per 100 leukocytes. We also find approximately 30 or at most 40 erythrocyte precursors per 100 leukocytes, 2 to 6 plasma cells, and approximately 10 reticulum cells, the exact count varying, as noted, with the smear technique. It is very difficult to state figures for megakaryocytes, but this is not essential for routine clinical tests. A better way to obtain comparable absolute figures, however, is by counting all bone marrow cells (excluding megakaryocytes) sequentially, continuing until at least 200 cells have been counted. Table 4 shows the distribution that Bain obtained by counting 500 nucleated cells in the bone marrow smears from 50 healthy subjects.

Table 5 shows the changes in differential cell counts that are associated with certain common diseases. *Cytochemical procedures* have gained major importance in the diagnosis of hematologic disorders in recent years. Cytochemical staining methods are described on pp. 7 – 16, and the staining characteristics of the various blood cells and their precursors are reviewed in **Table 3** and in **Figs. 18 and 19** for the most common staining methods.

Morphologic, cytochemical, and immunologic techniques must be used for the accurate differentiation of leukemias and lymphomas.

Figure 21a – d illustrates the different degrees of cellularity that may be found in bone marrow smears in various pathologic conditions. These variations underscore the importance of examining the smear at low magnification before proceeding with a more detailed evaluation. Figure 22f, g shows the appearance of a normal bone marrow smear viewed at high magnification. Figure 22a, b illustrates the range of variation in the cellular and fat distribution that may be found in normal bone marrow (histologic sections). Figure 22c shows how the naphthol AS-D chloroacetate esterase method can be used to localize early neutrophilic granulocytopoiesis close to bony trabeculae. Figure 22d, e illustrates small intact vessels in a bone marrow smear demonstrated by the alkaline phosphatase method. Detached endothelial cells appear as "reticulum cells" when this method is used.

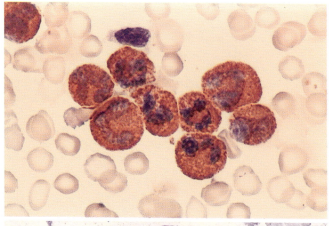

Fig. 18. a – d

a Peroxidase reaction
(POX of Graham-Knoll)

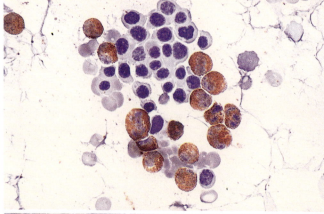

b POX in bone marrow. Mature granulocytes are positive, and erythroblasts are negative. Nuclei stained with hemalum

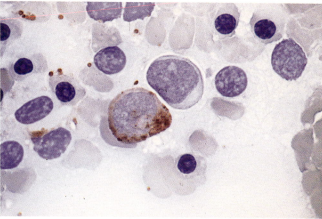

c POX in bone marrow. At *center* is a negative blast; next to it is a positive, isomorphic cell (promyelocyte)

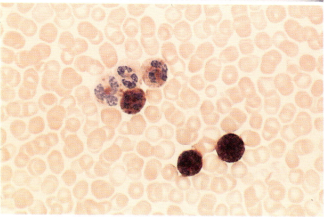

d Leukocyte alkaline phosphatase (LAP) with the substrate α-naphthyl phosphate and variamin blue salt B. Grades 1 – 4 in the peripheral blood

Fig. 18. e – h

e LAP (Sigma method). Very high activity levels (grades 3 and 4) are observed after G-CSF therapy

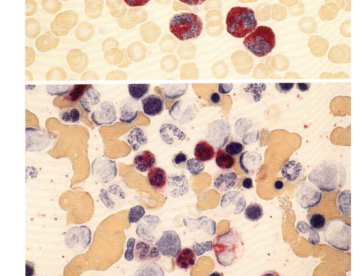

f LAP in bone marrow. Only mature granulocytes are positive (*red*)

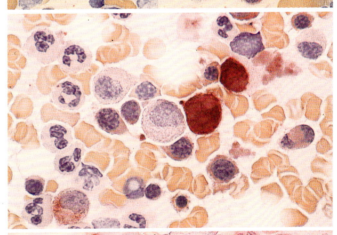

g Nonspecific esterase reaction (α-naphthyl acetate, hexazonium-pararosaniline) in bone marrow. Monocytes are strongly positive, and a weak reaction is seen in the cytoplasm of erythroblasts

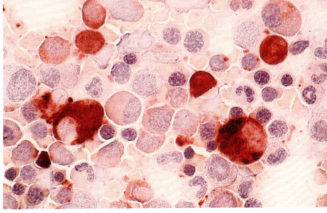

h Very strong nonspecific esterase reaction in macrophages and monocytes. A *dotlike* reaction pattern is seen in two lymphocytes

Fig. 19 a – d

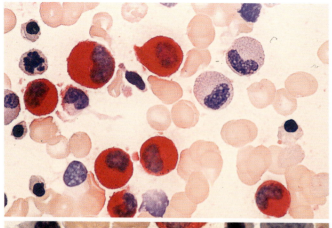

a Naphthol AS-D chloroacetate esterase (CE) in the bone marrow. Neutrophilic granulocytes are strongly positive (*red*), and two eosinophils are negative

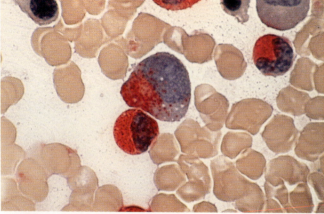

b CE: a promyelocyte with a positive reaction (*red*) in the nuclear indentation is visible. Below it is a positive myelocyte

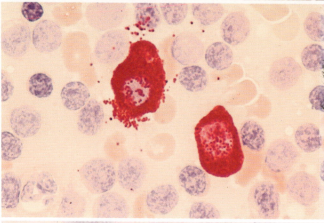

c CE in a lymph node smear shows two tissue mast cells with strongly positive granules, also negative lymphocytes

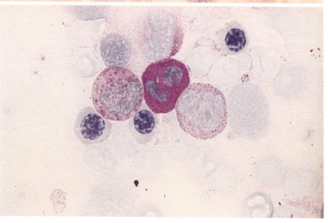

d PAS reaction: strong diffuse staining in a neutrophil, weak intergranular staining in an eosinophil (*left*), and fine positive granules in a monocyte (*right*). Neutrophils show an increasing reaction as they mature. Some lymphocytes contain fine PAS-positive granules

Fig. 19 e–h

e Acid phosphatase (Sigma method) in a macrophage

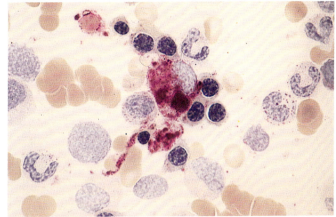

f Berlin blue reaction for detecting iron: a "reticulum cell" at the *center* of an erythroblast cluster shows strong, diffuse cytoplasmic staining

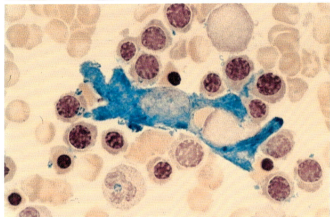

g Iron detection: coarse granular iron deposits in a macrophage

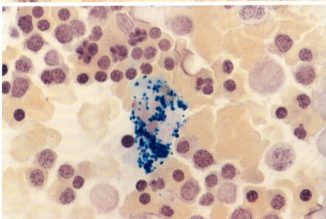

h Iron detection: fine granular cytoplasmic reaction in an endothelial cell (may be seen after the intravenous administration of iron)

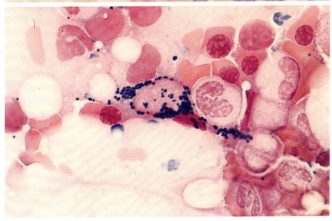

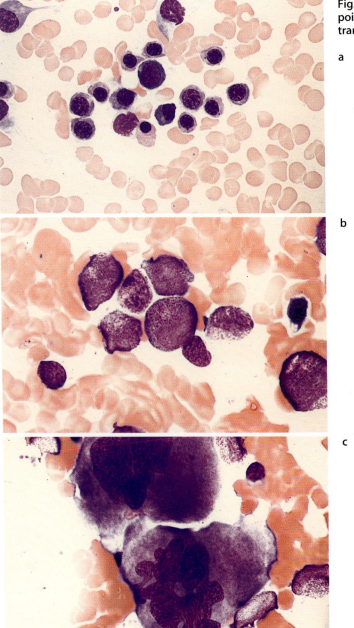

Fig. 20 a–c. Mature cells of hematopoiesis following peripheral stem cell
transplantation

a

b

c

Fig. 21 a–d. Variations in the cellularity of bone marrow smears

a Normal bone marrow

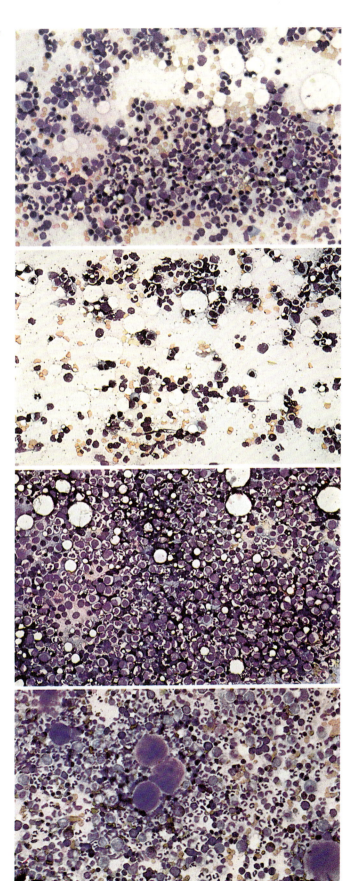

b Hypocellular bone marrow

c Hypercellular bone marrow

d Hypercellular bone marrow with numerous megakaryocytes

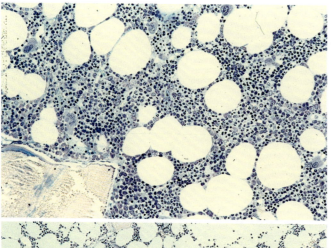

Fig. 22 a–d

a, b Range of variation in the cellular and fat distribution of normal bone marrow

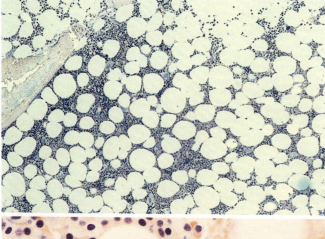

b

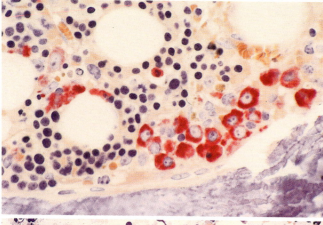

c Localization of early neutrophilic granulocytopoiesis (naphthol AS-D chloroacetate esterase method)

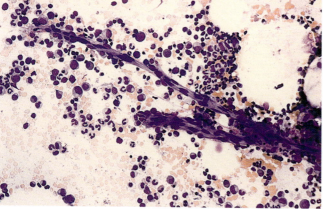

d, e Small intact vessels in the bone marrow smear (**e** demonstrated by alkaline phosphatase method)

Fig. 22 e–g

e

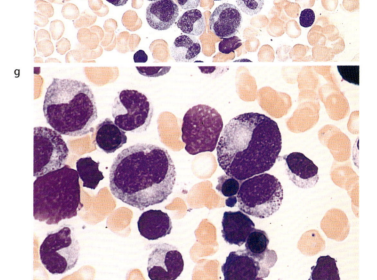

f, g Normal marrow smear viewed at
high magnification

g

Table 4. Percentage of bone marrow cells found in smears from 50 healthy subjects (slightly modified from Bain BJ 1996) Br J Haematol 14:206–209

	Observed range	95 % range	(Average)
Blasts	0–3.2	0–3.0	(1.4)
Promyelocytes	3.6–13.2	3.2–12.4	(7.8)
Myelocytes	4.0–21.4	3.7–10.0	(7.6)
Metamyelocytes	1.0–7.0	2.3–5.9	(4.1)
Band and segmented forms			
Men	21.0–45.6**	21.9–42.3	(32.1)
Women	29.6–46.6**	28.8–45.9	(37.4)
Eosinophils	0.9–7.4	0.7–6.3	(3.5)
Basophils	0–0.8	0–0.4	(0.1)
Erythroblasts			
Men	18.0–39.4**	16.2–40.1	(28.1)
Women	14.0–31.8**	13.0–32.0	(22.5)
Lymphocytes[a]	4.6–22.6	6.0–20.0	(13.1)
Plasma cells	0–1.4	0–1.2	(0.6)
Monocytes	0–3.2	0–2.6	(1.3)
Macrophages	0–1.8	0–1.3	(0.4)
Myeloid:erythroid ratio			
Men	1.1–4.0*	1.1–4.1	(2.1)
Women	1.6–5.4*	1.6–5.2	(2.8)

Significance of the difference between men and women: $*p = 0.01$, $**p = 0.001$.

[a] The percentage of lymphocytes in small children may reach approximately 35 %, and isolated lymphatic blasts ("hematogones") are found which express CD 19.

Table 5. Changes in differential counts of bone marrow in various diseases

	Normal	Iron deficiency anemias	Hemolytic anemias	Megaloblastic anemias	Infection	Chronic myeloid leukemia	Chronic lympho-cytic leukemia	Agranulocytosis
	20 40 60 80	20 40 60 80	20 40 60 80	20 40 60 80	20 40 60 80	20 40 60 80	20 40 60 80	20 40 60 80
Reticulum cells								
Plasma cells								
Megaloblasts								
Basophilic proerythroblasts								
Polychromatic erythroblasts								
Orthochromatic normoblasts								
Myeloblasts								
Neutrophilic promyelocytes								
Neutrophilic myelocytes								
Neutrophilic metamyelocytes								
Band neutrophils								
Segmented neutrophils								
Immature eosinophils								
Mature eosinophils								
Basophils								
Monocytes								
Lymphoblasts								
Lymphocytes								
Megakaryocytes	+	+–++	+	(+)	+	++	(+)	+

(+) = weakly positive; + = positive; ++ = markedly positive

Disturbances of Erythropoiesis

Hypochromic Anemias (Fig. 23a–d)

Hypochromic anemias are the morphologic prototype of all anemias that arise from a disturbance of hemoglobin synthesis in erythrocytes. In cases of severe iron deficiency, the erythrocytes are small, flat, and feature a large area of central pallor (anulocytes) (**Fig. 23a**). Typically there is a *"left shift" of erythropoiesis*, meaning that there is a predominance of younger basophilic forms. *Nuclear-cytoplasmic dissociation* is also present, i.e., the nucleus is relatively mature while the cytoplasm still appears strongly basophilic and may be poorly marginated (**Fig. 23b, c**).

The quantitative changes in erythropoiesis can be quite diverse. *Iron deficiency* due to an acute or chronic blood loss is usually associated with a marked increase of erythropoiesis, with a shift in the balance of erythropoiesis and granulocytopoiesis in favor of red cell production. Additionally, the megakaryocytes are usually increased in number.

By contrast, there is often an absolute reduction of erythropoiesis in *toxic-infectious processes* and *neoplastic diseases* ("chronic disease anemias"), although there are no hard and fast rules.

The bone marrow changes found in *iron utilization disorders* (sideroachrestic anemia, "iron deficiency without iron deficiency") are similar to those observed in iron deficiency. They can be differentiated by iron staining (see p. 9).

In the iron deficiency anemias (**Fig. 23a–d**) it is rare to find siderocytes and sideroblasts, and iron deposits are never detected in macrophages (**Fig. 23d**). On the other hand, sideroachrestic anemias are characterized by numerous sideroblasts with coarse granular iron deposits (*ringed sideroblasts*, **Fig. 61**) and massive iron storage in the macrophages [see myelodysplastic syndromes, refractory anemia with ringed sideroblasts (RARS)]. Iron-storing cells can also be found in infectious and neoplastic anemias. The various forms of iron deficiency and their pathogenesis are reviewed in Scheme 1.

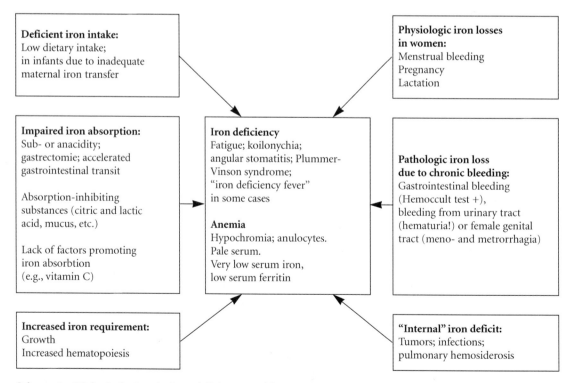

Scheme 1. Etiologic factors in iron deficiency and its symptoms.
[From Begemann H, Begemann M (1989) Praktische Hämatologie, 9th ed. Thieme, Stuttgart]

Fig. 23 a – d

a Erythrocytes in severe iron deficiency. The large area of central pallor (anulocytes) is typical. The erythrocytes are flat, small, and appear pale

b Group of bone marrow erythroblasts in iron deficiency. The basophilic cytoplasm contrasts with the relatively mature nuclei (*nuclear-cytoplasmic dissociation*)

c In severe iron deficiency, even the cytoplasm of some mature erythroblasts is still basophilic and has indistinct margins

d Iron stain reveals absence of iron stores in bone marrow fragments due to severe iron deficiency

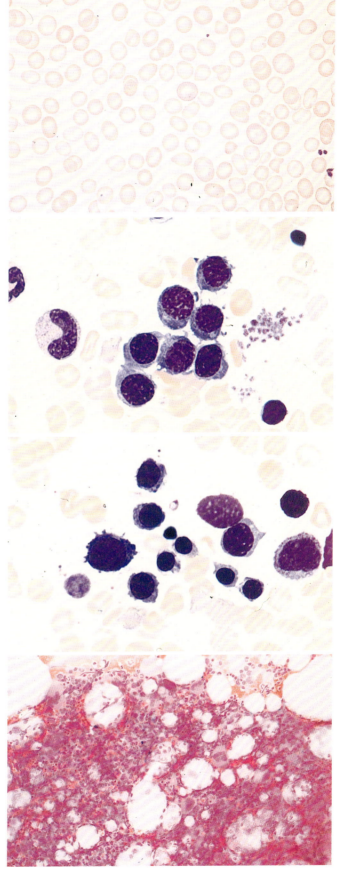

Hemolytic Anemias

Hemolytic anemias (HA) are characterized by a shortening of the erythrocyte life span, which normally is about 120 days. Anemia will develop, however, only if the bone marrow is unable to increase red cell production sufficiently to compensate for the increased rate of destruction. If the erythropoietic response is adequate, *"compensated hemolytic disease"* is present. *"Decompensated hemolytic disease"* exists when there is a disproportion between the destruction and production of erythrocytes. The best way to detect shortened erythrocyte survival is by chromium radiolabeling of the cells (^{51}Cr). This technique can also identify the preferential site of erythrocyte destruction (e.g., the spleen).

When functioning normally, the bone marrow will respond to an increase in hemolysis with *erythroid hyperplasia*, which is manifested by a predominance of mature, nucleated red cell precursors (normoblasts). Usually these precursor cells do not show significant qualitative abnormalities. But if the hemolysis is of long duration, megaloblastic changes can develop mainly as a result of folic acid deficiency, which can be detected in the serum. *Granulocytopoiesis* is qualitatively and quantitatively normal in most cases. It is common to find increased numbers of phagocytized red cells (*erythrophagocytosis*) and iron deposits in the macrophages (see **Fig. 14a**). Examination of the peripheral blood may show an increased *reticulocyte count* (usually by several hundred per thousand), *basophilic stippling* of red cells, occasional normoblasts (**Fig. 24a**), especially in acute hemolysis, and leukocytosis, depending on the rate of red cell destruction and the level of bone marrow activity. Besides these nonspecific changes, there are findings considered pathognomonic for specific entities [spherocytes (**Fig. 24b**), ovalocytes (**Fig. 24c**), and sickle cells (**Fig. 25d, e**)]. In addition, Heinz body formation is characteristic of a number of enzymopenic HA, and methemoglobin is increased in toxic HA.

Several groups of hemolytic anemias are recognized on the basis of their *pathogenetic mechanisms*, as shown in Scheme 2.

Hemolytic anemias may also be classified clinically as acute (acute hemolytic crisis) or chronic. It is common for the chronic course to be punctuated by episodes of acute disease.

The absolute increase of erythropoiesis that occurs during the course of regenerative hemolytic anemias is illustrated in **Fig. 24e, f**.

The most common corpuscular HA in Central Europe is spherocytic anemia or *microspherocytosis*, which is easily recognized by the typical morphology of the red blood cells (**Fig. 24b**) (see also Price-Jones curves, Scheme 3).

The principal hematologic features of *thalassemia* are anisocytosis, hypochromic erythrocytes, poikilocytosis, schistocytes, and especially target cells (see **Fig. 24g**). The marked elevation of HbF in thalassemia major can be demonstrated by staining (see **Fig. 24h**; for method, see p. 9). Examination of the bone marrow in thalassemia shows, in addition to increased erythropoiesis, iron-storing macrophages along with scattered pseudo-Gaucher cells (**Fig. 25a, b**). Some mature erythroblasts contain PAS-positive granules, and some macrophages show a bright red PAS reaction (**Fig. 25c**, left and right).

Sickle cells are most easily detected by the direct examination of a deoxygenated blood sample (see **Fig. 25d, e**; for method, see p. 5). CO hemoglobin also can be visualized by staining.

One class of toxic HA is characterized by erythrocytes that contain deep-blue, rounded, often eccentrically placed inclusion bodies that were first described by Heinz. These *Heinz bodies* display a special affinity for vital stains (Nile blue sulfate, brilliant cresyl blue) (see p. 8 and **Fig. 24d**). They occur almost exclusively in mature erythrocytes and are very rarely found in normoblasts and reticulocytes. Heinz body formation results from the oxidative denaturation of hemoglobin and is particularly common in glucose-6–phosphate dehydrogenase deficiency.

However, this phenomenon occurs only after the ingestion or administration of substances that are harmless in persons with a normal erythrocyte metabolism, such as antimalarial drugs, anticonvulsants, analgesics, sulfonamides, nitrofuran, sulfones, certain vegetables, fava beans, and a number of other drugs and chemicals.

Heinz bodies can also occur in the absence of primary erythrocyte metabolic defects following intoxication with phenols, aniline, phenacetin, salicylazosulfapyridine, and many other substances. Again, this probably results from the dose-dependent blocking of various intraerythrocytic enzymes by the offending compound.

Very rarely, Heinz body formation is seen in congenital hemolytic anemias following splenectomy (hereditary Heinz body anemia). Since the presence of an abnormal hemoglobin with a pathologic thermal stability has been demonstrated in this anemia, the disease has been classified as a hemoglobinopathy.

The principal serogenic HA caused by isoantibodies is *hemolytic disease of the newborn* (HDN), a consequence of fetomaternal Rh incompatibility. Examination of the infant's blood usually reveals large numbers of erythroblasts. These cells

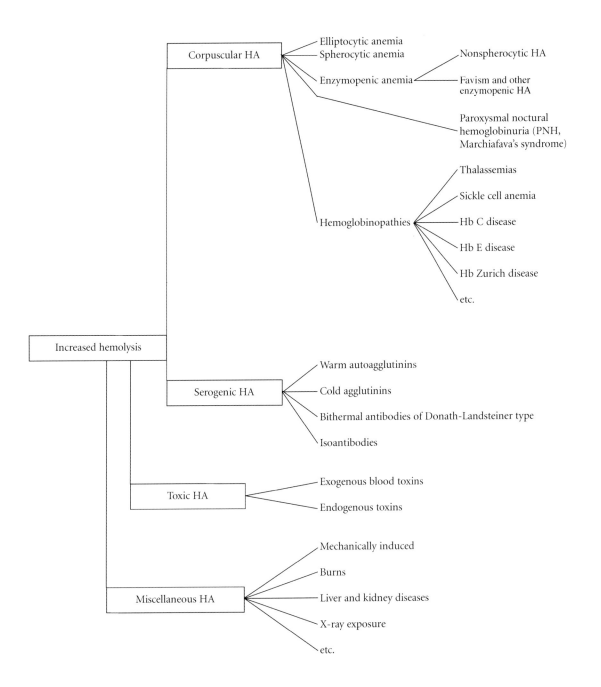

Corpuscular HA
- Elliptocytic anemia
- Spherocytic anemia
- Enzymopenic anemia
  - Nonspherocytic HA
  - Favism and other enzymopenic HA
- Paroxysmal noctural hemoglobinuria (PNH, Marchiafava's syndrome)
- Hemoglobinopathies
  - Thalassemias
  - Sickle cell anemia
  - Hb C disease
  - Hb E disease
  - Hb Zurich disease
  - etc.

Increased hemolysis

Serogenic HA
- Warm autoagglutinins
- Cold agglutinins
- Bithermal antibodies of Donath-Landsteiner type
- Isoantibodies

Toxic HA
- Exogenous blood toxins
- Endogenous toxins

Miscellaneous HA
- Mechanically induced
- Burns
- Liver and kidney diseases
- X-ray exposure
- etc.

Scheme 2. Classification of hemolytic anemias (HA)

probably originate from extramedullary hematopoietic foci, which can be quite extensive in newborns. The example in **Fig. 25f** shows a number of normoblasts.

Erythrocyte-storing macrophages (*erythrophagocytosis*) are a very common finding in *autoimmune hemolytic anemia* caused by warm-reactive, cold-reactive and bithermal antibodies (see **Fig. 25i**, left). In cold agglutinin disease, the agglutination of erythrocytes is observed on a cold microscope slide but is inhibited on a warm slide (**Fig. 25i**, right).

In acute alcoholic HA with associated lipidemia (Zieve syndrome), examination of the bone marrow reveals abundant fat cells in addition to increased erythropoiesis.

Hemolytic anemias due to mechanical causes are marked by the presence of characteristic erythrocyte fragments (fragmentocytes, schizocytes). Erythroblasts are also found if hemolysis is severe (**Fig. 25g**).

Finally, reference should be made to the H chains (β-chain tetramers) that can be demonstrated by supravital staining. When these chains are present, densely stippled erythrocytes are found (**Fig. 25h**, center).

Fig. 24 a–d

a Blood smear in autoimmune hemolytic anemia (AIHA) with three normoblasts and polychromatic erythrocytes (reticulocytes)

b Blood smear in spherocytic anemia shows small, round erythrocytes packed with hemoglobin (microspherocytes). These cells are characteristic but not specific, as they also occur in autoimmune hemolytic anemias

c Elliptocytes: the narrow elliptical form, as shown here, is specific for hereditary elliptocytosis

d Heinz bodies demonstrated by Nile blue sulfate staining. These bodies occur mainly in association with enzymopenic hemolytic anemias or hemoglobin instability

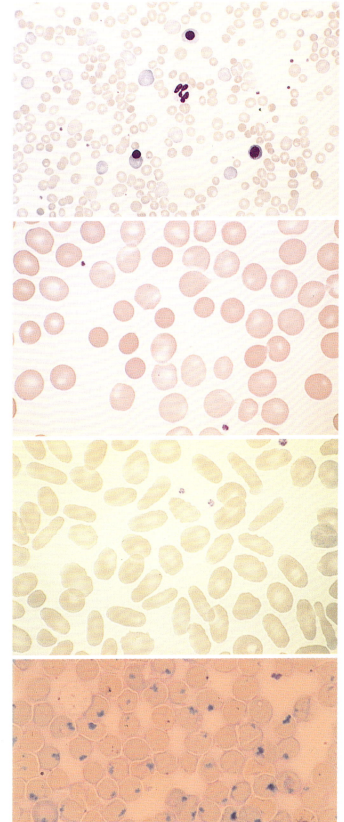

Fig. 24 e – h

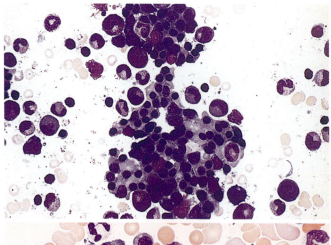

e Greatly increased, predominantly normoblastic erythropoiesis in hemolytic anemia

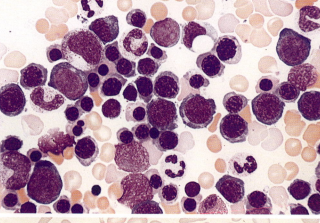

f Predominantly mature, morphologically normal erythroblasts in hemolytic anemia

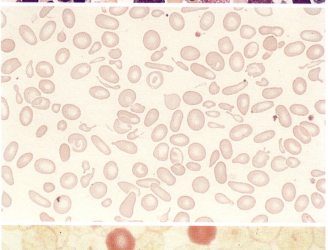

g Blood smear in β-thalassemia with marked anisocytosis, poikilocytosis, and several typical target cells

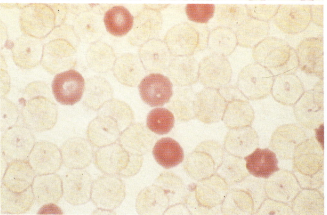

h Detection of HbF in the peripheral blood. Erythrocytes that contain HbF are stained red

Fig. 25 a–d

a Bone marrow smear in β-thalassemia. Increased erythropoiesis is accompanied by hemosiderin-containing macrophages

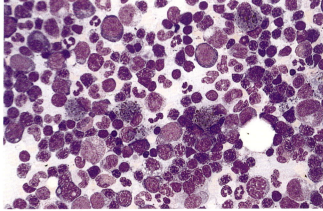

b Storage cell in the bone marrow in β-thalassemia

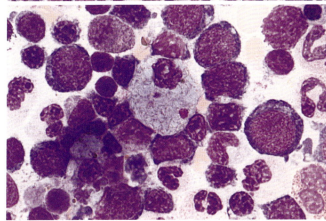

c **Left:** two normoblasts in the bone marrow with a granular PAS reaction in thalassemia. **Right:** macrophage in which bright red-staining material is interspersed with yellow-gold hemosiderin (PAS reaction)

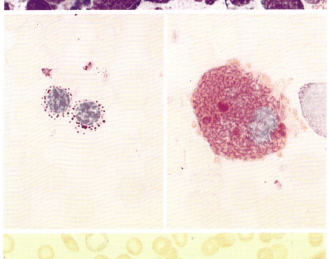

d Sickle cells in the peripheral blood in sickle cell anemia

Fig. 25 e–h

e Sickling test with sodium metabisulfite in Hb S disease

f Normoblasts in a blood smear in fetal erythroblastosis

g Fragmentocytes and a freshly expelled erythroblast nucleus (still adherent) in thrombotic thrombocytopenic purpura (TTP)

h Reticulocytes and large Heinz bodies adjoined at *center* by a finely stippled erythrocyte with H chains

Fig. 25 i Cold agglutinin disease, peripheral blood. *Left:* smear on a *cold* slide; *right:* smear on a *warm* slide

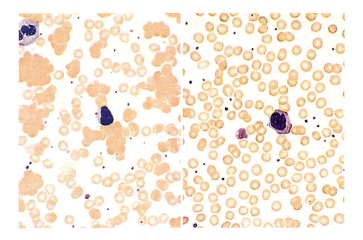

Megaloblastic Anemias

This term is applied to a class of anemias whose major representative in Europe is the cryptogenic *pernicious anemia*. They are characterized morphologically by the appearance of megaloblasts in the bone marrow – erythropoietic cells that differ from normal erythroblasts in their size and especially in their nuclear structure. But the disease process does not affect erythropoiesis alone; the *granulocytes and their precursors* as well as the *megakaryocytes* also display typical changes.

These disturbances of hematopoiesis are manifested by anemia (usually hyperchromic) and by a reduction of leukocytes and platelets in the peripheral blood. Examination of the blood smear shows marked anisocytosis and poikilocytosis with large, usually oval erythrocytes well filled with hemoglobin. These *megalocytes* (**Figs. 26, 27**), as they are called, result in a broad-based *Price-Jones curve* whose peak is shifted to the right (see Scheme 3). Nucleated red cell precursors that may show basophilic stippling are also occasionally found in the peripheral blood. Leukocytopenia results from a decreased number of granulocytes, some showing hypersegmentation.

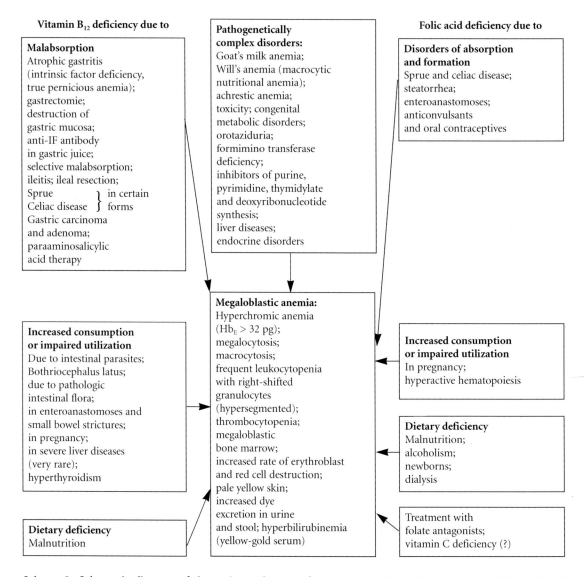

Scheme 3. Schematic diagram of the major pathogenic factors in megaloblastic anemias and their clinical symptoms. [Slightly modified from Begemann H, Begemann M (1989) Praktische Hämatologie, 9th ed. Thieme, Stuttgart]

Besides their hematologic manifestations, megaloblastic anemias affect various organ systems. Gastrointestinal changes are well known and consist mainly of *Hunter's glossitis* and *atrophic gastritis. Central nervous system involvement* is present in a high percentage of cases, usually in the form of degenerative spinal cord disease with its associated symptoms. The extent and severity of organ involvement and the various hematologic manifestations depend on the nature, duration, and degree of the underlying avitaminosis as well as on individual, possibly genetic factors.

In the last four decades we have learned much about the *pathogenesis* of megaloblastic anemias. The great majority of these diseases are based on a deficiency of either vitamin B_{12} or folic acid. Both vitamins play a crucial role in the nucleic acid metabolism of the cell, and each complements but cannot replace the other. A deficiency of either vitamin (in the absence of adequate stores) will lead to a disturbance of DNA synthesis and to a megaloblastic anemia. Disease in a different organ system may even precede and precipitate the anemia. Once a megaloblastic anemia has been diagnosed, it is imperative that its cause be identified. Two large etiologic groups are recognized: anemias caused by a vitamin B_{12} deficiency and anemias caused by a folic acid deficit (see Scheme 3). In most cases the cause of the underlying vitamin deficiency can be determined. In "cryptogenic" pernicious anemia, the type most common in Europe, the gastric juice lacks an intrinsic factor necessary for the absorption of ingested vitamin B_{12} (extrinsic factor) in the small bowel. The gastric lesion responsible for the failure of intrinsic factor formation is also manifested in a "histamine-refractory" anacidity, which is a typical symptom of the disease. The absent or deficient absorption of orally administered vitamin B_{12} can be accurately detected in the Schilling urinary excretion test. Today it has become routine practice to determine the serum vitamin B_{12} level or measure the folic acid content of the erythrocytes.

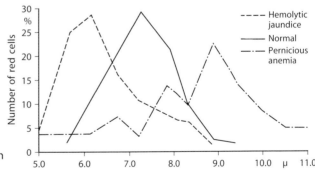

Scheme 4. Price-Jones curves in hemolytic jaundice (microcytic anemia), in health, and in pernicious anemia (megalocytic anemia)

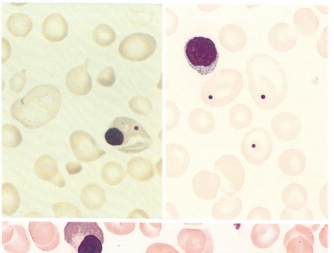

Fig. 26 a – h. Megaloblastic anemias

a Blood smears in pernicious anemia: at *left*, severe anisocytosis, poikilocytosis, a very large megalocyte, and a normoblast with an extra Howell-Jolly body. At *right* are three megalocytes with Howell-Jolly bodies

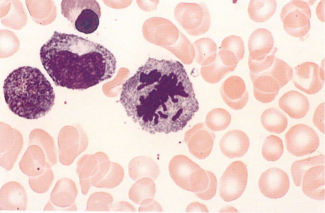

b Mitotic megaloblast with a chromosome fragment that will develop into a Howell-Jolly body

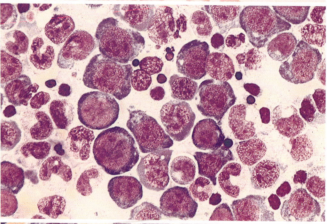

c Very cellular bone marrow in megaloblastic anemia, here showing a predominance of immature megaloblasts and the typical fine, loose chromatin structure. Incipient hemoglobin formation in the cytoplasm signals a decrease in basophilia

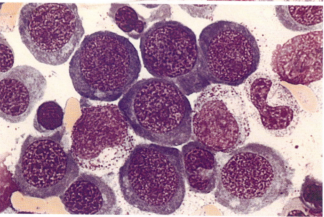

d Group of promegaloblasts showing a typical nuclear structure. The appearance of the cells reflects the disturbance in DNA synthesis

Fig. 26 e–h

e Megaloblasts at various stages of maturity, also metamyelocytes and segmented forms showing a loose chromatin structure

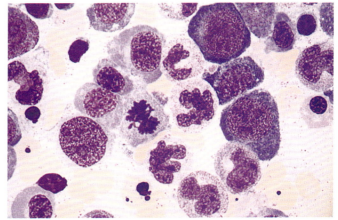

f Very pronounced nuclear abnormalities in megaloblasts

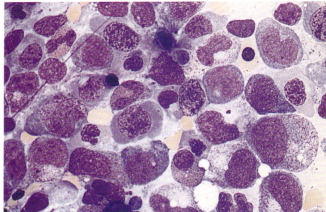

g Megaloblasts showing incipient apoptosis. At *lower right* is a giant metamyelocyte

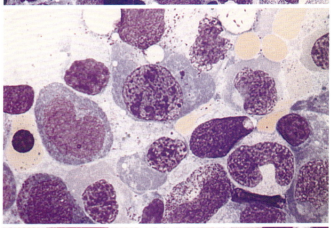

h Very large megaloblast with unusually broad cytoplasm already showing partial hemoglobination. Below it and to the right are giant forms in the granulocytopoiesis series

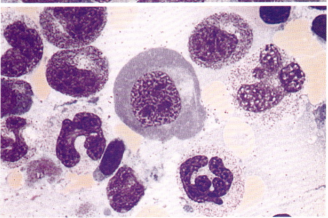

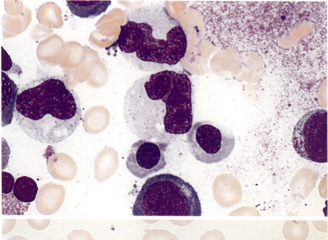

Fig. 27 a–d

a Two giant metamyelocytes in pernicious anemia

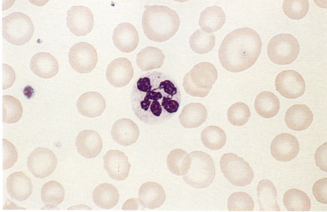

b Hypersegmented neutrophil in a blood smear in pernicious anemia

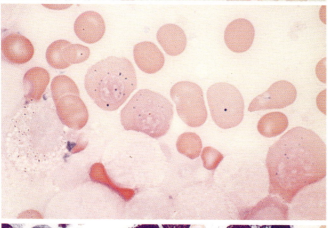

c Iron stain demonstrates two sideromegaloblasts and one sideromegalocyte containing coarse iron granules

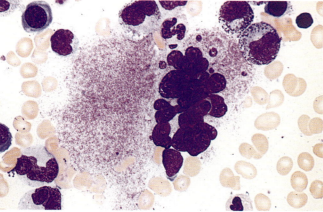

d Hypersegmented megakaryocyte in megaloblastic anemia

Fig. 27 e–h

e Hypersegmented megakaryocyte with a bizarre-shaped nucleus in megaloblastic anemia

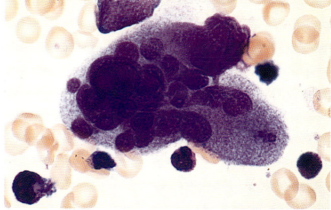

f, g Nonspecific esterase (α-naphthyl acetate, pH 7.2): megaloblasts show strong esterase activity that is most pronounced in the perinuclear area

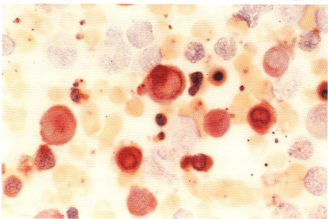

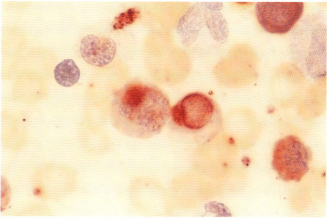

h Subtle megaloblastic change (transitional form) like that seen in mild megaloblastic anemia or shortly after the institution of vitamin B$_{12}$ therapy

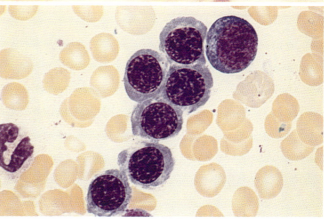

Toxic Disturbances of Erythropoiesis

In cases of chronic alcohol abuse, examination of the bone marrow may show vacuolation of both the red and white cell precursors (**Fig. 28c, d**). Chloramphenicol is among the drugs that can impair erythropoiesis. Once widely used as an antibiotic, this drug leads to the increased formation of abnormal sideroblasts and to vacuolation of the cytoplasm in erythroblasts (**Fig. 28a, b**). Rare cases of irreversible aplastic anemia (panmyelophthisis) have been reported as a fatal side effect.

Fig. 28 a–d

a, b Conspicuous vacuolation in the cytoplasm of early proerythroblasts following treatment with chloramphenicol

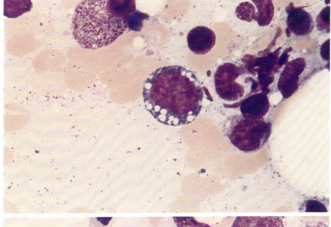

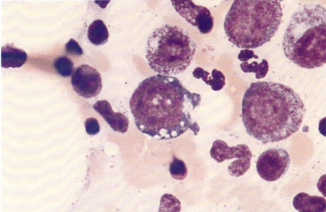

c Vacuolation in the cytoplasm of proerythroblasts due to alcohol abuse

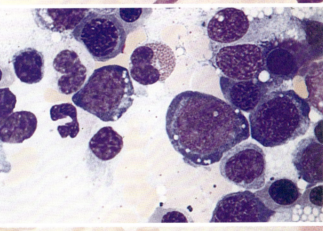

d Iron in the cytoplasm of a plasma cell, demonstrated by iron staining. At *upper left* is a vacuolated proerythroblast (alcohol abuse)

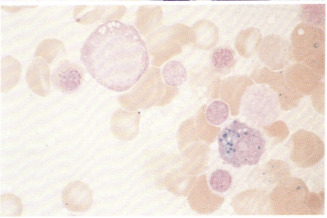

Acute Erythroblastopenia

This severe reduction of erythropoiesis in the bone marrow occurs mainly in children but may also develop in hemolytic anemias (aplastic crisis). Parvovirus B19 infection has been identified as the causal agent for the decreased erythropoiesis and consequent reticulocytopenia. The diagnosis is established by the presence of giant proerythroblasts in the bone marrow, which reach the size of megakaryocytes (**Fig. 29a–h**). Most cases resolve spontaneously in 1 to 2 weeks.

Transient erythroblastopenia in children may occur in the absence of parvovirus B19 infection, but these cases do not present with giant erythroblasts in the bone marrow.

Fig. 29 a – d

a Bone marrow smear in acute erythro-blastopenia. At the *center* of the field is a giant proerythroblast with intensely basophilic cytoplasm, a loose nuclear chromatin structure, and very large nucleoli. This cell is several times larger than a normal erythroblast and is roughly the size of a megakaryocyte

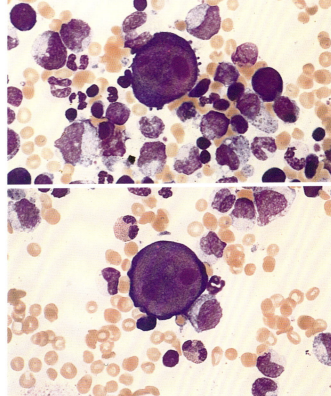

b Another giant proerythroblast

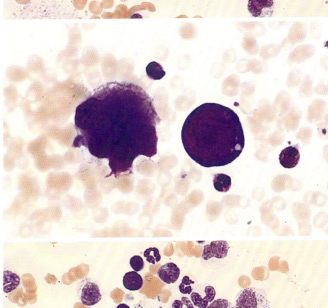

c Giant proerythroblast next to a mature megakaryocyte

d Giant proerythroblast in a group of granulocytopoietic cells, three plasma cells, and lymphocytes

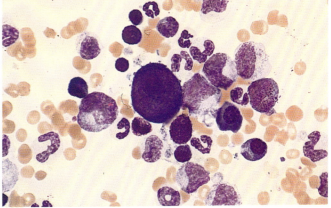

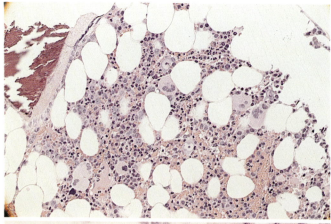

Fig. 29 e–h

e Histologic bone marrow section in acute erythroblastopenia. Two giant proerythroblasts, each with a pale nucleus and very large nucleolus, appear at *upper center* and *lower right of center*. Hematoxylin-eosin

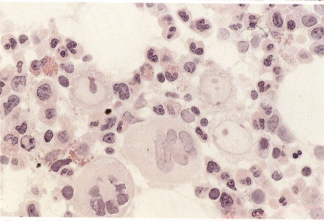

f Bone marrow section. Three giant proerythroblasts with large nucleoli and very pale chromatin are visible to the *left* and *right of center*. Below them are two mature megakaryocytes and granulocytopoietic cells. Hematoxylin-eosin

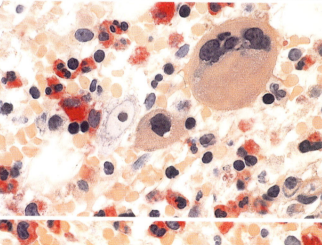

g Bone marrow section. At *left center* is a giant proerythroblast with a pale nucleus and very large nucleolus. To the right of it is a megakaryocyte with a round nucleus, and above that is a mature segmented megakaryocyte. CE stain

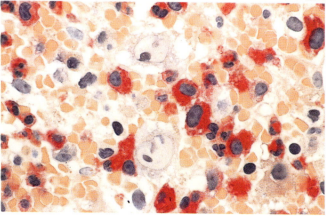

h Bone marrow section. A pair of giant proerythroblasts are visible in the upper and lower central part of the field. Granulocytopoiesis with red cytoplasmic stain. CE reaction

Chronic Erythroblastopenia (Pure Red Cell Aplasia)

This is an *"aplastic anemia in the strict sense"* involving a profound disturbance of erythropoiesis. It is characterized by an absence or *severe reduction of red cell precursors* in the bone marrow. Granulocytopoiesis and thrombocytopoiesis are essentially normal. Reticulocytes are either absent from the peripheral blood or present in very small numbers. The result is a severe anemic state that dominates the clinical picture. Giant proerythroblasts are absent.

Congenital Dyserythropoietic Anemias

These rare disorders are characterized by a *severe disturbance of erythropoiesis*, which leads to conspicuous morphologic changes. *Type I* congenital dyserythropoietic anemia (CDA) shows a hazy nuclear structure with fine chromatin strands interconnecting the nuclei of separate erythroblasts (**Fig. 30a**, ultrastructure **Fig. 30b**). Multinucleated erythroblasts characterize the *type II* form of CDA (**Fig. 30c – e**). Approximately 15 % – 20 % of all red cell precursors contain 2 – 4 nuclei, found mainly in the more mature forms, and there are bizarre aberrations of nuclear division (karyorrhexis). The blood film shows aniso- and poikilocytosis, basophilic stippling, and Cabot rings. In *type III* CDA, bone marrow examination reveals erythroid hyperplasia with a multinucleation of erythroblasts affecting all maturation stages (**Fig. 30f – h**). Giant cells with 10 – 12 nuclei are observed.

Fig. 30 a

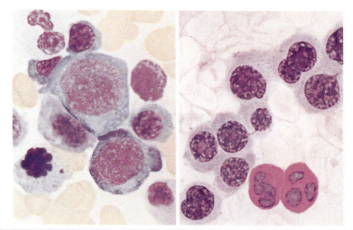

Fig. 30 b

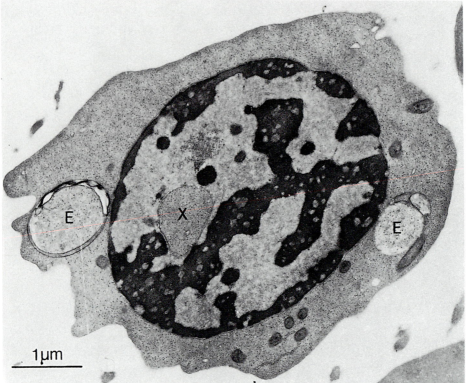

Fig. 30 a – b. Dyserythropoietic anemia.

a Type I bone marrow, containing erythroblasts with an indistinct chromatin structure. **Right:** chromatin strands interconnecting the erythroblast nuclei. Bottom: two neutrophils nuclei showing a positive PAS reaction

b Normoblast in Type I dyserythropoietic anemia. Note the typical morphologic features of this rare disease: cordlike condensations of chromatin with many small, rounded clear zones; invagination of cytoplasm into the nucleus (**X**) and disruptions in the nuclear membrane; tiny iron deposits in the mitochondria; and cytoplasmic inclusions (**E**) that probably represent phagolysosomes

Fig. 30 c – f

c Type II dyserythropoietic anemia, characterized by mature erythroblasts with very small nuclei, often duplicated, or with bizarre nuclear shapes (karyorrhexis)

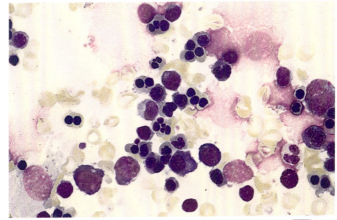

d Binucleated erythroblast and "daisy forms"

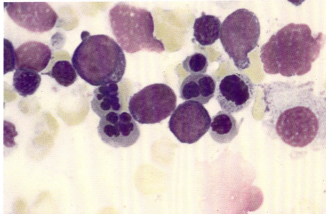

e Erythroblasts with very small or duplicated nuclei

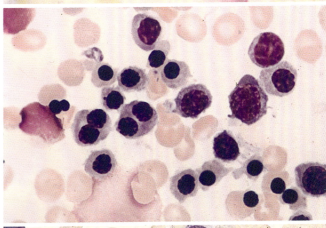

f Proerythroblast with six nuclei in type III dyserythropoietic anemia

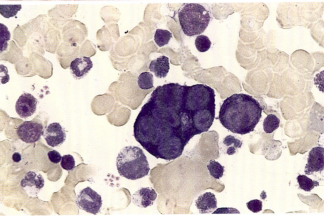

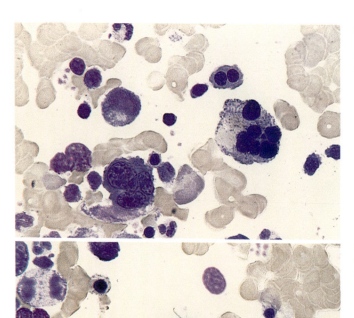

Fig. 30 g – h

g Erythroblasts with two, three, and six nuclei in type III dyserythropoietic anemia

h Multinucleated erythroblast with mature cytoplasm and a bizarre-shaped nucleus

Synartesis. Figure 31 illustrates the phenomenon of *synartesis* in a case showing marked dyserythropoietic disturbances of erythropoiesis (Type II). This phenomenon involves a syncytium-like aggregation of erythroblasts, which form pale cytoplasmic bridges at points of contact between the individual cells.

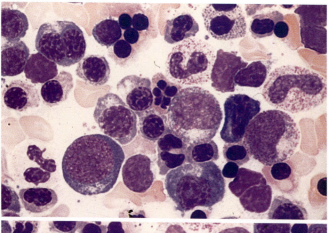

Fig. 31 a–d. Dyserythropoietic anemia with synartesis.

a At *upper left* is a binucleated erythroblast, and at *center* is a karyorrhectic figure. Below that is another binucleated erythroblast with deformed nuclei

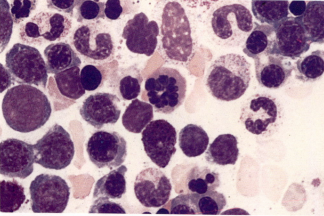

b A karyorrhectic figure is visible at *center*. Note the abnormal nuclear shape at *lower left*

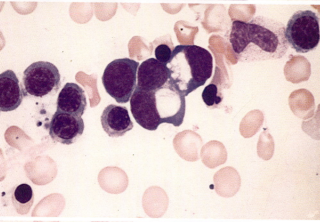

c At *center* are three erythroblasts, apparently clustered and featuring very large perinuclear halos

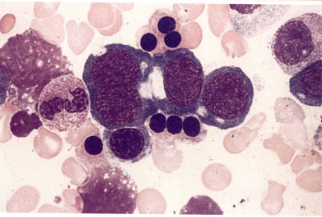

d A cluster of four proerythroblasts at the *center* of the field appear to be closely connected and contain large perinuclear clear zones

Reactive Blood and Bone Marrow Changes

The response of the bone marrow to *infection* consists of an increase in granulocytopoiesis and a relative decrease in erythropoiesis (**Fig. 32a**). If an abnormality of iron distribution coexists with the infection, as is frequently the case, some increase in erythropoiesis will also be seen. Usually the immature precursors of granulocytopoiesis are markedly increased as well and may lead to a predominance of promyelocytes (see **Fig. 32a**). Eosinophilia is also common. Qualitative changes in erythropoiesis and granulocytopoiesis are manifested by nuclear-cytoplasmic dissociation, persistent cytoplasmic basophilia, toxic granulations, and nuclear abnormalities. The plasma cells also are increased in number and in extreme cases can mimic a plasmacytoma (**Fig. 32b**; see **Table 7**). This is most common in chronic inflammatory processes involving the liver (chronic hepatitis, cirrhosis) and biliary tract (cholangitis, cholecystitis, etc.). Whether the individual picture is dominated by a left shift in granulocytopoiesis or a proliferation of plasma cells depends on the virulence and toxicity of the causative infectious organism. HIV infection can lead to very severe "toxic bone marrow changes" that may be associated with significant plasmacytosis and even dysplastic changes as in MDS (**Figs. 32c, d** and **67d, e**).

The bone marrow responds to *neoplastic diseases* in much the same way as to infection and various toxic insults. The most common morphologic findings in the blood and bone marrow of patients with infections and neoplastic disease are summarized in **Table 6.** The anemia that develops in these conditions has been referred to as "anemia of chronic disease." In cases where the serum iron level is low but there is a normal or elevated ferritin and adequate bone marrow stores, an abnormality of *iron distribution* exists rather than a true iron deficiency. The reactive changes consist of plasma cell alterations (Russell bodies), monocytosis, and small granulomas formed by monocytes or epitheloid cells as well as circumscribed lymphocytic foci (polyclonal) in chronic inflammatory or immunologic diseases (**Fig. 33a–d**).

Occasionally the response of the *eosinophils* is so pronounced that they come to dominate the blood picture. This pattern can be difficult to interpret etiologically. It is most commonly seen in allergic reactions, certain infectious diseases, insect bites, skin diseases, parasitic infections (helminths!), collagen diseases (hypereosinophilic syndrome), blood diseases, and endocrine disorders. Eosinophils tend to be increased in the presence of carcinoma, especially if the tumor has already metastasized. Eosinophilia is also seen in patients on hemodialysis. If the eosinophils are sufficiently numerous to produce a more or less pronounced leukocytosis, *hypereosinophilia* is said to be present (**Fig. 34a–h**).

Eosinophilia with splenomegaly and *eosinophilia persistans,* in which splenomegaly usually coexists with diffuse enlargement of the lymph nodes are special disorders. Apparently these conditions represent severe allergic disorders of

---

Table 6. Reactive bone marrow changes (findings in the blood and bone marrow)

Peripheral blood	Bone marrow
Anemia (aplastic, hemolytic) Abnormal erythrocytes Basophilic stippling of erythrocytes	*Erythropoiesis:* Maturation defects Cytoplasmic vacuoles Megaloblastoid forms Reduction → Erythroblastophthisis Hyperplasia
Pancytopenia — Granulocytopenia Agranulocytosis Toxic granulations Cytoplasmic vacuoles Doehle bodies	*Panmyelopathy-Granulocytopoiesis:* Maturation defects Cytoplasmic vacuoles Left shift Eosinophilia Reduction → Agranulocytosis *Monocytopoiesis* Monocytes Granuloma formation
Thrombocytopenia Abnormal platelets	*Thrombocytopoiesis:* Maturation defects Reduction → Absence of megakaryocytes

varying etiology. It can be difficult to differentiate the *hypereosinophilias* (**Fig. 34a – h**) from the very rare eosinophilic leukemias, in which the peripheral blood is flooded with large numbers of mature eosinophils (see **Fig. 112**). Often this distinction can be accomplished only by observing the clinical course, but eosinophilic leukemias can be confirmed by the detection of chromosomal abnormalities.

Hypereosinophilic syndrome (HES) is often difficult to distinguish from the eosinophilic leukemias and other hypereosinophilias. Diagnostic criteria include the persistence of eosinophilia for at least 6 months with leukocyte counts of 10,000 to 30,000/μL and a 30 % to 70 % proportion of eosinophils. Most patients manifest signs and symptoms of organ involvement such as hepatosplenomegaly, congestive cardiomyopathy, pulmonary fibrosis, etc. Frequently the eosinophils show morphologic abnormalities (enlarged cells with a decreased number of weakly staining granules, vacuolation, multisegmentation). Immature forms are often present in the peripheral blood. The bone marrow is dominated by eosinophils (25 % – 75 %) with a shift to the left and qualitative changes.

"Tropical eosinophilia" is associated with lymph node enlargement, splenomegaly, pulmonary infiltration, and severe asthmatic complaints. *B. malayi* or *W. bancrofti* microfilariae (see **Figs. 198, 199d**) have been identified in the enlarged lymph nodes of most patients. None have been detected in the blood, although a high titer against filariae has been demonstrated in the serum by complement fixation. The term "tropical eosinophilia" should no longer be used to designate a separate disease entity. Severe eosinophilia diagnosed in persons returning from the tropics is usually the result of a helminthiasis.

Administration of the hematopoietic growth factors G-CSF and GM-CSF stimulates the proliferation and differentiation of progenitor cells. While GM-CSF also leads to the stimulation of monocytes and eosinophils, the administration of G-CSF leads only to an increase in neutrophils. This is accompanied by a left shift and in some cases by mild atypias that do not adversely affect cellular function. Neutrophilic alkaline phosphatase is maximally activated. Bone marrow examination following chemotherapy shows a more rapid regeneration of neutrophilic granulocytopoiesis (**Fig. 35a – d**). The more rapid and increased recruitment of stem cells has proven to be a very useful phenomenon in the practice of bone marrow transplantation and especially in peripheral stem cell transplantation.

Table 7. Differential diagnosis of a plasma cell increase in the bone marrow

	Number	Morphology	Remarks
Normal bone marrow	< 5 %	Almost exclusively small, mature plasma cells	
Reactive bone marrow changes (toxic-infectious or neoplastic process)	5 %-10 %	Predominantly small, mature plasma cells	Very strong increase after HIV infection, in chron. inflammatory processes of the liver, biliary tract, etc., frequent bone marrow eosinophilia
Multiple myeloma	> 10 %	Marked pleomorphism of plasma cells ("immature forms," atypical nucleoli)	Strong acid phosphatase activity in the myeloma cells
Lymphoplasmacytoid immunocytoma (Waldenströms disease, Waldenströms macroglobulinemia)	> 10 %	Marked pleomorphism	Marked lymphatic infiltration, mast cells
Monoclonal gammopathy of undetermined signifance (MGUS)	> 10 %	Slight pleomorphism	Transition to multiple mycloma is possible
Concomitant paraproteinemia	> 10 %	Slight pleomorphism	Especially in systemic lymphoreticular disease, carcinoma

Fig. 32 a–d. Reactive blood and bone marrow changes

a Greatly increased granulocytopoiesis with a left shift and markedly reduced erythropoiesis due to an acute infection

b Marked proliferation of mature plasma cells with eosinophilia, scattered basophils, and a slight increase in lymphocytes

c Bone marrow in HIV infection, showing significant "toxic" abnormalities

d Marked plasmacytosis in the bone marrow of an HIV-infected patient

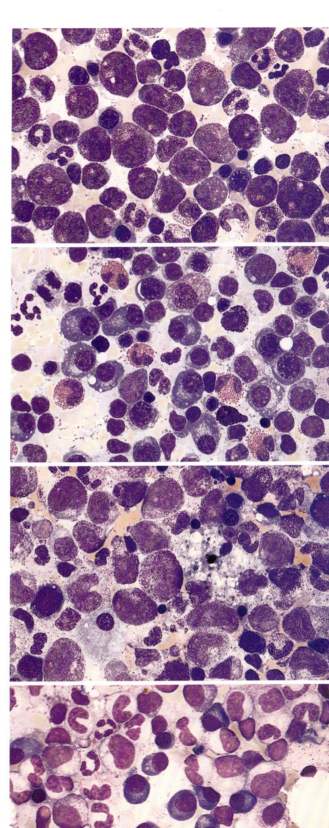

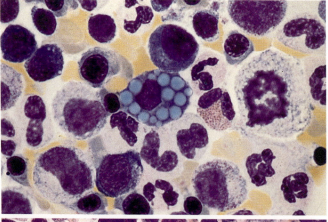

Fig. 33 a–d Reactive bone marrow changes

a Plasma cell with numerous Russell bodies (reactive change)

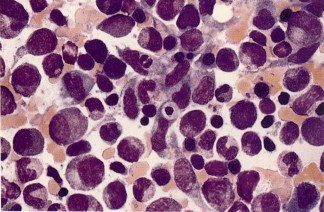

b At *center* is a granuloma-like aggregation of monocytes, and below that is a cell containing phagocytized material in rheumatoid arthritis

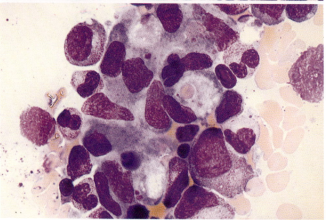

c High-power view of a monocytic granuloma. One cell contains a phagocytized erythrocyte

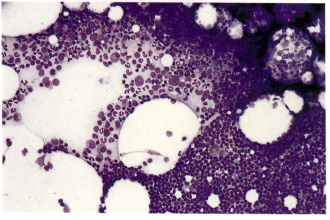

d Lymphocytic focus in the bone marrow. Note the relatively sharp demarcation of the focus from the hematopoietic background (*lower right* and *side of field*)

Fig. 34 a–d. Reactive eosinophilia and hypereosinophilic syndrome

a, b Pronounced eosinophilia in the peripheral blood, with typical eosinophils that generally contain bilobed and occasionally trilobed nuclei

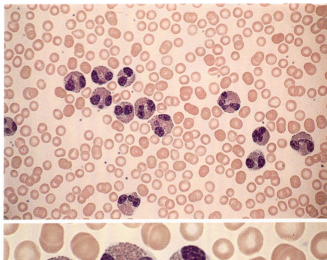

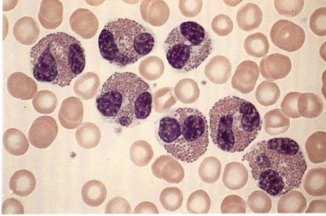

c Pronounced eosinophilia in the bone marrow, with immature precursors containing small numbers of purple-stained granules

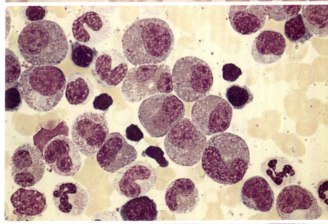

d At *center* is an eosinophilic promyelocyte with immature purple granules along with scattered mature granules. The cytoplasm is basophilic

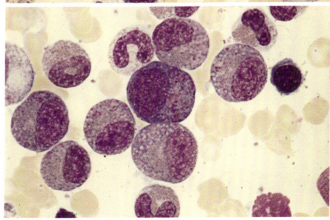

Fig. 34 e–h

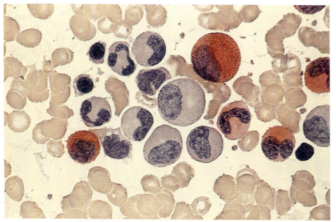

e Naphthol AS-D chloroacetate esterase in the bone marrow in reactive eosinophilia. Only the neutrophilic granulocytes are positive; the eosinophils are negative

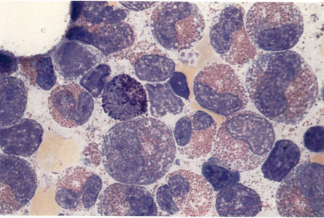

f Various maturation stages in reactive eosinophilia. The cell at *center left* is a basophilic granulocyte

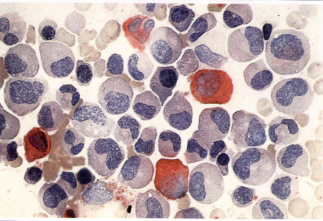

g Extreme eosinophilia of the bone marrow in hypereosinophilic syndrome. The eosinophils are negative for naphthol AS-D chloroacetate esterase, and four neutrophils in the field are positive

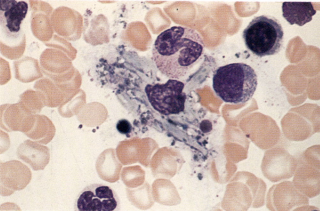

h Macrophage containing Charcot-Leyden crystals in eosinophilia. The crystals develop from the eosinophilic granules

Fig. 35 a – d. Effect of hematopoietic growth factors

a Peripheral blood smear after the administration of G-CSF

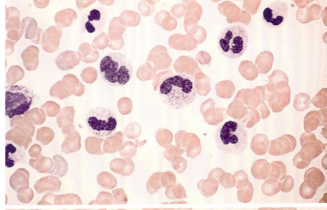

b Left shift following G-CSF

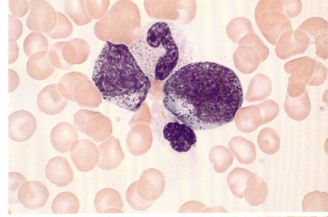

c Maximum leukocyte alkaline phosphatase activity following G-CSF

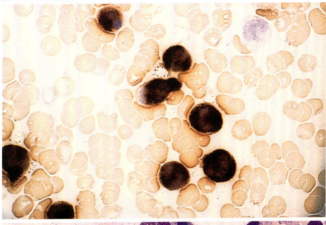

d Bone marrow following chemotherapy and the administration of G-CSF demonstrates promyelocytes and myelocytes, some showing mild atypia

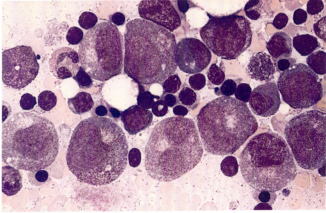

Agranulocytosis

Agranulocytosis is a collective term applied to diseases associated with an extreme reduction or complete absence of granulocytes in the peripheral blood. A more accurate and descriptive term is granulocytopenia, which in fact has been adopted for most diseases in this category. Agranulocytosis in the strict sense is reserved for diseases that are based on a *specific, individual hypersensitivity* to exogenous or (rarely) endogenous agents and usually have an acute onset. (This does not include "cyclic agranulocytosis," whose pathogenesis is not yet fully understood.) Potential exogenous offenders include almost all chemicals and especially drugs, the most notorious being pyrazolone. The causal agent incites an immune response in which antigen-antibodies complexes are formed and bring about the destruction of granulocytes. The cytolytic process affects not only granulocytes in the peripheral blood but also precursors in the bone marrow, including promyelocytes in some cases. The pathogenetic mechanism underlying the agranulocytosis is unrelated to the formation of antibodies directed against endogenous granulocytes. Thus, a strict distinction must be drawn between allergic agranulocytosis and the true autoimmune granulocytopenias.

The morphologic substrate of the antibody-mediated agranulocytosis depends on the timing of the examination. If bone marrow is sampled early in the course, granulocytopoiesis may be almost completely absent; if later, the characteristic promyelocytic marrow is found (**Fig. 36e**). Examination during the remission phase shows only an increase in granulocytopoiesis. Erythropoiesis is not impaired in uncomplicated agranulocytoses, and often it is relatively increased due to the overall reduction in granulocytopoiesis. Septic complications can also lead to changes in red cell precursors and megakaryocytes. If there is an arrest of normal granulocytopoiesis, the bone marrow findings may closely resemble those in aplastic anemias and acute leukemias, with a potential for confusion. In particular, it may be possible to distinguish hypoplastic acute leukemias only by observing their course.

Fig. 36 a – h. Bone marrow in agranulocytosis

a Overall decrease in cellularity with scattered early promyelocytes and relatively numerous lymphocytes

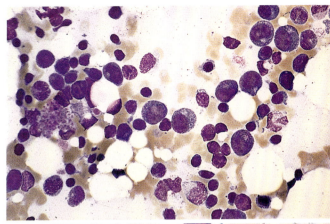

b Bone marrow in agranulocytosis in a very early regenerative stage. Small numbers of early transitional forms between blasts and promyelocytes are intermingled with lymphocytes. An acute hypoplastic leukemia should also be considered at this stage. The diagnosis is established by serial examinations

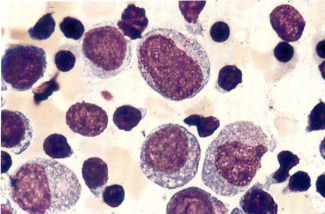

c Bone marrow in agranulocytosis. In this early regenerative phase, some neutrophils are already peroxidase-positive. A neutrophil mitotic figure is seen at *upper right*

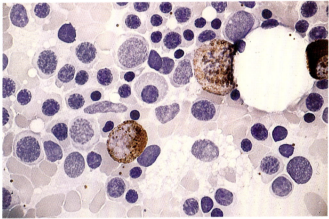

d Early regenerative phase with "promyelocytic marrow," clearly recognized here by its granularity

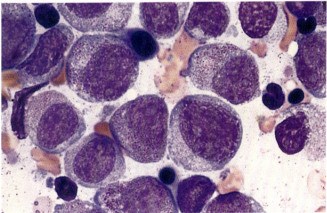

Fig. 36 e–h

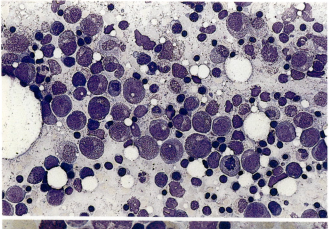

e Overview of the regenerative stage: promyelocytes are predominant but are already accompanied by small numbers of mature forms

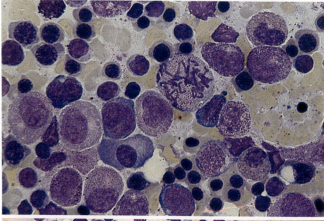

f Promyelocytic marrow in agranulocytosis. At *center* is a mitotic figure. In contrast to promyelocytic leukemia, the cells are quite regular and have uniformly distributed granules with an absence of Auer rods

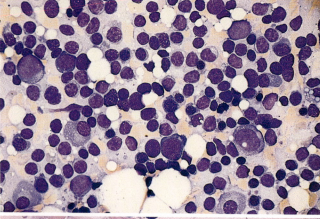

g Lymphocytic focus in the marrow in agranulocytosis. Usually these foci are clearly demarcated from their surroundings

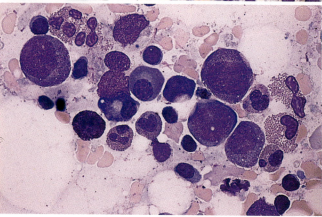

h Severe granulocytopenia following chemotherapy, virtually indistinguishable from agranulocytosis. This specimen contains relatively large numbers of eosinophilic granulocytes

Kostmann Syndrome

Kostmann syndrome (severe congenital neutropenia) is inherited as an autosomal recessive trait. Affected children are born with an extreme paucity or absence of granulocytes. Granulocytopoiesis in the bone marrow becomes arrested at the promyelocyte stage, rarely progressing to the myelocyte stage; more mature forms are absent.

Shwachman syndrome, which has the same mode of inheritance, is characterized by neutropenia in addition to various malformations. Granulocytopoiesis in the bone marrow is diminished.

Thrombocytopenias and Thrombocytopathies

Hemorrhagic disorders rarely present obvious morphologic clues that permit a diagnosis, doing so only when they are associated with quantitative or qualitative changes in the blood platelets. Two major disease groups can be identified: those in which the platelets are reduced in number, and those in which the platelets are present in normal numbers but do not function normally. Diseases of the first group are called *thrombocytopenias;* those of the second, *thrombocytopathies.* Both groups have similar effects on blood coagulation, and both lead to similar clinical manifestations.

The most important of the diseases in which platelet counts are reduced is *idiopathic thrombocytopenic purpura* (Werlhof disease, Werlhof syndrome). It is associated with a thrombocytopenic hemorrhagic diathesis. The pathogenesis is based on an *acceleration of platelet destruction due to an autoimmune response.* No characteristic changes are found in the bone marrow (**Fig. 37a**). The megakaryocytes may be normal but usually are markedly increased. There are large numbers of young basophilic forms with a round or minimally lobulated nucleus. Eosinophilia may be present in the bone marrow. A compensatory increase in erythrocytopoiesis is usually present due to prior blood losses. The abnormalities of platelet morphology seen in this disease result from the acceleration of thrombocytopoiesis. Giant platelets with a dense granulomere are a frequent finding and may approach the size of leukocytes. Marked platelet anisocytosis is also common.

Deficient platelet production is causative of thrombocytopenia in cases where bone marrow function has become severely compromised in the setting of a lymphoma, plasmacytoma, leukemia, or by elements extrinsic to the marrow (e.g., bone marrow metastases from solid tumors). Occasionally, however, essential thrombocytopenias are encountered that must result from a depopulation of the megakaryocyte compartment of the bone marrow (amegakaryocytic thrombocytopenia).

One way to determine whether a thrombocytopenia is caused by deficient platelet production or increased platelet turnover is by the use of *radiolabeled platelets.* In *hemorrhagic diatheses due to platelet dysfunction,* there is rarely a characteristic morphologic correlate that can be demonstrated by panoptic staining. While these diseases are usually diagnosed at an early age, they do not always present overt hemorrhagic symptoms. The most important of these disorders are the May-Hegglin anomaly (with an autosomal dominant mode of inheritance), congenital thrombocytic dystrophy (Bernard-Soulier syndrome) (**Fig. 37b**), and Glanzmann-Naegeli thrombasthenia.

Glanzmann-Naegeli thrombasthenia is not associated with abnormalities of platelet count or morphology. By contrast, giant platelets are characteristic of Bernard-Soulier syndrome (**Fig. 37b**) and May-Hegglin syndrome. Bernard-Soulier syndrome is also associated with concomitant platelet dysfunction (autosomal recessive inheritance). The giant platelets and thrombocytopenia in the May-Hegglin anomaly are accompanied by specific pale dirty-blue leukocyte inclusions, which are seen most clearly in neutrophilic granulocytes but are difficult to detect in eosinophils and monocytes. They are distinguishable from the "Doehle bodies" of infectious conditions by electron microscopy (see **Fig. 12a–d**).

Pseudothrombopenia

A reduced platelet count in EDTA-treated blood (pseudothrombopenia) may result from platelet aggregation or from platelet adhesion to leukocytes. This laboratory phenomenon can be identified as such by the microscopic examination of smears (**Fig. 37c**).

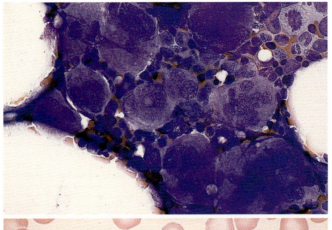

Fig. 37a – c. Thrombocytopenias and thrombocytopathies

a Accumulation of megakaryocytes in the bone marrow in idiopathic thrombocytopenia. The increase is not always dramatic, and a large proportion of immature megakaryocytes is sometimes found

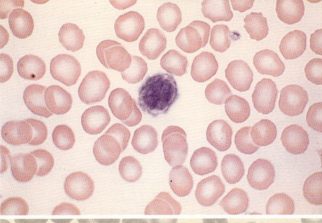

b Giant platelet in Bernard-Soulier syndrome

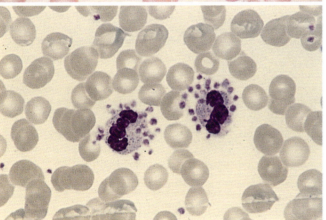

c Neutrophil surrounded by adherent platelets in EDTA-induced pseudothrombocytopenia. Pseudothrombocytopenia may result from the autoagglutination of platelets (platelet aggregate) or from the adherence of platelets to neutrophils or monocytes (satellitism). It is a laboratory phenomenon that does not occur when other anticoagulants are used (citrate, heparin) because it requires a calcium-poor medium

Bone Marrow Aplasias (Panmyelopathies)

Bone marrow aplasias are conditions in which the bone marrow is acellular or severely hypoplastic, resulting in peripheral cytopenia. Hyperplastic bone marrow with peripheral cytopenia should raise suspicion of a myelodysplasia and excludes bone marrow aplasia. The old term "panmyelopathy" covers such a range of conditions involving bone marrow injury that it should no longer be used.

Bone marrow aplasia can result from various hematopoietic disturbances, which fall into the following groups (see also **Table 9**):
1. Aplastic anemia, primary or secondary
2. Bone marrow aplasia secondary to cytostatic therapy or irradiation
3. "Displacement" of normal hematopoietic tissue by hematologic or nonhematologic tumor cells or by myelofibrosis or myelosclerosis

Regarding group 1, aplastic anemia, which is equivalent to a panmyelophthisis when fully developed, may be congenital (very rare in children) or acquired. Congenital Fanconi anemia and Diamond-Blackfan syndrome are known to occur in children along with a few extremely rare conditions that involve other congenital anomalies or metabolic disorders. Aplastic anemia is classified into three grades of severity on the basis of hematologic findings:

Table 8.

	Granulo-cytes	Platelets	Reticulo-cytes
Aplastic anemia (AA)	$< 1 \times 10^9/l$	$< 50 \times 10^9/l$	$< 40 \times 10^9/l$
Severe aplastic anemia (SAA)	$< 0,5 \times 10^9/l$	$< 20 \times 10^9/l$	$< 20 \times 10^9/l$
Very severe aplastic anemia (VSAA)	$< 0,2 \times 10^9/l$	$< 20 \times 10^9/l$	$< 20 \times 10^9/l$

A diagnosis of aplastic anemia requires at least two of the above criteria in the peripheral blood in addition to hypoplastic or aplastic bone marrow.

Groups 2 and 3 above must be excluded before aplastic anemia is diagnosed. Whenever bone marrow aspiration yields insufficient material for a positive diagnosis or if the aspiration is unsuccessful (dry tap), the diagnosis should be established by biopsy and histologic examination.

Besides the idiopathic form of aplastic anemia, the secondary acquired forms are most frequently caused by drugs, particularly analgesic and antirheumatic agents. Viral hepatitis (< 1 % of patients) and exposure to chemicals are rarely implicated. Finally, it should be noted that aplastic phases may occur during the course or even at the onset of paroxysmal nocturnal hemoglobinuria (PNH). Acute leukemia (particularly ALL) may also run through a preliminary aplastic stage.

Table 9. Classification of panmyelopathies.
[After Begemann and Rastetter (eds.) (1986) Klinische Hämatologie, 3rd ed., Thieme, Stuttgart]

I. Idiopathic or primary forms
II. Symptomatic or secondary forms
  a) Injurious physical or chemical agents in sufficient doses to produce sustained hypo- or aplasia of the bone marrow
    1. Ionizing radiation (X-rays, radium, radiophosphorus, radiogold, etc.)
    2. Cytostatic drugs
    3. Benzene
    4. Other toxic substances (e.g., arsenic compounds, inorganic gold preparations)
  b) Agents that occasionally cause hypo- or aplasia of the bone marrow
    1. Chemical agents (e.g., chloramphenicol, anticonvulsants, antithyroid drugs, analgesics, insecticides, sulfonamides, etc.)
    2. Infectious insults (hepatitis, etc.)
  c) Proliferation of neoplastic processes in the marrow spaces (medullary carcinomatoses and sarcomas including hemoblastoses and malignant lymphomas).

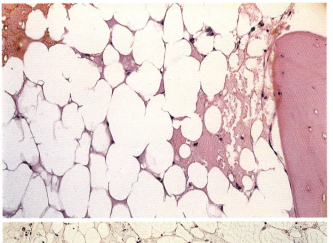

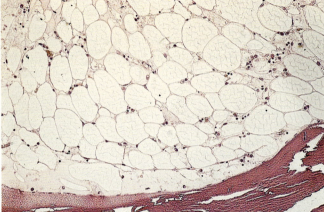

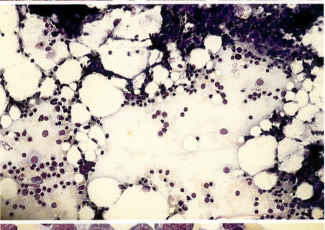

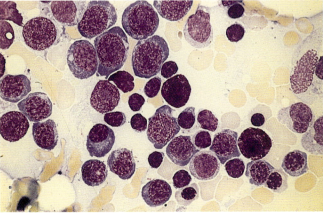

Fig. 38 a–f. Bone marrow aplasia

a Complete absence of hematopoiesis in aplastic anemia (AA). The bone marrow contains only fat cells embedded in a proteinaceous fluid (*right edge of field*)

b Another case of AA, also showing panmyelophthisis. Isolated plasma cells and lymphocytes are still interspersed among the fat cells

c–f Smears and histologic sections from a patient with aplastic anemia. All samples were taken at the time of diagnosis

c Predominance of fat cells in a bone marrow smear. An erythropoietic area is seen at *lower left*

d Higher-power view of an erythropoietic area shows interspersed lymphocytes and two tissue mast cells (*center and lower right*). The incidental aspiration of an erythropoietic area may cause misinterpretation

Fig. 38 e – h

e Typical features of panmyelophthisis in a histologic section

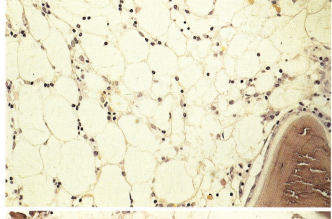

f In this section, a nest of proerythroblasts is visible at *upper center*

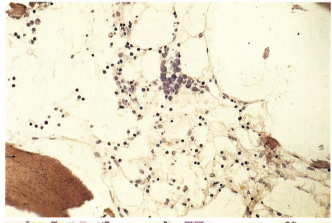

g, h Bone marrow at different stages of paroxysmal nocturnal hemoglobinuria (PNH)

g Initial sample shows typical picture of AA, consisting almost entirely of lymphocytes, plasma cells, two tissue mast cells, and increased numbers of fat cells

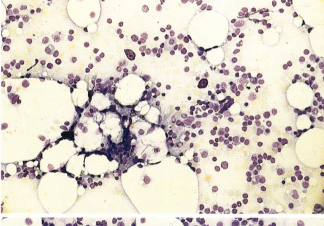

h Bone marrow smear 3 years later shows a very cellular marrow with increased erythropoiesis. One megakaryocyte is visible in the field. This pattern is suspicious for hemolytic anemia

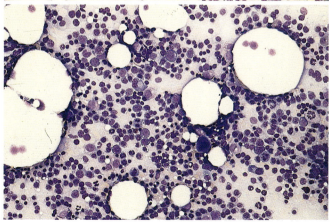

Storage Diseases

Gaucher Disease

Gaucher disease is a cerebroside storage disease caused by a deficiency of β-glucocerebrosidase. It is a familial disorder that is usually diagnosed in children after 1 year of age (juvenile form), but infantile and adult forms are also known. It presents clinically with splenomegaly and occasional hepatomegaly. A yellowish brown skin discoloration is typical in adults. Leukopenia is frequent, and a moderate normochronic anemia may be seen in later stages. Today the disease can be diagnosed by detecting the enzyme deficiency in the blood. If there is no known family history, the presumptive diagnosis can usually be confirmed by bone marrow aspiration. Gaucher cells can also be demonstrated in splenic and liver aspirates or biopsies. Gaucher cells are very large storage cells (up to 60 μm in diameter) with small central or eccentric nuclei that show a round or irregular outline and little if any internal structure. The abundant cytoplasm stains a pale grayish blue with panoptic stain and has a characteristic wispy or fibrillary appearance (like crumpled paper). Rarely the cells may contain two or more nuclei. Gaucher cells have extremely high tartrate-resistant acid phosphatase activity, they give a diffusely positive PAS stain, and some show a diffuse iron reaction.

Isolated pseudo-Gaucher cells may be found in bone marrow samples from patients with chronic myeloid leukemia, where they have no particular diagnostic or clinical significance. They are doubly refractive under polarized light, a feature that distinguishes them from true Gaucher cells. Pseudo-Gaucher cells are also found in thalassemias (strongly PAS positive).

Figure 39a–h illustrates the appearance of Gaucher cells in bone marrow.

Fig. 39 a – h. Gaucher disease

a Bone marrow smear in Gaucher disease. Numerous typical storage cells show distinctive crumpled, fibrillary cytoplasm with a bluish-gray tinge. The nuclei have a loose, sometimes moth-eaten appearance

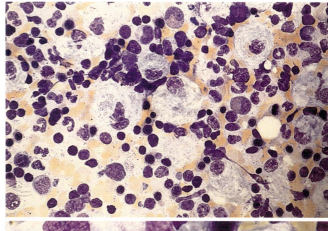

b High-power view of Gaucher cells

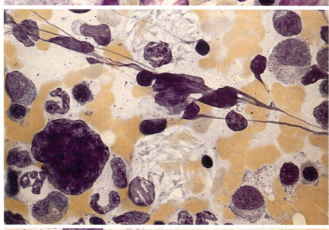

c Gaucher cells still containing erythrocyte remnants are seen above and below the *center* of the field

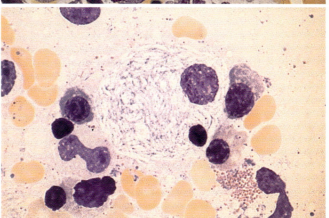

d Prominent fibrillary cytoplasmic structure in a Gaucher cell

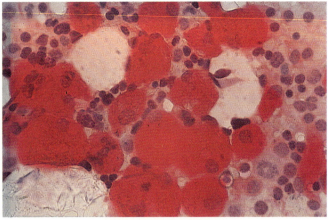

Fig. 39 e–h

e Very intense acid phosphatase reaction in Gaucher cells

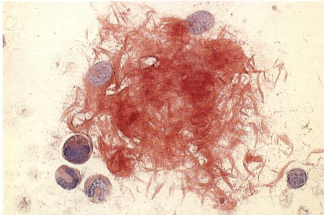

f Acid phosphatase. The fibrillary structure of the cytoplasm is apparent in the slightly crushed cells

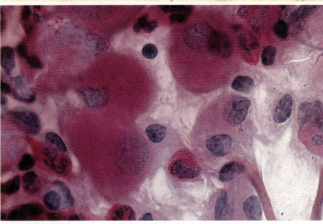

g Strong diffuse PAS reaction

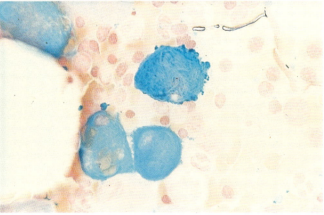

h Iron stain produces marked diffuse staining of the cytoplasm

Niemann-Pick Disease

Niemann-Pick disease is a sphingomyelin storage disease (sphingolipoidosis) that is based on a deficiency of sphingomyelinase. It is inherited as an autosomal recessive trait and produces clinical manifestations during childhood. Five different biochemical subtypes have been identified. Characteristic foam cells are found in the bone marrow, liver, spleen, and lymph nodes.

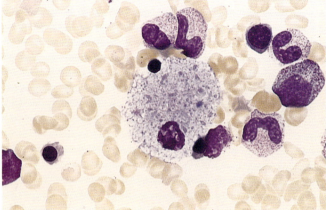

Fig. 40 a – d. Niemann-Pick disease

a, b Storage cells with very small nuclei and fine, closely spaced, partially confluent pale bluish-gray inclusions, some of which are dislodged during staining and appear as vacuoles (foamy cytoplasm)

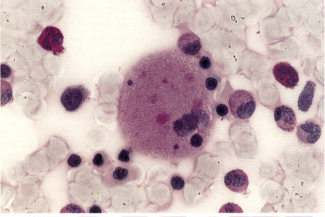

c Relatively weak PAS reaction

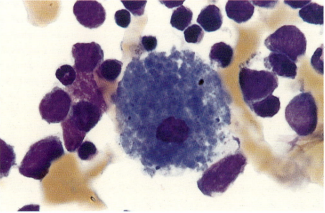

d The inclusions may show marked basophilic staining like the storage cells in sea-blue histiocytic disease, considered a variant of Niemann-Pick disease. These "sea-blue histiocytes" may also occur as storage cells when cellular breakdown is increased (as in this case)

Glycogen Storage Disease Type II
(Acid Maltase Deficiency, Pompe Disease)

In our examination of an adult with severe muscular dystrophy, we noted severe vacuolation in the plasma cells of the bone marrow (**Fig. 41a–d**). The PAS reaction demonstrated coarse positive inclusions. Electron microscopy of semithin sections and cytochemical analysis revealed the presence of a polysaccharide- and protein-containing material in the "vacuoles."[1]

---

[1] Pralle H, Schröder R, Löffler H (1975) New kind of cytoplasmic inclusions of plasma cells in acid maltase deficiency. Acta Haematol 53:109–117

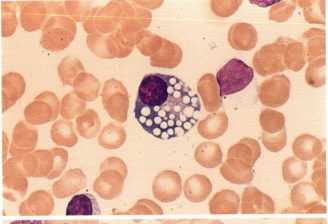

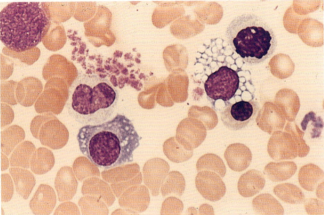

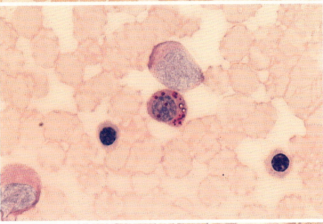

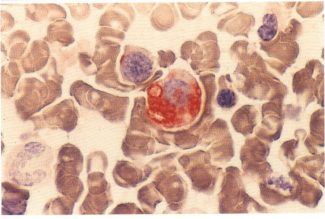

Fig. 41 a–d. Type II glycogen storage disease (acid maltase deficiency, Pompe disease)

a, b Plasma cells contain closely spaced vacuoles of varying size, found on electron microscopy and cytochemical analysis to contain glycopeptide

b

c Coarse PAS-positive inclusions in the plasma cells

d The "vacuoles" are strongly positive for acid phosphatase

Hemophagocytic Syndromes

The phagocytosis of blood cells by macrophages may occur in the setting of inflammatory processes, immune responses, or malignant diseases. An hereditary form, familial hemophagocytic lymphohistiocytosis, predominantly affects infants, with 80 % of cases occurring before the second year of life. Marked phagocytic states with greatly increased numbers of macrophages were formerly described as malignant histiocytoses or histiocytic medullary reticuloses. Many of these states may be caused by viruses (e.g., cytomegalovirus) and other infectious organisms. They are most common in immunosuppressed patients but also occur in the setting of malignant diseases. The "malignant histiocytoses" probably consist mainly of different forms of monocytic leukemia, and some may represent misidentified forms of large-cell malignant lymphoma. True neoplasias with a macrophagic phenotype are probably quite rare.

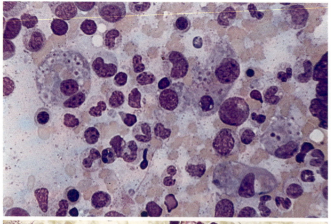

Fig. 42 a–h. Hemophagocytic syndrome

a Low-power view of bone marrow shows several macrophages that have phagocytized platelets and erythrocytes. The cause in this case is unknown

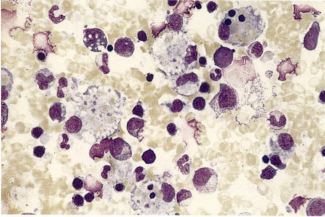

b Macrophages with erythrocytes, platelets, and (*at top*) a small nucleus in the cytoplasm

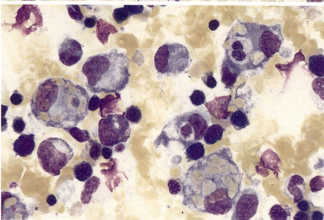

c Bone marrow from the same patient shows a phagocytized neutrophil at *upper right*

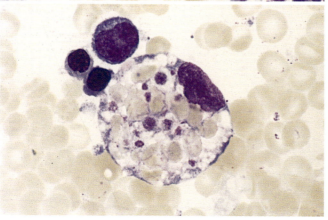

d Phagocytized erythrocytes and platelets have displaced the macrophage nucleus to the edge of the cell

Fig. 42 e–h

e Macrophage with phagocytized normoblasts

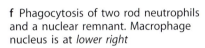
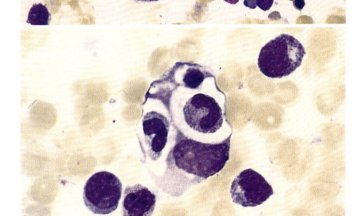

f Phagocytosis of two rod neutrophils and a nuclear remnant. Macrophage nucleus is at *lower right*

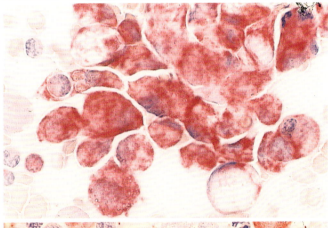

g Macrophages preserved in air-dried smears for 15 months still show strong acid phosphatase activity

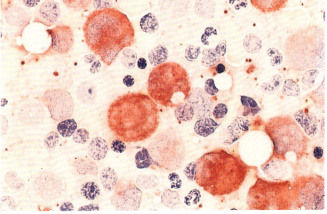

h Sample from the same patient (fresh smear) shows strong esterase activity in the macrophages

Histiocytosis X

Histiocytosis X (Langerhans cell histiocytosis, **Fig. 43**) is characterized by large cells with abundant grayish-blue cytoplasm and round to oval nuclei. CD11c, CD1, and S-100 protein serve as markers. The Birbeck granules that are specific for Langerhans cells can be demonstrated by electron microscopy. Multinucleated giant cells are characteristic.

Fig. 43 a–d

a, b Bone marrow involvement by histiocytosis X (Langerhans cell histiocytosis). Note the large cells with broad, bluish-gray cytoplasm and round to oval nuclei

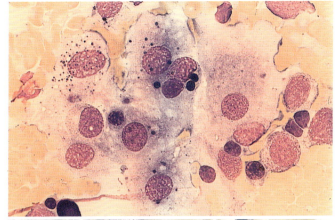

b

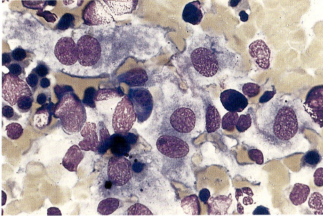

c Nonspecific esterase reaction (ANAE) demonstrates fine positive granules in the cytoplasm

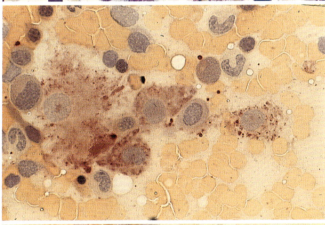

d Demonstration of acid phosphatase in the cytoplasm of malignant cells. The reaction is weaker than in the macrophages

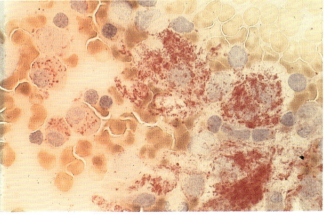

Chronic Myeloproliferative Disorders (CMPD)

Dameshek introduced the "myeloproliferative syndrome" as a collective term encompassing essential thrombocythemia, polycythemia vera, osteomyelosclerosis, and chronic myeloid leukemia. Since the detection of the Philadelphia chromosome (Ph) by Nowell and Hungerford in 1960 and later the underlying BCR/ABL translocation by Bartram et al., a sharp distinction must be drawn between chronic myeloid (granulocytic) leukemia and the other chronic myeloproliferative disorders. The concept of CMPD is justified by certain similarities in the course of these diseases. Several apparent transitions between the different forms have been elucidated using molecular genetic techniques and have been classified as various manifestations of chronic myeloid leukemia. Many questions remain unanswered, however, and it is necessary to provide an accurate description of individual cases.

The diagnosis of *essential thrombocythemia* is based on a consistently elevated platelet count (higher than $6 \times 10^9/L$), the exclusion of a different cause (including chronic inflammatory disease), and an increase of megakaryocytes in the bone marrow, which often show only subtle abnormalities (hypersegmented nuclei) and are grouped in clusters. The peripheral blood film may show a mild leukocytosis with slight basophilia and eosinophilia in addition to thrombocytosis. These cases require a chromosomal and/or molecular genetic evaluation to exclude chronic myeloid leukemia. *Polycythemia vera* can be diagnosed only when findings meet the criteria defined by the Polycythemia Vera Study Group. The cellularity of the bone marrow is markedly increased, and fat cells are completely absent in fully established cases. There is a significant increase in megakaryocytes, which show an extreme diversity of sizes. Erythropoiesis and usually granulocytopoiesis are markedly increased, and iron stores are absent from the marrow. A slight increase of basophils is observed in the blood and bone marrow. Histologic examination is necessary for an accurate quantitative evaluation of bone marrow structures. An increase in leukocyte alkaline phosphatase activity is detected in blood smears. *Osteomyelosclerosis* or *myelofibrosis* is characterized by an increase in reticular fibers and/or cancellous bone ranging to the complete obliteration of the bone marrow and by extramedullary hematopoiesis. The differential blood count may be very similar to that in chronic myeloid leukemia, but there are significant erythrocyte abnormalities that include teardrop-shaped cells and the presence of erythroblasts in the blood smear. Leukocyte alkaline phosphatase is usually elevated or normal.

Transient Myeloproliferation

In newborns with Down syndrome, an increase in blast cells in the peripheral blood may occur that spontaneously disappears within months. However, in some cases an acute megakaryoblast leukemia (M7) may develop after an average of 1–2 years. The blast cells of the transient form are monoclonal, very immature and may differentiate themselves into the neutrophilic, monocytic, basophilic, erythrocytic, and megakaryocytic series.

In patients with Down syndrome and AML, in addition to the constitutive trisomy 21, complete or partial trisomies of chromosomes 8 and 1 are found.

An isolated proliferation of megakaryocytes (**Fig. 46g, h**) is as rare as tumorlike megakaryoblastomas (see **Fig. 104d, e**).

Fig. 44 a – d. Essential thrombocythemia (ET)

a Blood smear reveals anisocytosis and a greatly increased number of platelets

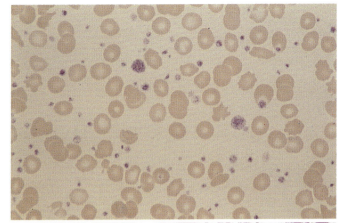

b Bone marrow smear in ET shows large masses of platelets and scattered megakaryocytes

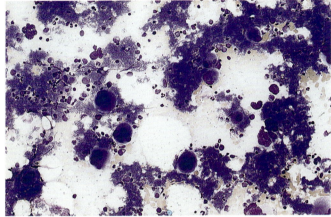

c Three mature megakaryocytes and large platelet aggregations

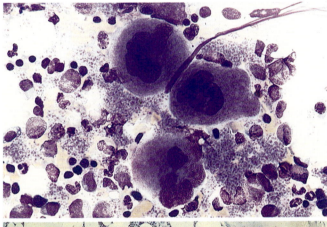

d Histologic section in ET shows a substantial increase in moderately pleomorphic megakaryocytes, some arranged in clusters. There is a normal proportion of fat cells. Giemsa stain

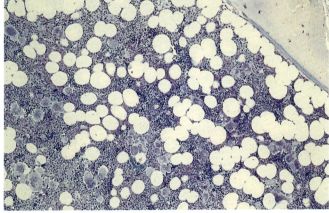

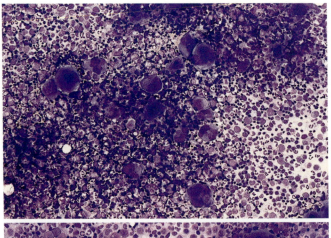

Fig. 45 a–e. Polycythemia vera

a Bone marrow smear shows marked hypercellularity with a significant increase in megakaryocytes, which vary markedly in size and maturation

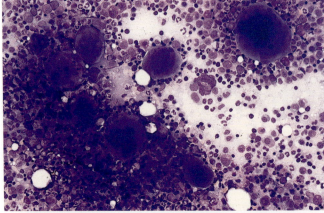

b High-power view shows the size variation of the megakaryocytes

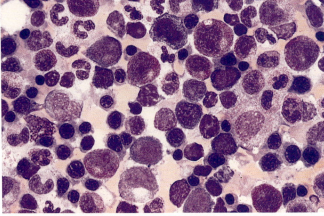

c Bone marrow area with increased erythropoiesis and granulocytopoiesis. At *left* is a basophil

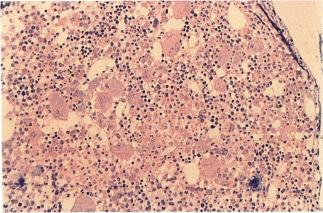

d Histologic section shows residual fat cells, a typical increase in megakaryocytes of varying size, and increased erythropoiesis. Giemsa stain

Fig. 45 e – h

e Blood smear shows a substantial increase in leukocyte alkaline phosphatase activity (*red*)

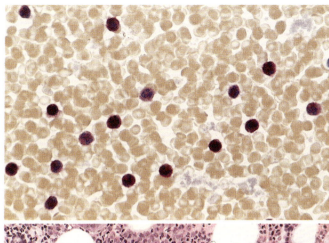

f Bone marrow in myelofibrosis. Note the clustering of the pleomorphic megakaryocytes. Hematoxylin-eosin stain

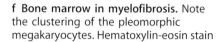

g Bone marrow section in myelofibrosis. Silver stain demonstrates heavy fiber proliferation. At *lower left* is a cluster of megakaryocytes

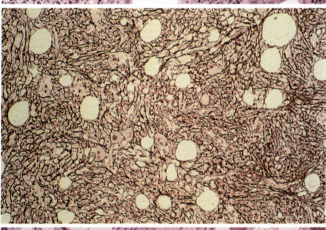

h Bone marrow in osteomyelosclerosis (OMS). The marrow cavity is almost completely obliterated by collagen and increased cancellous trabeculae. Hematoxylin-eosin stain

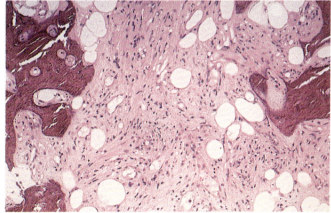

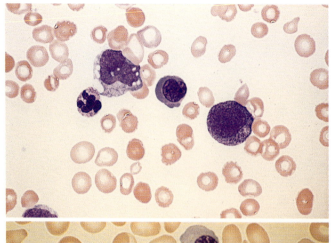

Fig. 46 a–d

a Blood smear in osteomyelosclerosis (OMS). Monocyte and segmented cell at *left*, erythroblast at *center*, and promyelocyte at *right*

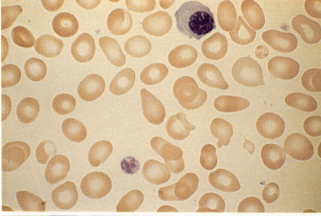

b Blood smear in OMS shows significant poikilocytosis with teardrop-shaped erythrocytes. At *top* is a normoblast

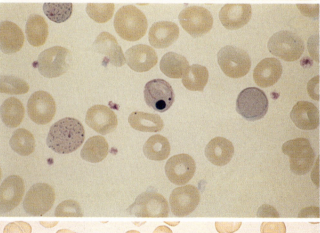

c Blood smear in OMS shows heavy basophilic stippling and two erythrocytes with Cabot rings. At *center* is an erythrocyte with Howell-Jolly bodies and a nuclear remnant

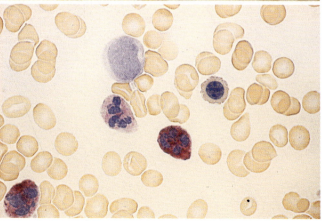

d Increased leukocyte alkaline phosphatase (LAP) in OMS. There is one grade 1 and one grade 4 neutrophil, a normoblast, and a negative blast at *upper left*

Fig. 46 e–h

e Blood smear in chronic myeloprolife-rative disease (CMPD) shows five erythroblasts and, at the *center of the field*, basophilic stippling. Such cases were once termed "chronic erythremia." Erythroblastosis can occur in various forms of CMPD

f Blood smear in chronic myeloid leuke-mia (CML) during the accelerated phase after splenectomy. At *center* is a mega-karyocyte nucleus, at *right* are two megakaryoblasts, and at *left* is a myelo-blast

g Histologic section from an iliac crest biopsy in "pure" megakaryocytic myelosis consists almost entirely of megakaryo-cytes at various stages of maturity. Giemsa stain

h Silver-stained specimen from the same patient clearly shows the darkly stained nuclei of the megakaryocytes and fiber proliferation

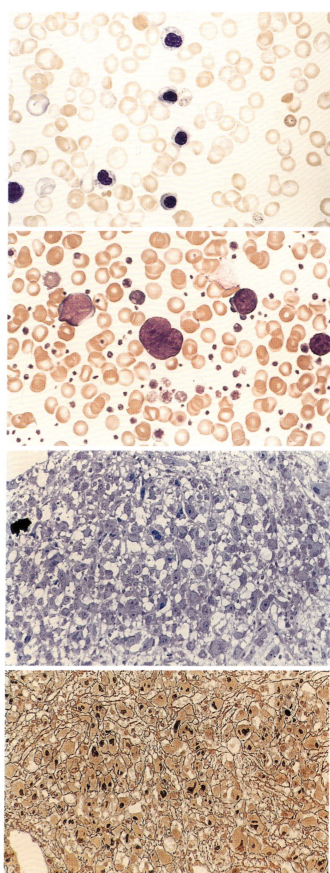

The pure malignant proliferation of megakaryocytes (Fig. **46g** and **h**) is as rare as tumorous megakaryoblastoma (Fig. **104d** and **c**)

In one case with an exceptional increase in megakaryoblasts and promegakaryocytes and a very high proportion of mitoses, we were able to classify the disease as promegakaryocytic-megakaryoblastic leukemia (megakaryocyte precursor cell leukemia). The cells and mitoses could be positively identified by the immunocytochemical detection of the megakaryocyte markers CD41 and CD61. This case is more characteristic of a CMPD than an acute leukemia (**Fig. 47a–h;** joint observation with D. Müller, Hof).

Figure 48a–c shows an example of familial polyglobulia with positive erythrocyte alkaline phosphatase. Cytochemical and biochemical tests in four family members (three generations) showed that some of the erythrocytes and 100 % of the erythroblasts contained alkaline phosphatase, which differs from the phosphatase in neutrophils. It is likely that the increased breakdown of 2,3-diphosphoglycerate plays a role in the pathogenesis of the erythrocytosis.

Fig. 47 a – h. Promegakaryocytic-mega-karyoblastic leukemia (after Löffler and Müller, unpublished)

a Six megakaryocytic mitoses and numerous small megakaryoblasts

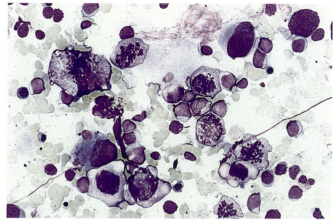

b Higher-power view of megakaryo-blasts and four mitoses

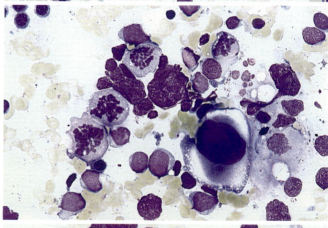

c Four mitoses, blasts, and a promega-karyocyte in the *lower half* of the field

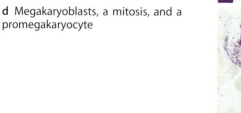

d Megakaryoblasts, a mitosis, and a promegakaryocyte

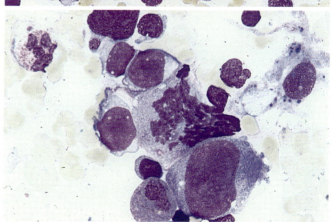

Fig. 47 e–h

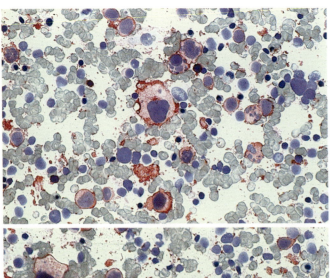

e Immunocytochemical detection of CD41. A large proportion of the megakaryoblasts and promegakaryocytes are positive

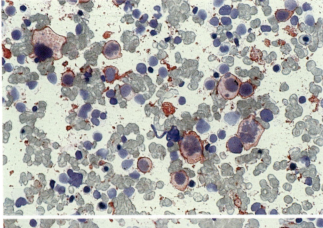

f CD41: three positive mitoses are seen at *upper left* and *lower right*. Other features are the same as in **e**

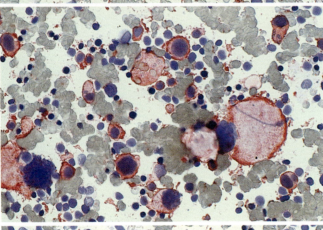

g CD41: besides blasts and promegakaryocytes, a positive mature megakaryocyte is visible at *right*

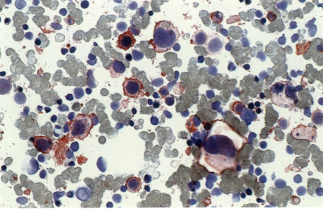

h CD61: the result is the same as with CD41

Fig. 48 a – c. Familial erythrocytosis. Cytochemical detection of alkaline phosphatase

a Blood smear. Erythrocytes show weak diffuse reaction with fine positive granules

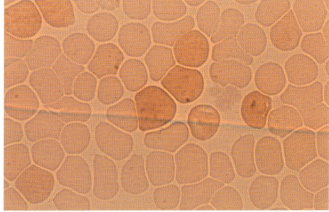

b Erythroblast cluster in bone marrow smear with marked cytoplasmic reaction (substrate α-naphthyl phosphate)

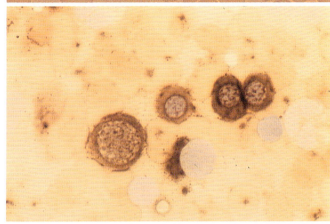

c Marked reaction (*red*) in erythroblasts with the substrate naphthol-AS-Bi phosphate

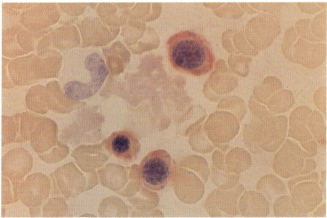

Chronic Myeloid (Granulocytic) Leukemia

The blood picture in chronic myeloid leukemia (CML) often contributes more to the diagnosis than the bone marrow. Besides the high leukocyte count and a pathologic left shift with the appearance of immature granulocytopoietic forms at all stages (including promyelocytes and myeloblasts), eosinophilia and basophilia are present in the *peripheral blood* and corroborate the diagnosis of CML. In addition, individual granulocytes show qualitative changes such as anisocytosis, nuclear-cytoplasmic asynchrony, and hyposegmentation ("pseudo-Pelger forms"). These changes are largely absent during the early chronic phase. The same changes may be found in severe reactive leukocytoses. The *bone marrow* is very cellular. Erythropoiesis is greatly suppressed in favor of granulocytopoiesis, which dominates the cell picture. The granulocytopoietic line include a great many immature forms, producing a marked shift to the left. Marrow basophils and eosinophils are usually increased and show qualitative changes involving asynchronous maturation of the nucleus, cytoplasm, and granulation. Despite these findings, it can be difficult to distinguish the bone marrow changes from those associated with severe reactive leukocytoses. The behavior of the plasma cells is often helpful in these cases. These cells are usually increased in reactive leukocytoses, whereas they are generally decreased in CML. The cytochemical detection of *leukocyte alkaline phosphatase* activity (LAP, see p. 13) is of key importance. Generally, LAP activity is very low or even negative in CML while it is high or at least normal in reactive leukocytoses. A rise of LAP activity during the course of CML may herald the onset of an acute myeloblastic phase. LAP activity also increases in response to complicating infections, but the activity index remains within normal limits. The diagnosis is established by detection of the Philadelphia chromosome (Ph). It represents a reciprocal translocation between the long arms of chromosomes 9 and 22 [i.e., t(9;22)], resulting in a translocation of the BCR and ABL genes. This creates a new fusion gene called the BCR-ABL gene. The corresponding proteins, which have molecular weights of 210 (p210) and 190 (p190), can be detected in very low concentration by PCR. Thus, molecular biology and its combination with cytogenetic analysis in the FISH technique provide highly sensitive detection methods that complement morphology and cytogenetics in the diagnosis and especially the follow-up of CML after intensive therapy.

The differentiation of CML from chronic myelomonocytic leukemia (CMML), which is sometimes included among the myelodysplasias, can be difficult to accomplish by morphology alone, since there are "intermediate forms" that the FAB group has classified as atypical CML. The most reliable differentiating method is the cytogenetic detection of the (9;22) translocation or the molecular genetic detection of the BCR-ABL translocation. The absence of these changes precludes a diagnosis of CML (CGL).

Almost all chronic myeloid leukemias progress to an acute phase (*acute blast phase, blast crisis*) during the course of the disease. This acute phase may arise by transformation from the chronic phase, or an accelerated phase may precede it. The accelerated phase can be diagnosed by its clinical manifestations (fever, bone pain, splenomegaly) and an increasing left shift of the granulocytes. There may also be an increase in basophilic granulocytes, which are already numerous in this disease. An increase in leukocyte alkaline phosphatase activity is occasionally detected during the blast phase. Sometimes the acute phase has its onset in a particular organ such as the spleen or lymph nodes.

The blasts consist predominantly of cytochemically and immunologically identifiable myeloblasts and less commonly (20 % – 30 %) of lymphoblasts, which may be PAS-positive and display the immunologic features of common ALL. Megakaryoblast or erythroblast transformation is less frequent, but mixed blast phases are somewhat more common. Besides the t (9;22) translocation, the accelerated phase or blast phase is often characterized by other cytogenetic changes that mainly consist of an extra Ph chromosome, an isochromosome 17, trisomy 8, or a combination of these.

Because the BCR-ABL translocation occurs in early stem cells, CML affects a portion of the T lymphocytes and may affect all hematopoietic cells, although the involvement need not be complete. It is not surprising, therefore, when a high percentage of eosinophils or basophils are discovered in variants of CML. As long as the typical cytogenetic or molecular genetic abnormality is present, there is no need to classify the leukemia as "eosinophilic" or "basophilic." True eosinophilic and basophilic leukemias do exist, but they are more aptly classified as acute leukemias and are discussed under that heading.

Table 10. Stages of CML

a) Chronic phase		
Blood smear		*Bone marrow*
GP:	Pathologic left shift Increased eosinophils Increased basophils	GP: Very hyperplastic Shift to the left Increased eosinophils Increased basophils
EP:	Scattered normoblasts Anisocytosis, polychromatophilia	EP: Decreased (absolute or relative)
ThP:	Platelets usually increased Anisocytosis, giant platelets Scattered megakaryocyte nuclei	ThP: Megakaryocytes usually increased, some abnormal forms (microkaryocytes)

b) Accelerated phase		
Blood smear		*Bone marrow*
GP:	Pathologic left shift, pseudo-Pelger forms Increased numbers of N.C. or "blasts," < 20 % Basophils may be markedly increased, < 30 %	GP: Pathologic left shift Increased numbers of N.C. or "blasts," < 20 % Basophils may be markedly increased
EP:	Scattered normoblasts anisocytosis, polychromatophilia	EP: Decreased
ThP:	Platelets normal or decreased Anisocytosis, scattered megakaryocyte nuclei	ThP: Normal or decreased

c) Acute phase (blast crisis)		
Blood smear		*Bone marrow*
GP:	Practically all cells are N.C. (blasts)	GP: Practically all cells are N.C. (blasts), > 30 %
EP:	Pronounced anisocytosis Polychromatophilia, normoblasts	EP: Greatly decreased
ThP:	Platelets absent or greatly decreased Anisocytosis, megakaryocyte nuclei	ThP: Greatly decreased

N.C., nonclassifiable cells;
GP, granulocytopoiesis;
EP, erythropoiesis;
ThP, thrombocytopoiesis, megakaryocytopoiesis

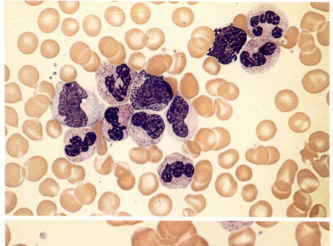

Fig. 49 a–h. Chronic myeloid leukemia (CML)

a Blood smear shows a preponderance of mature neutrophilic granulocytes. Myelocyte at *center*, basophil at *upper right*

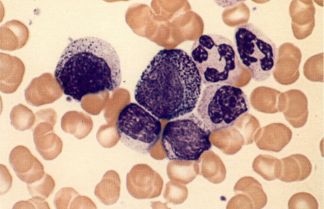

b Promyelocyte (*center*) in a blood smear

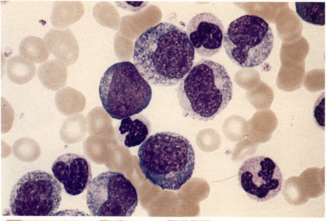

c Blood smear showing a greater left shift. At *center* is a myeloblast

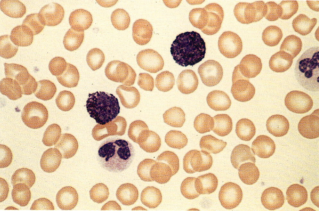

d Two basophils in blood smear

Fig. 49 e – h

e Two blasts in blood smear – an unusual finding during the chronic phase

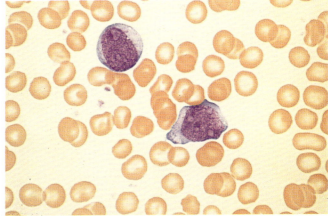

f Increased granulocytopoiesis in a bone marrow smear. Neutrophilic granulocytes, two basophils, and four eosinophils

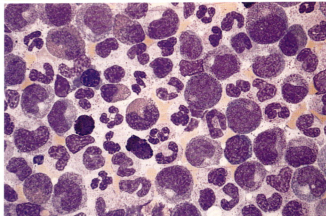

g Bone marrow smear in CML shows greatly increased numbers of megakaryocytes, including many with round nuclei and mature cytoplasm

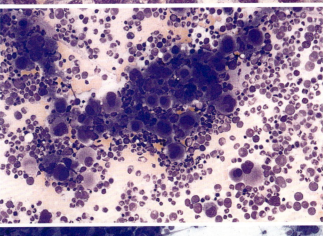

h Bone marrow smear. Despite the presence of a large megakaryocyte cluster, the patient had typical CML with BCR/ABL translocation

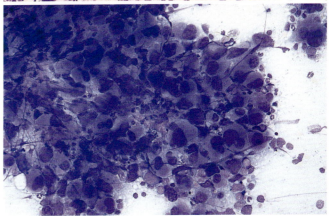

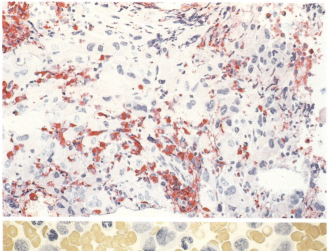

Fig. 50 a – d. Chronic myeloid leukemia (CML)

a Megakaryocytes are greatly increased and interspersed with (*red*) neutrophilic granulocytes. Histologic section, naphthol AS-D chloroacetate esterase reaction

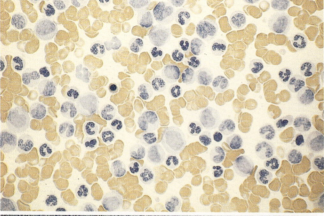

b Blood smear in untreated CML. All cells are negative for leukocyte alkaline phosphatase (index 0)

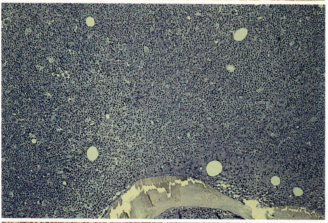

c Histologic section from an iliac crest core biopsy (Giemsa stain) illustrates the extremely high cellular density and paucity of fat cells

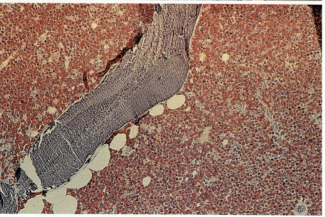

d Histologic section during chronic phase of CML. Naphthol AS-D chloroacetate esterase reaction shows an extreme increase in neutrophilic granulocytopoiesis

Fig. 51 a–f. Chronic myeloid leukemia (CML)

a Bone marrow smear shows two storage cells with abundant cytoplasm (pseudo-Gaucher cells) against a background of increased granulocytopoiesis

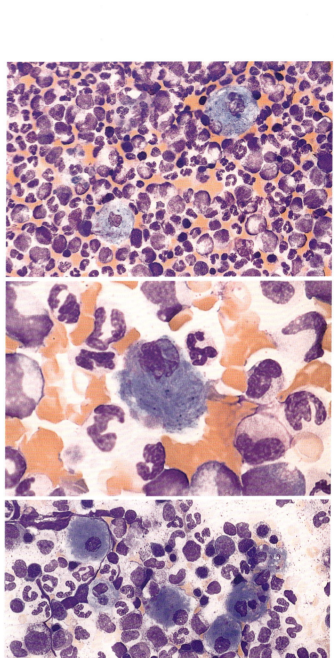

b Pseudo-Gaucher cell, virtually indistinguishable from a true Gaucher cell in its cytologic features

c Several pseudo-Gaucher cells with a slightly bluer cytoplasmic tinge. The double refraction in the cytoplasm of the pseudo-Gaucher cells under polarized light distinguishes them from true Gaucher cells

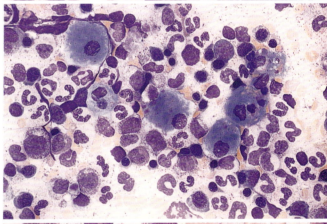

d Blasts, promyelocytes, and atypically maturing forms with nuclear atypia; also several small basophils in the accelerated phase of CML

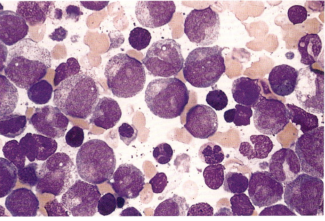

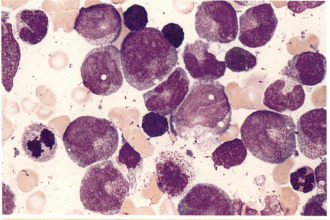

Fig. 51 e–f

e Higher-power view in accelerated phase of CML shows atypical forms and basophils

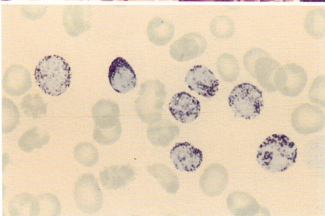

f Blood smear in accelerated CML shows a marked increase in basophilic granulocytes. Toluidine blue stain

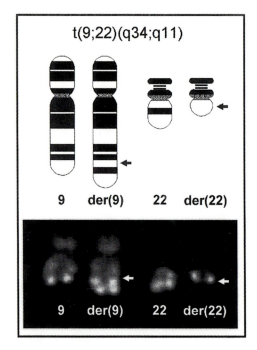

Fig. 52. Schematic diagram and partial karyotype of the typical Philadelphia translocation t(9;22)(q34;q21) in chronic myeloid leukemia

Fig. 53. BCR/ABL (Philadelphia) translocation in a megakaryocyte, demonstrated by fluorescence in situ hybridization (FISH) combined with fluorescent immunophenotyping (FICTION). The Philadelphia translocations in the cell are identified by the co-location of a green (BCR) and red (ABL) signal. The blue cytoplasmic stain indicates CD41 positivity. (Figure in cooperation with T. Haferlach et al.)

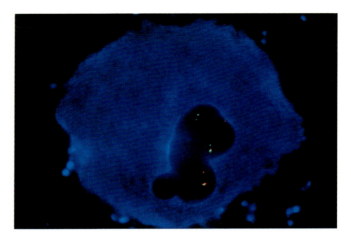

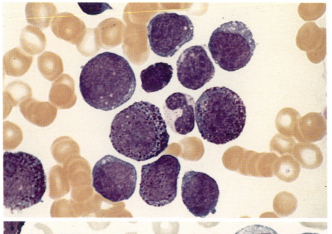

Fig. 54 a–g. Blast phases in CML

a Blood smear in myeloid blast phase of CML shows myeloblasts and promyelocytes with a rod form and basophil at the *center of the field*

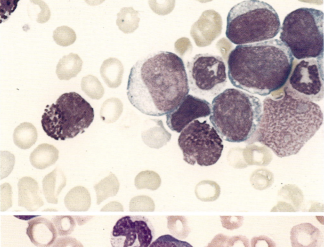

b Myeloid blast phase. Blasts and basophils

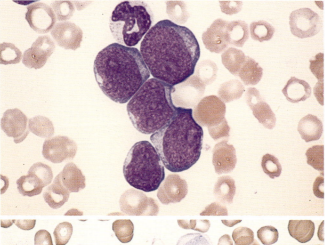

c Myeloid blast phase. Undifferentiated blasts

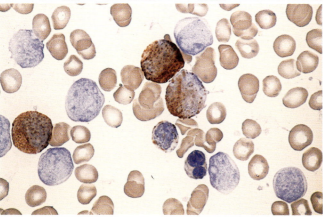

d Blood smear from the same patient shows two peroxidase-positive precursors at *upper center*

e Same smear series as in **c** and **d**, immunoperoxidase reaction. All the blasts are positive. If findings are equivocal, other myeloid markers such as CD13 and CD33 can also be used

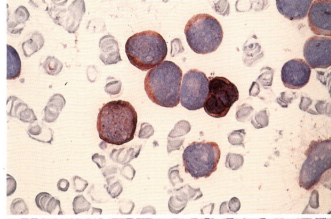

f Histologic section in blast phase. A nest of blasts (paler nuclei) is visible at *center* (HE stain)

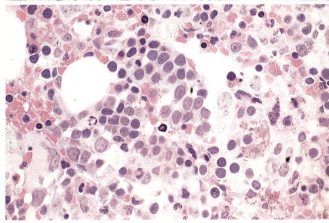

g Bone marrow smear in myeloblast phase shows predominant basophils and scattered eosinophilic granulocytes

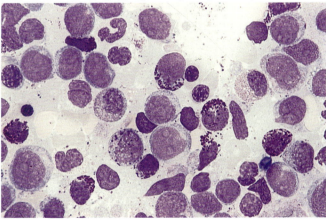

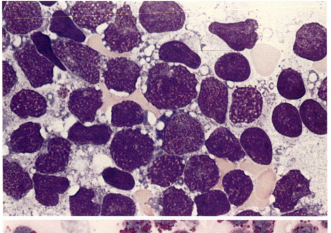

Fig. 55 a–d. Lymphoblast phase in CML. Immunophenotype of a C-ALL

a Blasts with numerous large vacuoles in the cytoplasm

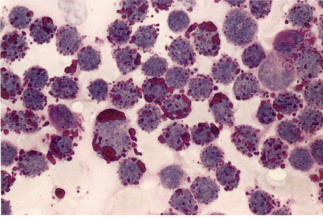

b Coarse PAS-positive clumps and granules in the vacuoles

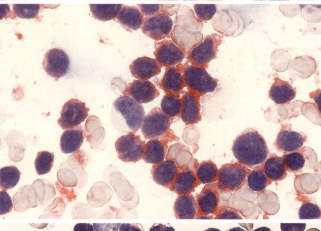

c Immunocytochemical detection of CD19. All blasts are positive

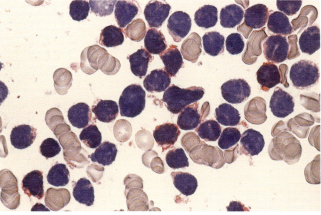

d Immunocytochemical detection of CD10. All blasts are positive (*red*)

Fig. 56 a – h. Megakaryocytic-megakaryoblastic and erythroblastic phases in CML

a Megakaryocytic-megakaryoblastic transformation

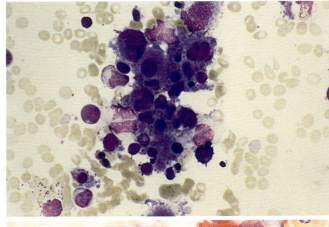

b Bone marrow from the same patient. Predominantly mature megakaryocytes are strongly esterase-positive

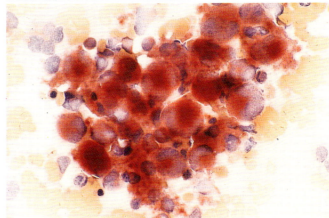

c Megakaryoblastic transformation in a different patient

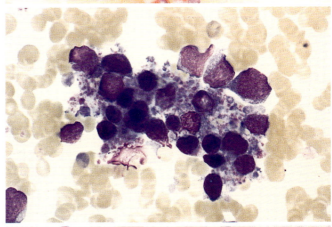

d Blood smear in megakaryoblast phase demonstrates three blasts

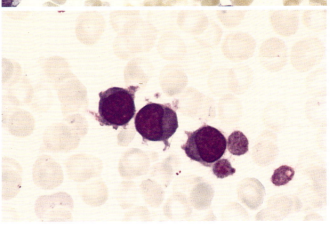

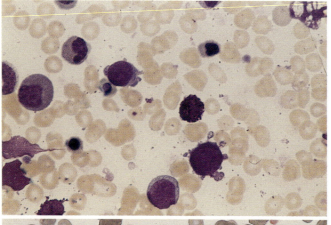

Fig. 56 e–h

e Three blasts in megakaryoblast phase

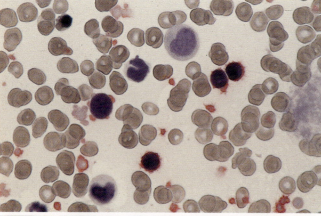

f Bone marrow smear from the patient in **e**. Immunocytochemical detection of CD61. The blasts are positive. Note the positive platelets

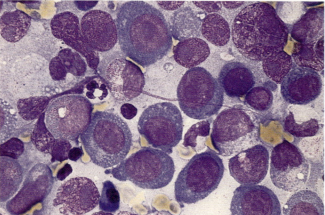

g Bone marrow from a patient in the erythroblast phase of CML shows very immature, partially megaloblastoid erythroblasts

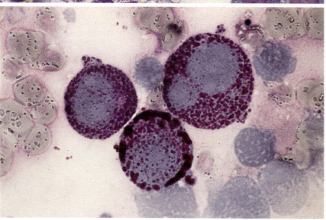

h Smear from the patient in **g** shows a very intense PAS reaction in coarse granules and clumps

Myelodysplastic Syndromes (MDS)

The diagnostic criteria for myelodysplastic syndromes (MDS) and a classification of these syndromes were presented by the FAB group in 1982. MDS are a class of subacute to chronic diseases that are associated with quantitative and qualitative blood and bone marrow changes.[1] The syndromes are seen predominantly in older patients, with some cases showing transformation to acute leukemia. An essential criterion is the number of blasts that can be detected in the bone marrow and/or the peripheral blood. Cytopenia is invariably present (anemia, granulocytopenia, or thrombocytopenia) despite normocellular or hypercellular bone marrow ("ineffectual hematopoiesis"). Disturbances of erythropoiesis (dyserythropoiesis) are reflected in quantitative and qualitative abnormalities of nucleated precursors in the bone marrow and of erythrocytes in the peripheral blood (see **Table 11**). The proportion of erythropoiesis in the bone marrow may be increased ($> 50\%$) or reduced ($< 5\%$). Disturbances of granulocytopoiesis (dysgranulocytopoiesis) are manifested in the bone marrow by abnormalities in granules or nuclei (pseudo-Pelger forms, ring forms, etc.). Occasionally the cytoplasmic basophilia is irregularly distributed, and a heavy basophilic rim is present at the cell periphery. Neutrophils in the peripheral blood are frequently agranular or hypogranular, and the mature forms sometimes show a basophilic cytoplasm. Disturbances of megakaryocytopoiesis lead to the appearance of abnormal cells (micromegakaryocytes, large mononuclear forms, hypersegmented forms, many single nuclei). Abnormal platelets (giant forms, conspicuous anisocytosis) are found in the peripheral blood (**Table 11**).

Two types of blast are observed in MDS (see **Fig. 68**):

Type I: The cells of type I range from forms indistinguishable from myeloblasts to cells of variable size that cannot be classified. The cytoplasm is agranular, and the nucleus shows distinct nucleoli and a loose chromatin pattern. The nuclear-cytoplasmic ratio is higher in smaller cells than in larger ones.

---

[1] Bennett JM, Catovsky D, Daniel MT, Flandrin G, Galton DA, Gralnick HR, Sultan C (1982) Proposals for the classification of the myelodysplastic syndromes. Brit. J. Haematol 51 : 189 – 199

Table 11. Signs of dysplasia

Erythropoiesis
Multinuclearity, megaloblastic nuclear changes, abnormal mitoses, karyorrhexis, ringed sideroblasts, coarse iron granules, cytoplasmic vacuoles.

Granulocytopoiesis
Pseudo-Pelger forms, hypersegmentation, giant forms, ring nuclei, hypogranulation, abnormal basophilia, peroxidase defect, atypical positive esterase in neutrophils and eosinophils.

Megakaryopoiesis
Micro(mega)karyocytes (small round nucleus, mature cytoplasm), large mononucleate forms, many small nuclei, hypersegmented nuclei, nuclear-cytoplasmic asynchrony, anisocytosis of platelets, giant platelets.

Type II: The cells contain few primary (azurophilic) granules, the nuclear-cytoplasmic ratio is smaller, and the nucleus is centrally located.

Five forms of MDS are recognized (**Table 12**):

1. Refractory anemia (RA). The cardinal symptom is anemia. Reticulocytes are diminished in the peripheral blood, and blasts are absent or do not exceed 1 %. The bone marrow is normo- or hyperplastic and usually shows a predominance of erythropoiesis, though there are cases in which erythropoiesis is reduced. Granulocytopoiesis and megakaryocytopoiesis may show evidence of dysplasia. The proportion of blasts is less than 5 %.

2. Refractory anemia with ringed sideroblasts (RARS). In contrast to RA, the proportion of ringed sideroblasts exceeds 15 %. The prognosis is most favorable in cases where granulocytopoiesis and megakaryocytes are unaffected. This form ("pure" sideroblastic anemia) should be distinguished from RARS, therefore.

3. Refractory anemia with excess blasts (RAEB). Cytopenia is usually present, and all three cell lines in the peripheral blood display abnormalities. Small numbers of blasts ($< 5\%$) may be found in the peripheral blood. The bone marrow is hypercellular with variable hyperplasia of erythropoiesis or granulocytopoiesis. Dyserythropoiesis, dysgranulocytopoiesis, and/or dysmegakaryocytopoiesis is invariably present. Ringed sideroblasts may be found. The percentage of blasts (types I and II) in the bone marrow is 5 % to 20 %.

4. Chronic myelomonocytic leukemia (CMML). The dominant feature is monocytosis, which must exceed $1 \times 10^9/L$ in the peripheral blood. Frequently this is associated with an increase in mature granulocytes, with or without dysgranulocytopoiesis (such as hypogranular or Pelger forms). The percentage of blasts in

Table 12. FAB criteria for the subtypes of MDS (key findings are in bold)

Diagnosis	Abbreviation	Bone marrow		Blood	
		Blasts[a]	Ringed sideroblasts[b]	Blasts	Monocytes ($\times 10^9$/l)
Refractory anemia	RA	< 5 %	< 15 %	≤ 1 %	< 1
Refractory anemia with ringed sideroblasts	RARS	< 5 %	$\geq 15\%$	≤ 1 %	< 1
Refractory anemia with excess blasts	RAEB	$5 - 20\%$	Variable	< 5 %	< 1
RAEB in transformation	RAEB-t	$> 20^c < 30$	Variable	≥ 5 %	< 1
Chronic myelomonocytic leukemia	CMML	< 20 %	Variable	< 5 %	≥ 1

[a] Percentage of all nucleated cells.
[b] Percentage of erythroblasts.
[c] 20 % is sufficient if peripheral blasts exceed 5 % or Auer rods are present

the peripheral blood is less than 5 %. The bone marrow findings are like those in RAEB, but usually there is a significant increase in monocytic precursors (promonocytes). There must be fewer than 30 % blasts. Monocytes are best demonstrated by esterase staining.

5. RAEB in transformation. The hematologic features resemble those of RAEB, except that the percentage of blasts in the peripheral blood exceeds 5 %, the marrow contains 20 % to 30 % blasts (types I and II), and conspicuous Auer rods are sometimes found in granulocytopoietic precursors. RAEB in transformation usually runs a brief course with a relatively swift progression to AML.

A separate biologic entity is the 5q-minus syndrome, which was formerly included in the RA or RARS subgroups. Occurring mainly in older women, it is characterized by a macrocytic anemia with normal or increased numbers of platelets. The bone marrow contains abundant megakaryocytes that mostly display round nuclei, nuclear hypolobulation, and a granular cytoplasm. Cytogenetic demonstration of the deletion on the long arm of chromosome 5 (5q-) establishes the diagnosis.

Another entity, which is characterized cytogenetically by a deletion or translocation of the short arm of chromosome 17 – del (17p) – and morphologically by pronounced dysgranulocytopoiesis with almost complete ("homozygotic") pseudo-Pelger transformation of the granulocytes, is usually associated with additional chromosome abnormalities. A very prominent clumping of the chromatin is often seen. Mutations of the p53 gene have been postulated as the cause.

Some cases of MDS do not fit into any of the subtype categories noted above. These cases present with bone marrow hypoplasia or fibrosis, which usually requires a histologic diagnosis, or with an increase in tissue or blood basophils. Many of these cases are secondary to treatment with cytostatic drugs.

Fig. 57 a – f. Myelodysplastic syndromes (MDS)

a Erythroblasts with megaloblastic changes. Binucleated form at *top center*. Refractory anemia (RA)

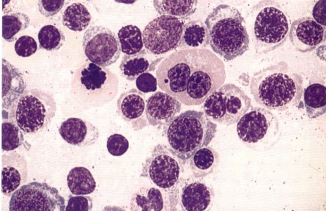

b Abnormal erythroblast mitoses with clumped and fragmented chromosomes

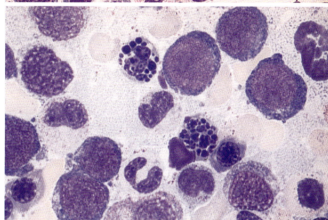

c Chromatin strands linking erythroblast nuclei in RA. Indistinguishable from the changes in type I form of CDA

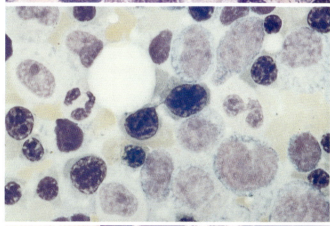

d Trinucleated proerythroblast at *top*, atypical mitosis at *lower right*, agranular pseudo-Pelger form at *center*, hypergranular pseudo-Pelger form at *bottom*, myeloblast at *lower left*. RAEB-t

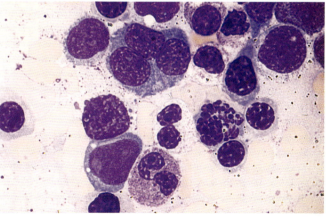

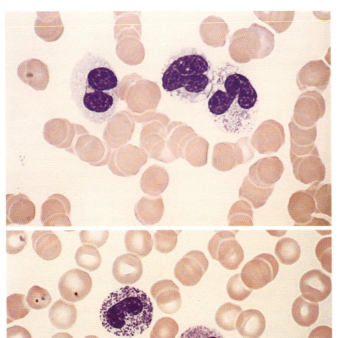

Fig. 57 e – f

e Pseudo-Pelger form without granules at *left*, vacuolated cytoplasm at *center*, vacuolation and unevenly distributed granules at *right* – typical of anomalies involving the short arm of chromosome 17 (17p)

f Two pseudo-Pelger forms, at *left* with "toxic" granules

Fig. 58 a – d Dysgranulocytopoiesis

a Bone marrow smear in RAEB-t shows hypogranular cells of granulocytopoiesis. Two myeloblasts appear at the *center* and *right edge of the field*

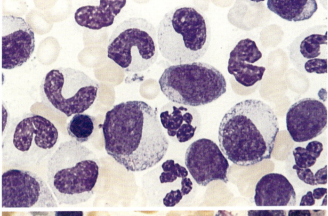

b Polyploid giant segmented form at *center*, below it a normal-appearing segmented neutrophil

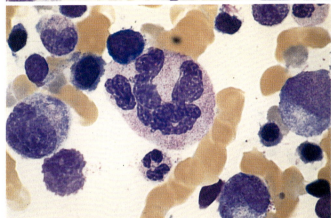

c Peroxidase reaction. One cell is positive at *top*, three neutrophils below it are negative: partial peroxidase defect

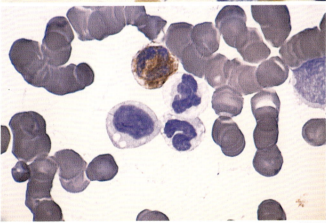

d Abnormal nonspecific esterase reaction (α-naphthyl acetate). Most of the neutrophils in the field show weak to moderate esterase activity; normally they are negative

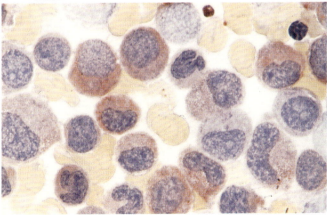

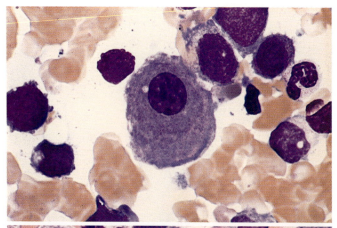

Fig. 59 a–d. Signs of megakaryocytic dysplasia in MDS

a Micro(mega)karyocyte with a typical small round nucleus and largely mature cytoplasm. RAEB-t

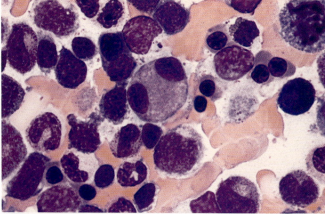

b Binucleated microkaryocyte at *center*. RAEB

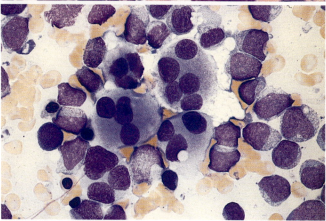

c Five abnormal megakaryocytes, each with multiple nuclei and an abnormal cytoplasmic stain. Cluster of myeloblasts at *right*. Transition from RAEB-t to AML

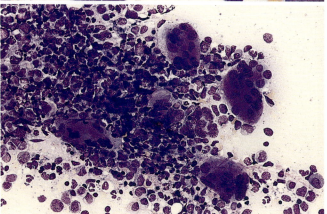

d Cluster of multinucleated megakaryocytes in CMML

Fig. 60–67. Subtypes of MDS
Fig. 60 a – h. RARS

a Bone marrow smear in RARS. Pappenheim stain. The cytoplasm is still mostly basophilic, shows some indistinct boundaries, and contains normal-shaped nuclei. Similar to findings in severe iron deficiency

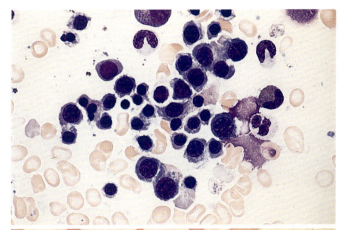

b Bone marrow smear from the same patient. Iron stain. Most erythroblasts contain coarse iron granules (blue) that encircle the nucleus like a ring. At *left* is a "normal" erythroblast with a prominent iron granule. The other erythroblasts are typical ringed sideroblasts

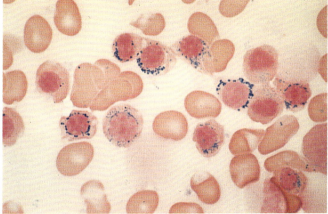

c Five, more mature ringed sideroblasts and one proerythroblast, also with iron granule rings. This finding is unusual, since iron granules normally are not detected in the proerythroblast stage

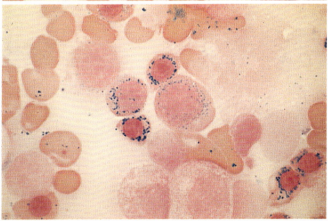

d Ringed sideroblasts with unusually large iron granules

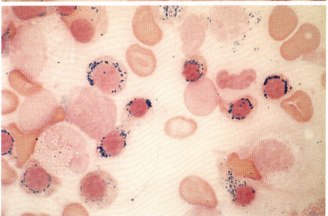

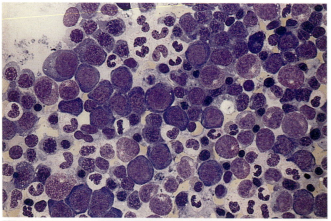

Fig. 60 e – h

e Another case of RARS. Erythropoiesis is mostly very immature and shows some megaloblastic changes

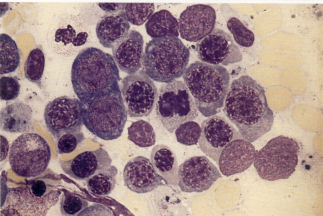

f Higher-power view more clearly demonstrates the megaloblastoid changes

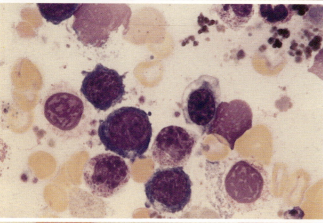

g Erythroblasts with vacuolated cytoplasm in RARS

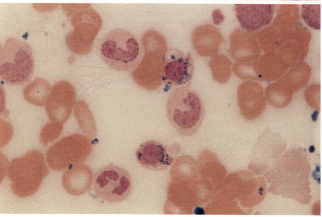

h Iron stain of same bone marrow as in **g** shows a ringed sideroblast (at *top*) with vacuolated cytoplasm

Fig. 61 a, b

a Electron microscopic view of iron deposition in the mitochondria, which encircle the nucleus (ringed sideroblast)

b Higher-power view of the iron-laden mitochondria. (Courtesy Prof. Dr. H. E. Schäfer, Freiburg)

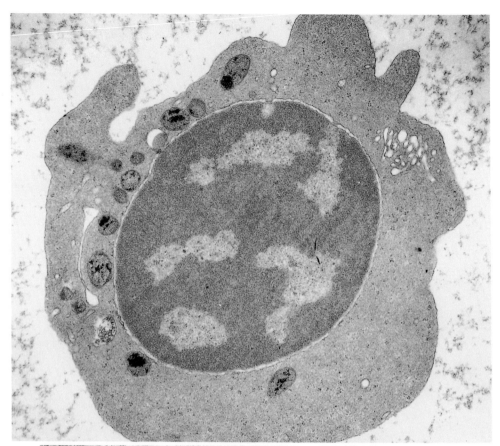

Fig. 61 a

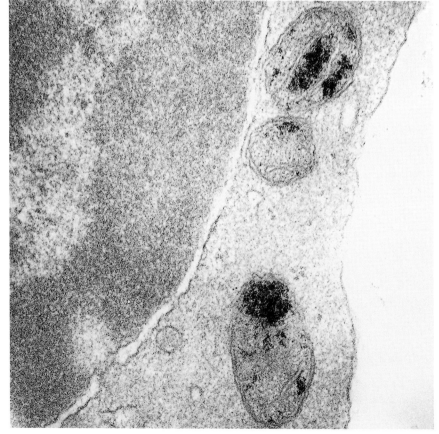

Fig. 61 b

Fig. 62 a – d

a Massive iron deposition, including coarse clumps, in a bone marrow fragment in MDS (partly transfusion-related)

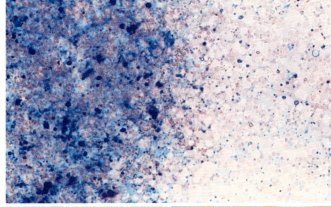

b Pappenheim stain shows hemosiderin deposition in a plasma cell (*left*). At *right* is iron-stained bone marrow from the same patient. Note the coarse granular iron deposition in the cytoplasm of a plasma cell in RARS. Nucleus is at *lower right*.

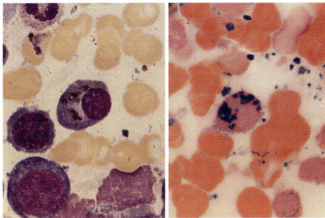

c – f The 5q-minus syndrome

c Two megakaryocytes with round nuclei and different stages of cytoplasmic maturity – a typical finding in this syndrome

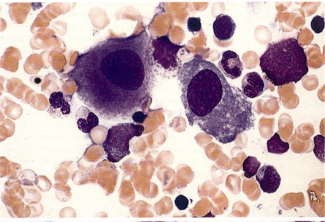

d Three typical megakaryocytes with round nuclei and relatively mature cytoplasm

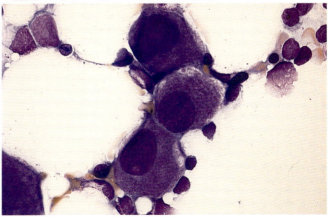

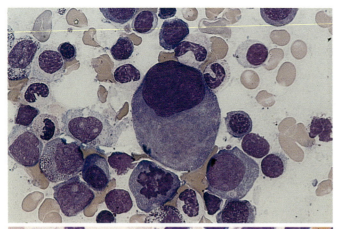

Fig. 62 e–f

e Large megakaryocyte with a nonsegmented nucleus. The cytoplasm is still partly basophilic. Below the megakaryocyte is an erythroblast in mitosis and a myeloblast

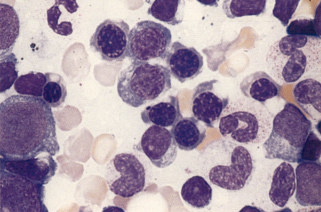

f Erythropoiesis showing subtle megaloblastic features in 5q-minus syndrome

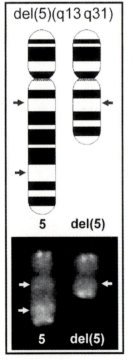

del(5)(q13 q31)

5   del(5)

5   del(5)

Fig. 63. Schematic diagram and partial karyotype of the deletion del(5)(q13;q31), which is found in the 5q-minus syndrome and in the setting of complex aberrant clones in secondary AML. The arrows indicate the breakpoints

Fig. 64 a – h. RAEB and REAB-t

a Bone marrow smear in RAEB. At *left* is a myeloblast, and below it is a lymphocyte. Most granulocytes in the myelocytic stage have no detectable granules. Note the absence of monocytes in the field!

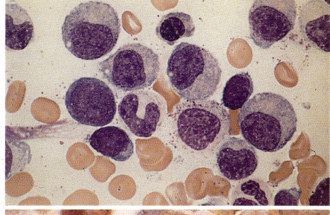

b Bone marrow from the same patient. Nonspecific esterase reaction shows abnormally high enzyme activity in granulopoietic cells as further evidence of dysplasia. No monocytes!

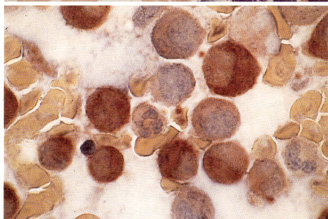

c Cluster of myeloblasts next to several maturing granulopoietic cells in RAEB-t

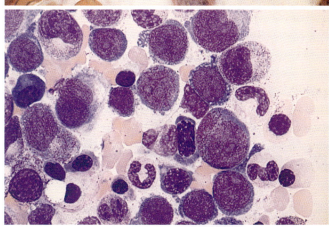

d Transition from RAEB-t to AML. The proportion of blasts is just below 30 %. Cluster of myeloblasts and one normal-appearing eosinophilic myelocyte

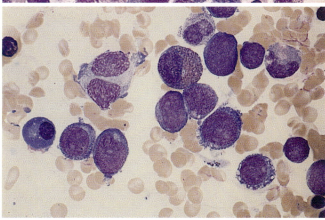

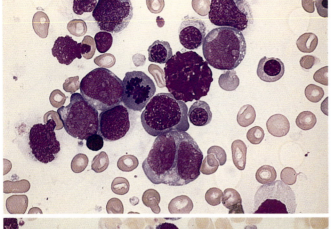

Fig. 64 e–h

e Myeloblasts and atypical erythroblasts in RAEB-t

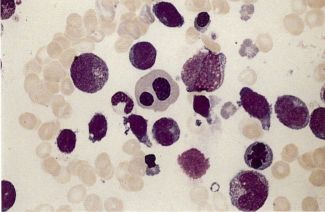

f Blasts and atypical binucleated erythroblast in the bone marrow in RAEB-t

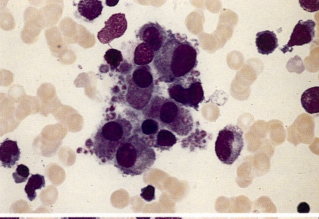

g Cluster of micro(mega)karyocytes in bone marrow from the same patient

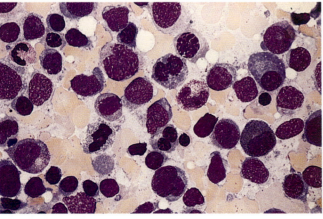

h Dysplastic erythropoiesis and blast increase in RAEB-t

Fig. 65 a – h. Chronic myelomonocytic leukemia (CMML)

a Blood smear shows a substantial increase in monocytes. To the *right of center* is an immature myelocyte

b Smear from the same patient. Nonspecific esterase. Most of the monocytes are strongly positive (brown stain)

c Blood smear. At *left* is a large promonocyte

d Bone marrow smear shows increased monocytes and some mild dysplastic changes in neutrophilic granulocytopoiesis

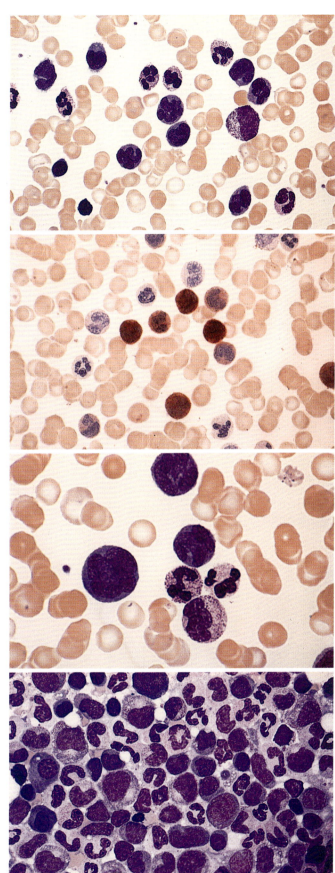

Fig. 65 e–h

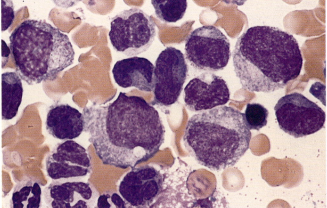

e Bone marrow from the patient in **d**. Nonspecific esterase reaction clearly differentiates the monocytes (often difficult with Pappenheim stain)

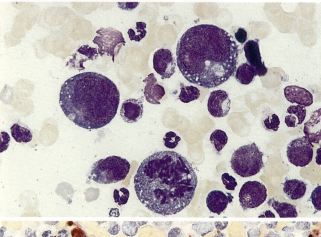

f Monocytes and dysplastic precursors of granulocytopoiesis in a bone marrow smear; granules are extremely sparse

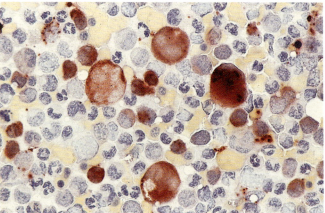

g Exceptionally large, strongly polyploid monoblasts in the blast phase of CMML. At *bottom* is a mitosis

h Bone marrow from the same patient. Nonspecific esterase reaction. The very large blasts and promonocytes are as strongly positive as the normal-sized monocytes

Fig. 66 a–h. Myelodysplasias with pseudo-Pelger changes

a Bone marrow smear. Nuclei of neutrophilic granulocytopoiesis show a coarse, clumped, dissociated chromatin pattern

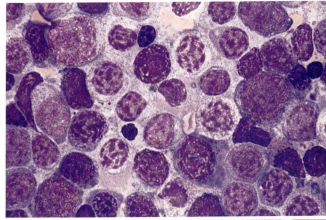

b Bone marrow from the same patient shows dysplastic megakaryocytes and erythroblasts. The round granulopoietic cells correspond to pseudo-Pelger forms of the homozygotic type

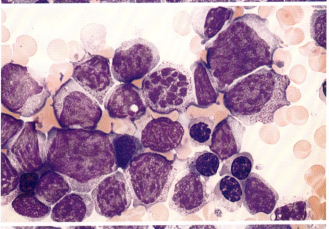

c Unusually strong chromatin fragmentation (*center*). Note the granules in the cytoplasm

d Homozygotic type of pseudo-Pelger forms in a different patient

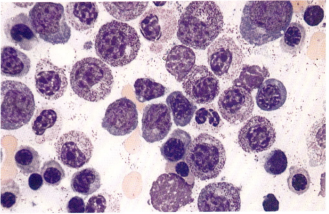

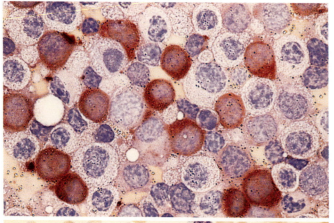

Fig. 66 e–h

e Bone marrow from the patient in **d**. Nonspecific esterase reaction shows a large proportion of strongly positive monocytes, most with round nuclei. The positive cells correspond to the round-nuclear forms in **d** with grayish-blue cytoplasm

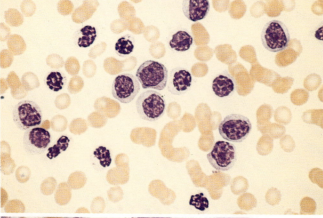

f Blood smear from a different patient shows abundant pseudo-Pelger forms of the homozygotic type

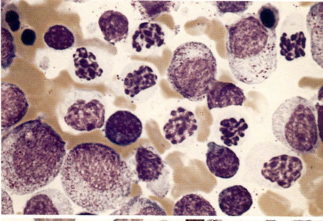

g Bone marrow from the patient in **f**. Obvious chromatin clumping is limited to the more mature forms

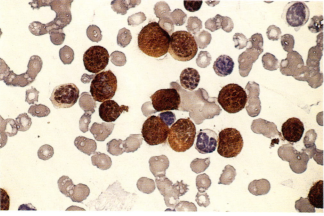

h Peroxidase reaction. Most of the homozygotic-type pseudo-Pelger forms are strongly peroxidase-positive

Fig. 66 i Schematic diagram and partial karyotype of the isochromosome 17q, which leads to loss of the short arm of chromosome 17 (17p) and changes in p53. The 17p structural changes are found in MDS and AML with the pseudo-Pelger anomaly, and isochromosome 17 occurs as a secondary aberration in Philadelphia-positive CML

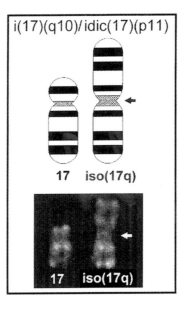

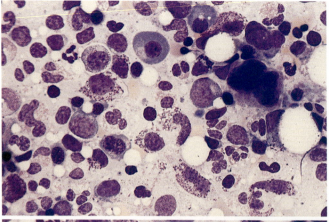

Fig. 67 a–d

a Bone marrow from a patient with atypical MDS shows a marked increase in tissue mast cells, some containing sparse granules

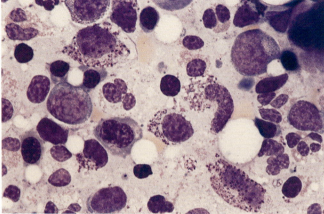

b Bone marrow from the same patient. Higher-power view of the atypical tissue mast cells

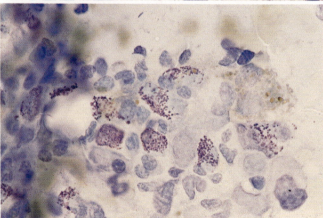

c Bone marrow from the same patient. Toluidine blue stain shows typical meta-chromasia of the tissue mast cell granules

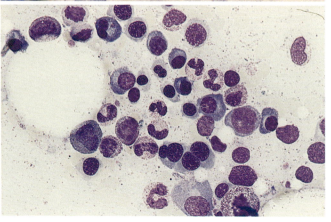

d Bone marrow in HIV infection. At the *bottom* of the field is a dysplastic erythroblast with four nuclei

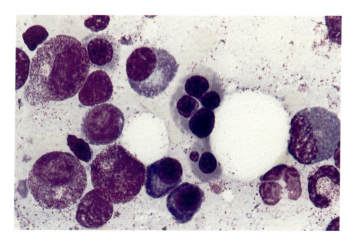

Fig. 67 e Higher-power view of dysplastic erythroblasts in the same patient. Panels **d** and **e** illustrate that HIV may present with significant dysplastic changes that are morphologically indistinguishable from MDS

Acute Leukemias

Acute leukemias are clonal diseases of hematopoietic precursors with molecular genetic abnormalities. All hematopoietic cell lines may be affected. Proliferation of the leukemic cell clone replaces normal hematopoiesis in varying degrees. In acute myeloid leukemia (AML), it is most common for granulocytopoiesis and monocytopoiesis to be affected. Erythropoiesis is less frequently affected, and megakaryopoiesis rarely so. The distribution of the subtypes varies according to age. Acute lymphocytic leukemia (ALL) occurs predominantly in children, while AML has its peak in adults. The involvement of several myeloid cell lines is relatively common, but the simultaneous involvement of myeloid and lymphoid cell lines is very rare (hybrid and bilinear acute leukemias). It is generally agreed that the percentage of blasts in the bone marrow must be approximately 30 % to justify a diagnosis of acute leukemia. The range of 20 % to 30 % blasts is considered borderline. Examination of the peripheral blood is not essential for diagnosis but can provide important additional information. The diagnosis and classification (subtype assignment) always rely on the bone marrow. The most widely accepted system at present for the classification of AML is based on the criteria of the French-American-British (FAB) Cooperative Group (**Table 13**). Because the quantity and quality of the blasts is of central importance in this classification, they should be defined as accurately as possible. The leukemic blasts include myeloblasts, monoblasts, and megakaryoblasts. The cells of erythropoiesis are generally counted separately, although in acute erythroleukemia (M6 subtype) the erythroblasts account for a preponderance of the leuke-

Table 13. FAB classification of akute myeloid leukemia (AML) (characteristic findings are in bold)

FAB type	Granulocytopoiesis [%]	Monocytopoiesis [%]	Erythropoiesis [%]	Immune markers
M 0	< 10 POX < 3	< 20	< 50	**Lymphoid neg. Myeloid pos.**
M 1	< 10 **POX > 3**	< 20	< 50	
M 2	**> 10**	< 20	<50	
M 3	**Hypergranular, Auer rods**	< 20	< 50	HLA-DR neg.
M 3v	**Microgranular, monocytoid nuclei**	< 20	< 50	HLA-DR neg.
M 4	> 20	**> 20**	< 50	
M 4Eo	> 20 **Abnormal Eo**	**> 20**	< 50	
M 5a	< 20	**>80, immature**	< 50	
M 5b	< 20	**>80, mature**	< 50	
M 6	>30% of NEC are blasts; variable	Variable	**> 50**	
M 7	> 30 megakaryoblasts	Variable	< 50	**CD 41 / CD 61 pos.**

☐ characteristic results

mic cells. Blasts are traditionally defined as immature cells that do not show signs of differentiation. But since French hematologists have always accepted blasts with granules, and cells having the nuclear and cytoplasmic features of classic blasts but containing granules are known to occur in leukemias, a distinction is now drawn between type I blasts, which are devoid of granules, and type II blasts, which contain scattered granules or Auer rods and do not show perinuclear pallor (**Fig. 68**). Occasional reference is made to "type III blasts," but we consider this a needless distinction except for the abnormal cells of promyelocytic leukemia (M3), which may be heavily granular but are still classified as blasts even though they do not strictly meet the criteria. Besides bone marrow and blood smears, histologic sections are required in cases where aspiration yields insufficient material. The standard stains (Pappenheim, Giemsa) are useful for primary evaluation, but a more accurate classification of the cells requires cytochemical analysis and immunophenotyping (flow cytometry and/or immunochemistry). In order to make a prognosis or define biological entities (**Table 14**), it is further necessary to perform cytogenetic and molecular genetic studies, fluorescence in situ hybridization (FISH), and combine FISH technology with immunocytochemistry.

As mentioned, the classification of AML essentially follows the recommendations of the FAB.

However, the experience of recent years in cooperative and prospective studies using modern methods supports the notion of a future-oriented, prognostic classification that takes into account the results of therapies and patient follow-ups. This will allow for a more individually tailored approach. At present this biological classification, or subdivision into biological entities, does not cover all the subtypes of AML or ALL, but in the future these gaps will be filled through the application of more sensitive methods.

Acute lymphocytic leukemias (ALL) are currently classified according to immunologic criteria (**Table 15**). The classification into three subtypes (L1–L3) originally proposed by the FAB no longer has clinical importance today except for the L3 subtype, which is virtually identical to the immunologic B4 subtype (mature B-ALL). Morphology and cytochemistry from the basis of diagnosis in ALL. The immunologic classification of ALL is based on two principal groups – the B-cell line and T-cell line with their subtypes. Cytogenetic and/or molecular genetic studies can also be used to define prognostic entities. These include c-ALL with t(9;22) and pre-B-cell ALL with t(4;11), which has a characteristic immunophenotype.

Besides morphologic analysis, the peroxidase technique is the most important basic method because lymphoblasts are always peroxidase-negative, regardless of their immunophenotype.

Table 14. Biological entities in acute myeloid leukemia

Morphology	FAB classification	Cytogenetics	Molecular genetics	Frequency (%)
Promyelocytic leukemia Hypergranular Microgranular	M3 } M3v ʃ	t(15;17) t(11;17)	PML/RARα PLZF/RARα	~5
Myeloblastic leukemia	M1/M2	t(8;21)	AML1/ETO	~10
Myelomonocytic leukemia with abnormal Eo	M4Eo	inv(16) t(16;16)	MYH11/CBFβ	~5
Myelomonocytic/monocytic-monoblastic leukemia	M4/5	t(9;11)	AF9/MLL	>5; more frequent in children
Myeloblastic leukemia etc., often with increased basophils	M1/2 MDS	t(6;9)	DEK/CAN	<1
Myelomonocytic leukemia with ery phagocytosis	M4/5 (5 ep)	t(8;16)	PLAT?	<0,1
Myeloblastic leukemia with dysmegakaryo-cytopoiesis	M1 etc.	3q21 and/or 3q26	e.g., EVI 1/ EAP/MDS1	~1
AML and MDS with pseudo-Pelger-Huet anomalies	AML u. MDS	17p with complex aberration	p53 alterations	3–5
Megakaryoblastic leukemia	M7	t(1;22)	?	~1 (small children)

Table 15. Immunologic classification of acute lymphoblastic leukemias (ALL) [after Bene, MC et al (1995) Proposals for the immunological classification of acute leukemias. European Group for the Immunological Characterization of Leukemias (EGIL). Leukemia. 1995 Oct;9(10):1783–1786]

ALL	Classification
1) B lineage (CD19 +) and/or CD 79a+ and/or CD22+	
a) B1 (pro-B) (no other differentiation antigens)	
b) B2 (common)	(CD10+)
c) B3 (pre-B)	Cytoplasmic IgM+
d) B4 (mature B)	Cytoplasmic surface kappa or lambda +
2) T lineage (cytoplasmic/membrane CD3+)	
a) T1 (pre-T)	CD7+
b) T2 (pre-T)	CD2+ and/or CD5+ and/or CD8+
c) T3 (cortical T)	CD1a+
d) T4 (mature T)	Membrane CD3+, CD1a-
T-α/β and T-γ/δ	anti-TCR α/β+, anti-TCR γ/δ+

All with expression of one or two myeloid markers (My + ALL)

CSF Involvement in Acute Leukemias and Malignant Non-Hodgkin Lymphomas

Involvement of the cerebrospinal fluid (CSF) is usually associated with clinical symptoms. The question of whether CSF involvement is present has major implications for further treatment, inasmuch as curative therapy in children with acute lymphoid leukemias has been possible only since the introduction of prophylacis against meningeal involvement. In this area as in others, the full arsenal of available analytic methods has been brought the bear. Decision-making can be particularly difficult in patients with mild CSF involvement, because cells in the CSF are subject to substantial changes. It is important, therefore, always to cerrelate the CSF findings with the findings in the blood or bone marrow (see Fig. 127).

Fig. 68 a – d. Acute myeloid leukemia (AML). Definition of blasts

a Two type I blasts. The cytoplasm is devoid of granules

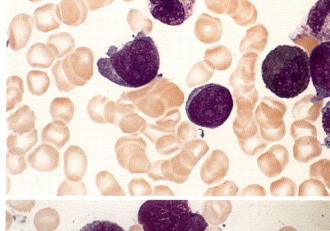

b Cytoplasmic granules distinguish this type II blast from type I. At *left* is a granulocyte in mitosis, above it is a promyelocyte

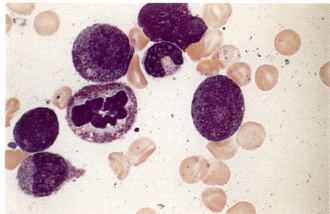

c At *left* are two type I blasts, at *right* is one type II blast with distinct granules. Below is a promyelocyte with very coarse primary granules. Between blasts I and II is an eosinophil

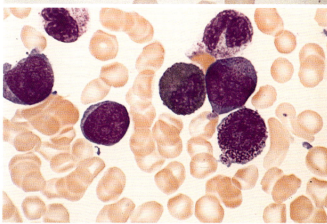

d At *left* is a type I blast. At *center* is an atypical promyelocyte with an eccentric nucleus and numerous granules occupying an area where a clear Golgi zone would be expected to occur

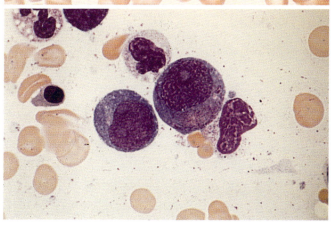

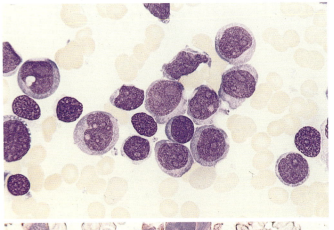

Fig. 69 a – h. AML, M0 subtype

a Morphologically undifferentiated blasts with distinct nucleoli are peroxidase-negative and do not show the esterase reaction typical of monocytes

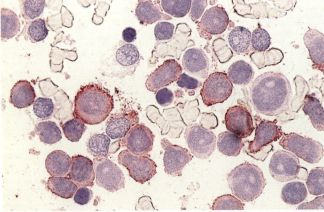

b Bone marrow smear from the same patient. Immunocytochemical detection of CD13. A large proportion of the blasts are positive (red). APAAP technique

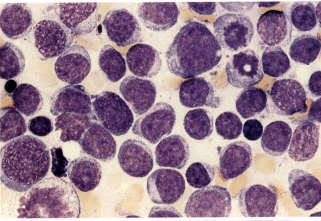

c Bone marrow smear from a different patient with the M0 subtype of AML. The blasts are difficult to distinguish morphologically from ALL

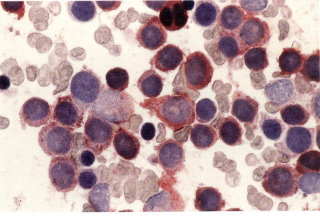

d Smear from patient in **c**. Demonstration of CD13

Fig. 69 e–h

e Same patient as in **c** and **d**. Esterase reaction shows a patchy positive reaction that is not sufficiently intense for monoblasts

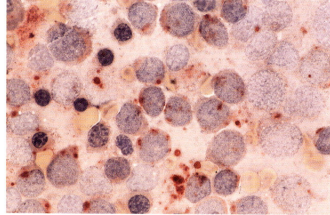

f Morphologically undifferentiated blasts in a smear from a different patient

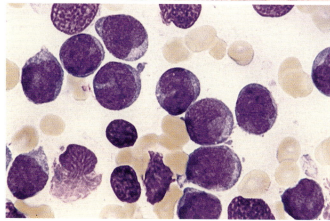

g Peroxidase reaction in the same patient. Blasts are negative, and among them is a positive eosinophil

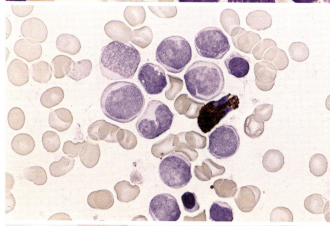

h Same patient as in **f** and **g**. Patchy esterase reaction is not sufficiently intense for monoblasts

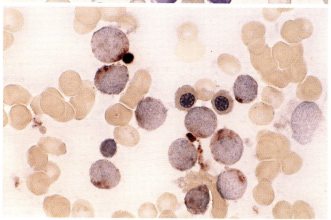

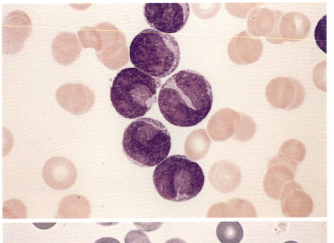

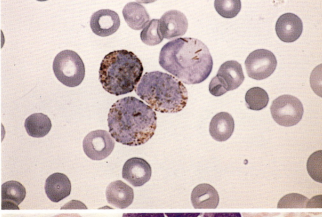

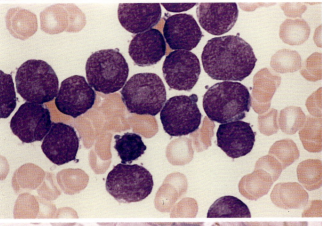

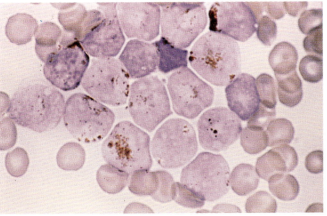

Fig. 70 a – h. AML, M1 subtype

a The pale blue areas in the nuclear indentation are caused by overlying cytoplasm (three lower blasts at *left of center*). This is a typical finding in AML-M1 and should not be confused with nucleoli

b Smear from the same patient. Peroxidase reaction. Positive Auer rods are visible in the nuclear indentation of the uppermost cell

c Pseudonucleoli in blasts from a different patient

d Same patient as in **c**. Positive peroxidase reaction

Fig. 70 e – h

e Small blasts appear morphologically undifferentiated

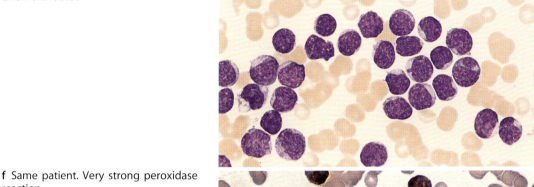

f Same patient. Very strong peroxidase reaction

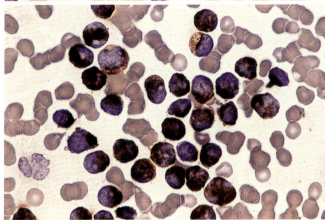

g Blasts appear undifferentiated except for purple inclusion

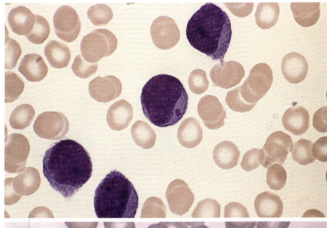

h Same patient. Peroxidase reaction. Numerous Auer rods, which often are very small (Phi bodies)

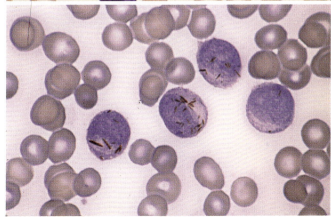

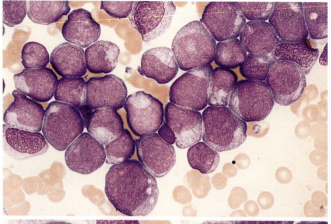

Fig. 71 a – h. AML, M1 and M2 subtypes

a Most of these blasts show no signs of differentiation, although the cytoplasm in some contains long, thin Auer rods

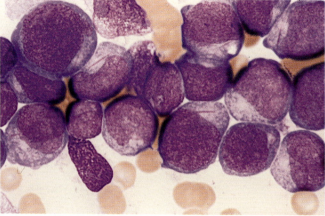

b High-power view of the same specimen. Long, thin Auer rods appear in the cytoplasm at *upper left* and *right* and *lower right*

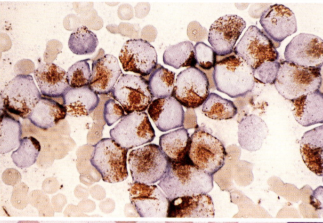

c Peroxidase reaction in the same patient shows an accentuated perinuclear reaction with conspicuous Auer rods. The (8;21) translocation was detected in this patient

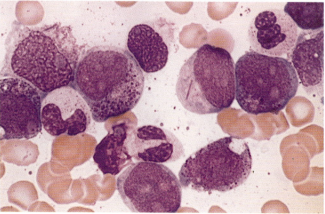

d Bone marrow from a different patient shows a long, thin Auer rod and pronounced maturation (more than 10 %). Chromosome findings were normal

Fig. 71 e–h

e Blood smear in AML. Undifferentiated blasts with scant cytoplasm

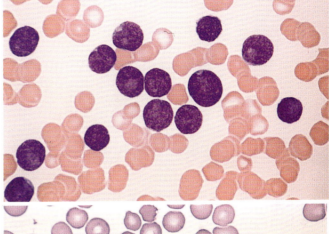

f Peroxidase reaction in the same patient. All blasts in the field are strongly positive

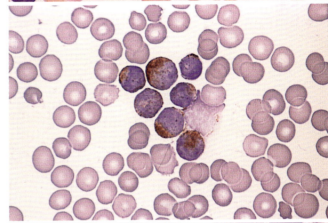

g Bone marrow from the same patient shows pronounced maturation (more than 10 %)

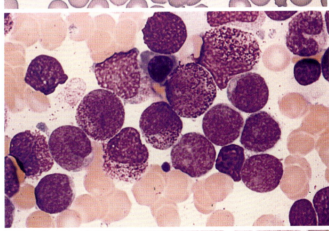

h Very strong peroxidase reaction in the same patient. This case demonstrates that bone marrow examination is necessary for an accurate classification

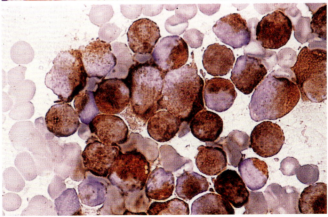

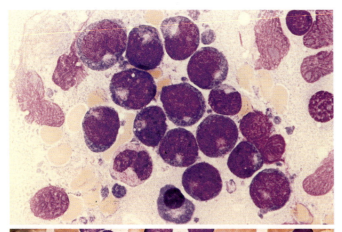

Fig. 72 a – g. AML, variants of M2 subtype

a Blasts with markedly basophilic cytoplasm and characteristic perinuclear pallor (Golgi zone). Cell at *lower left* shows atypical maturation. The FAB classifies this morphologic variant as M2. The (8;21) translocation is also present

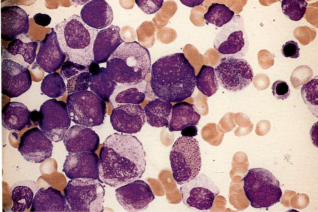

b Dysplastic maturation in M2. Several eosinophils are visible

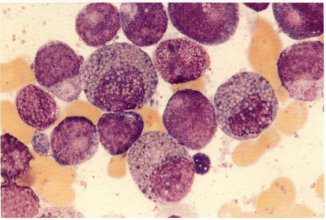

c M2 with eosinophilia. Three eosinophilic precursors contain scattered blue to violet immature granules and pale maturing granules. They differ from the eosinophils in inv(16)

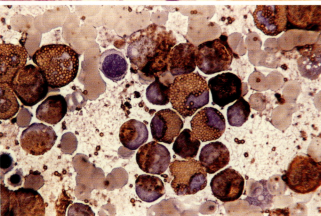

d Peroxidase reaction in the same patient. The eosinophils are distinguished by their characteristic granules. The blasts are also positive

Fig. 72 e–g

e CE reaction. Enzyme activity (*red*) is detected only in neutrophils. All the eosinophils are negative, in contrast to inv(16)

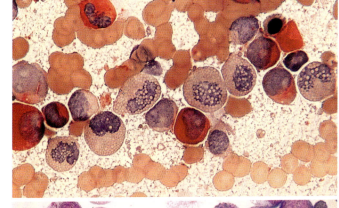

f Different case of M2 with eosinophilia. To the *right of center* is a blast with Auer rods. The t(8;21) is also found in this morphologic variant

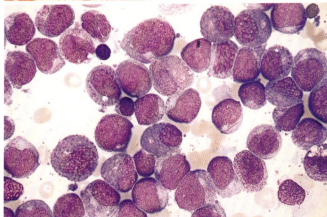

g M2 with eosinophilia. Peroxidase reaction. Auer rods appear above the nucleus of the cell at *center* (eosinophil?)

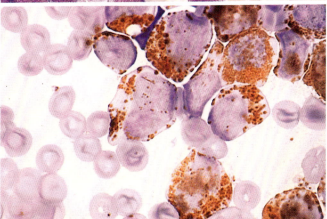

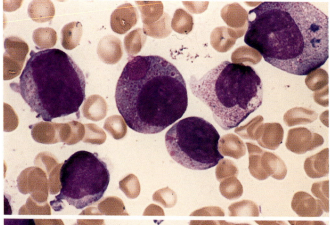

Fig. 73 a–h. Cytoplasmic inclusions in AML

a Secondary AML following chemotherapy for NHL with t(10;11). Unusually large reddish inclusions (pseudo-Chediak anomaly)

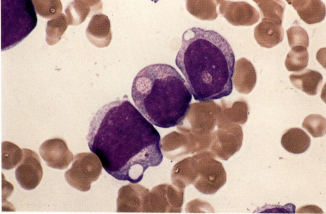

b Same patient. Large vacuoles with granular contents

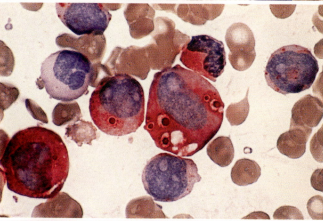

c CE reaction. At *center* are vacuoles with CE-positive inclusions in the cytoplasm

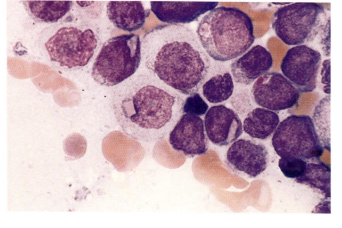

d Pink to red, round or angular inclusions in a different patient

Fig. 73 e–h

e Same patient as in **d**. At *center* is a pale, oblong inclusion over a binucleated cell

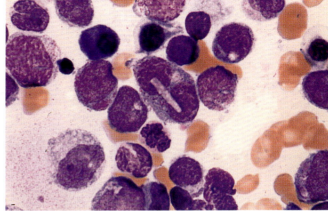

f Rounded and rod-shaped inclusions in the same patient. At *bottom* is an extracellular rod-shaped inclusion

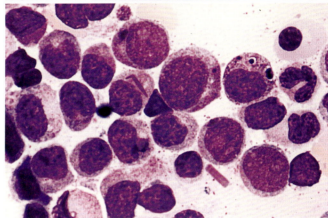

g PAS reaction. Positive rod-shaped inclusion at *center*, positive rounded inclusion above it

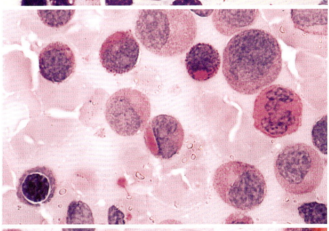

h CE reaction. Rod-shaped inclusion at *center* are strongly positive, like Auer rods. Cytogenetic analysis in this patient showed only a hyperdiploid clone without specific aberrations
(Prof. Fonatsch, then in Lübeck)

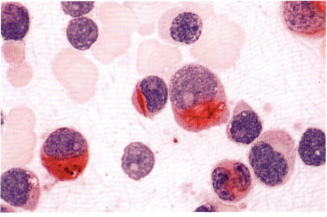

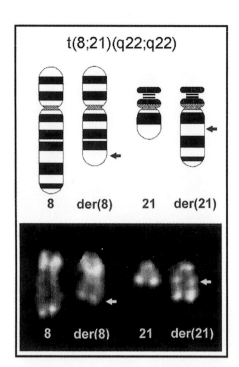

Fig. 74. Schematic diagram and partial karyotype of the translocation t(8;21)(q22;q22), found predominantly in the M2 subtype of AML

Fig. 75 a–h. AML, M2 subtype, characterized by increased numbers of tissue mast cells or basophilic granulocytes

a Bone marrow in M2 with t(8;21). The cytoplasm of two blasts (*left of center* and *upper right*) contains long, thin Auer rods

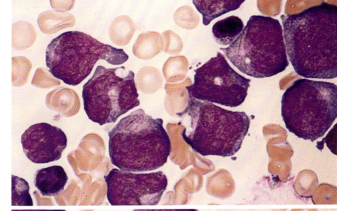

b Three tissue mast cells in the same patient. At *right* is a younger form with relatively few granules

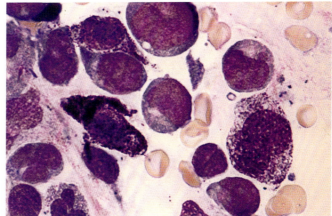

c Cytopenic bone marrow from the same patient following chemotherapy. The blasts have disappeared, and the marrow fragment contains abundant tissue mast cells

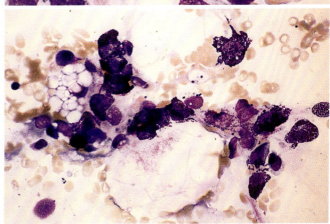

d Higher-power view of a group of tissue mast cells following chemotherapy. Increased tissue mast cells are found in a small percentage of patients with AML-M2 and t(8;21)

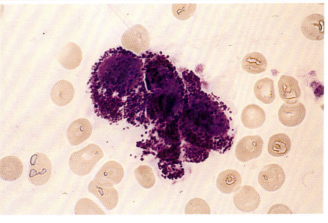

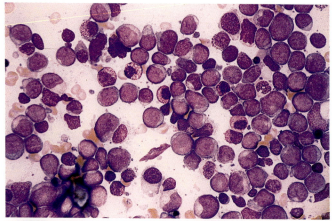

Fig. 75 e–h

e AML-M2 with t(6;9). Blasts and atypical-appearing basophilic granulocytes

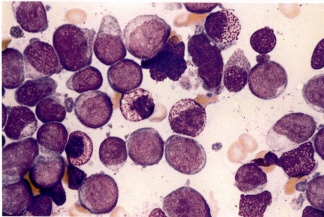

f High-power view in the same patient. The atypical basophils with predominantly fine granules are metachromatic after staining with toluidine blue

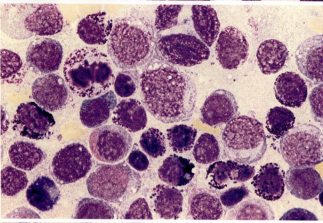

g Very strong increase of basophils in a different patient. At *upper left* is a basophil in mitosis. A (6;9) translocation could not be demonstrated

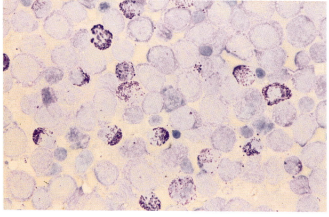

h Toluidine blue stain in same patient shows metachromatic reaction of basophilic granulocytes

Fig. 75 i Schematic diagram and partial karyotype of the t(3;12)(q26;p13), which is found in AML and MDS. Changes in the short arm of chromosome 12 (12p), like t(6;9), may be associated with increased basophilic granulocytes in the bone marrow. A similar increase is occasionally found in the M4 subtype in the absence of detectable anomalies

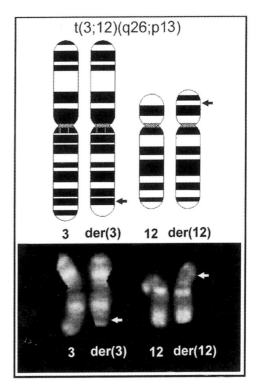

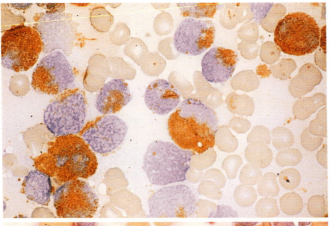

Fig. 76 a–g. AML, M2 subtype, with "Golgi esterase." In some cases of M2 with t(8;21), circumscribed nonspecific esterase activity in the perinuclear zone may cause the cells to be mistaken for monocytes. All the criteria of AML-M2 are present, however, including a marked peroxidase reaction.

a M2 with t(8;21). Peroxidase reaction. The blasts are peroxidase-positive, and a positive Auer rod is visible at *center* above the nucleus

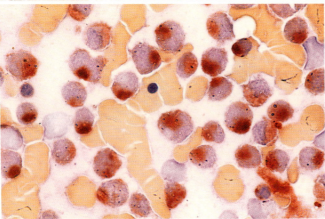

b Nonspecific esterase in the same patient. Strong "Golgi esterase"

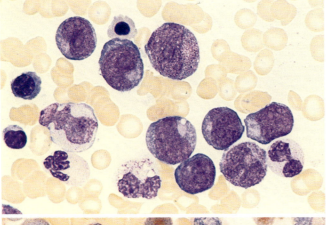

c Different case of M2. Pappenheim stain

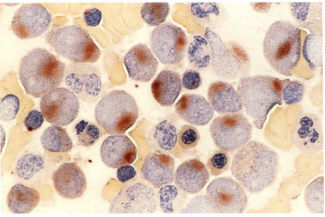

d Same as **c**. Nonspecific esterase. Typical "Golgi esterase"

Fig. 76 e – g

e Different case of M2 with t(8;21). Peroxidase reaction. At *top center* is a needle-shaped Auer rod above the nucleus

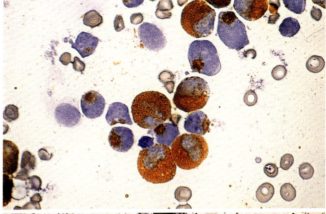

f Sudan black B reaction in the same case is identical to peroxidase

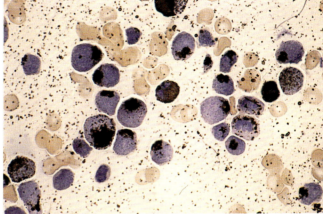

g Same as **e**. Typical "Golgi esterase"

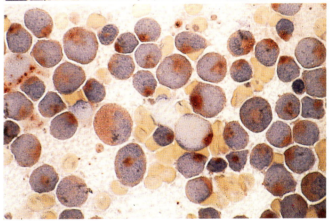

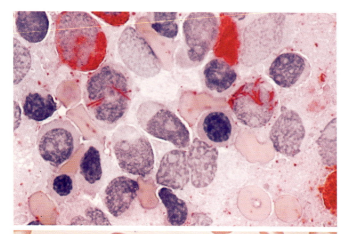

Fig. 77 a–h. Other atypias in AML

a CE reaction. Abundant Auer rods in two blasts in the M2 subtype of AML. This should not be confused with AML-M3

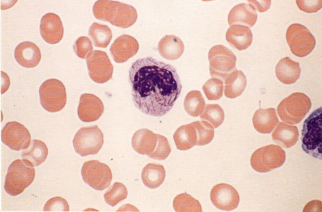

b Numerous Auer rods in a rod cell from the peripheral blood of a patient with AML-M4

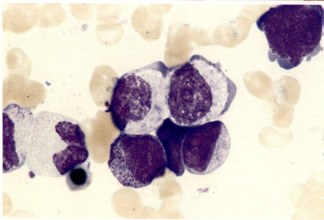

c Dysplastic cytoplasmic maturation with a peripheral basophilic zone in the two cells at *top*. AML-M2

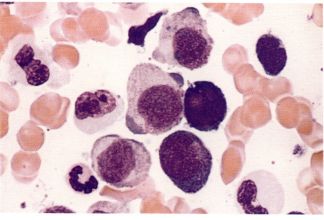

d Basophilic poles of cytoplasm at *top* and *center*, mature granulocytes devoid of granules. AML-M2

Fig. 77 e–h

e–g Polyploid giant forms of granulo-cytopoiesis, reaching the size of mega-karyocytes. **e** At *upper left* is a normal-sized atypical promyelocyte next to a giant form

f Normal-sized blast to the left of a giant promyelocyte

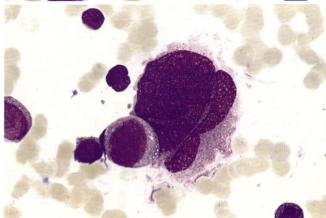

g Peroxidase reaction demonstrates three positive giant forms and, at *top*, three negative blasts

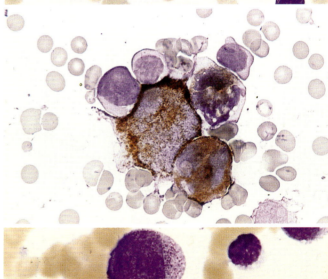

h Giant segmented form with central vacuolation of cytoplasm

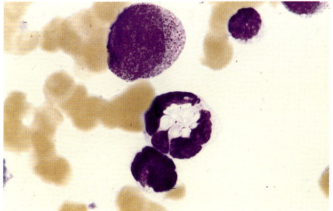

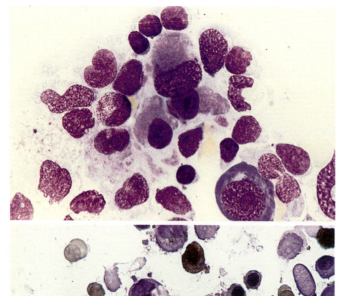

Fig. 78 a–c. Bone marrow smears in AML M1 and inv(3)(q21;q26) illustrate the morphologic changes that are associated with inversion or translocation anomalies of the long arm of chromosome 3

a At *center* is a cluster of micro(mega)-karyocytes

b Peroxidase reaction in the same patient. At *top* is a positive cell. At *center* and *below* is a group of negative microkaryocytes

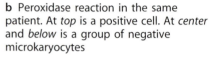

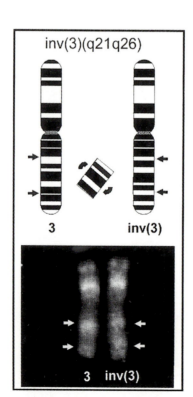

c Schematic diagram and partial karyotype of the inversion inv(3)(q21;q26), which is observed in AML with megakaryocytic abnormalities

Fig. 79 a – h. AML, M3 subtype

a Bone marrow smear with heavily granulated atypical promyelocytes and cells whose cytoplasm is packed full of Auer rods (faggots)

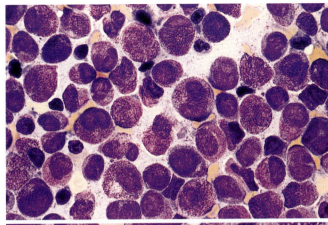

b Same patient. High-power view of the heavily granulated cells and cells with numerous Auer rods. The granules and Auer rods may coexist, or Auer rods may occur without other granules

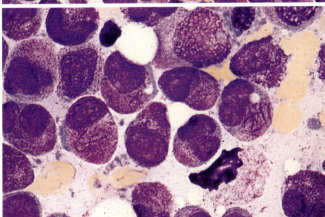

c At *left of center* is a cell with Auer rods and pale, agranular cytoplasm

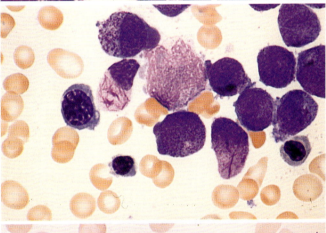

d Three atypical promyelocytes with Auer rods of various shapes

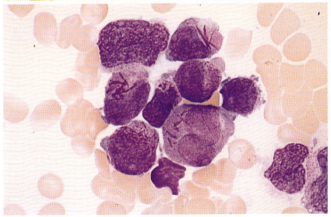

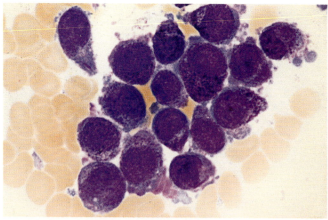

Fig. 79 e–h

e "Hyperbasophilic" variant with strongly basophilic ground substance and coarse granules

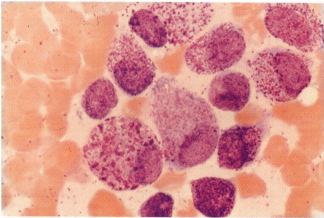

f Atypical promyelocytes with dispersed violet granules of exceptional size (like basophilic promyelocytes)

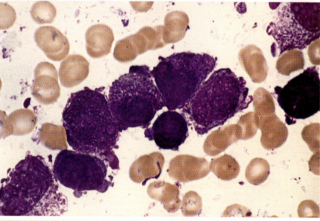

g Very dark violet granules in a different case

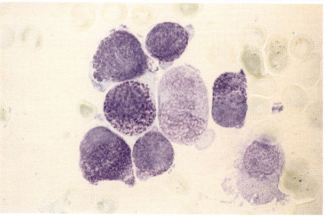

h Toluidine blue stain in the same patient shows a metachromatic reaction in some of the abnormal granules. Panels **g** and **h** illustrate the basophilic variant of M3

Fig. 80 a–d. AML, M3 V subtype

a Typical preponderance of bilobed nuclei with an apparently agranular cytoplasm, but a more extensive search of the bone marrow reveals heavily granulated cells or cells with Auer rods

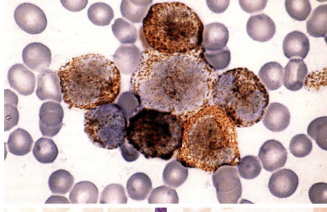

b Peroxidase reaction in the same patient demonstrates a marked granular reaction in all cells

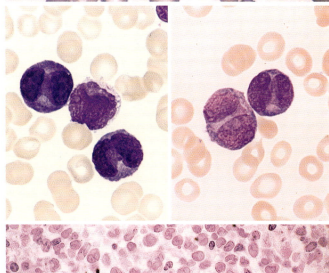

c Peripheral blood in AML-M3 V with typical bilobed or constricted nuclei and basophilic-appearing cytoplasm, found on electron microscopy to contain minute granules

d Histologic section in M3 V. HE stain. The monocytoid, frequently bilobed shape of the nuclei may cause confusion with monocytic leukemia. In all the cases shown in Figs. 79–84, the diagnosis has been established cytogenetically by detecting the t(15;17) translocation or by the molecular genetic demonstration of PML/RARA

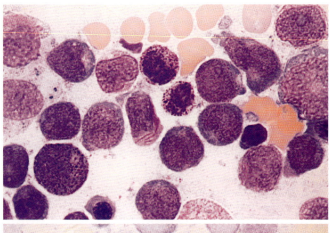

Fig. 81 a–d. AML, M3 V subtype with increase of Gasophilie granulocytes

a At *center* is an abnormal promyelocyte with Auer rods. Above it and to the right are two basophilic granulocytes

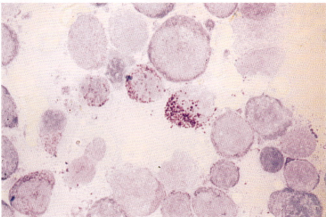

b Toluidine blue stain in the same case shows three basophilic granulocytes located along a diagonal at *center*

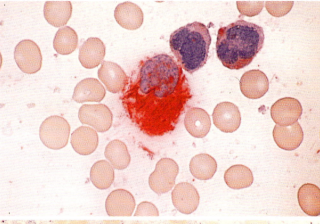

c CE reaction in the same patient. At *center* is a faggot cell with numerous positive Auer rods. Above it are two blasts with monocytoid nuclei showing a faint diffuse reaction

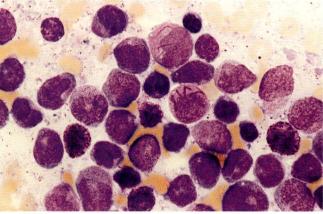

d Markedly increased basophilic granulocytes in a different case of M3 V. Two cells with Auer rods at *top* and *center*. Scattered basophilic granulocytes, some containing indistinct granules

Fig. 82 a – e. Cytochemical findings in M3

a Intense peroxidase reaction. It is common to find superimposition of the Auer rods

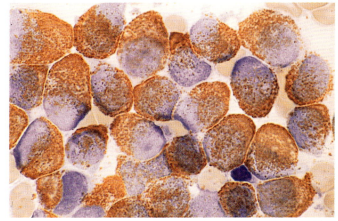

b CE reaction gives particularly clear visualization of the Auer rods

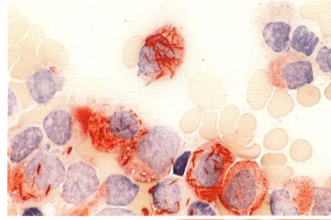

c Intensely CE-positive Auer rods and "Auer bodies."

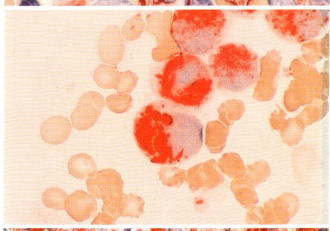

d Histologic section in untreated M3. CE reaction again shows coarse positive granules and scattered Auer rods. (Courtesy of Prof. R. Parwaresch, Kiel)

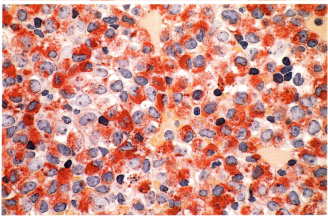

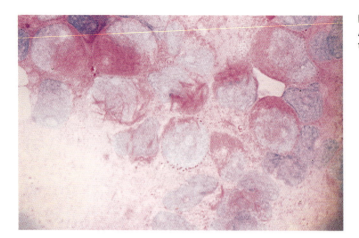

Fig. 82 e PAS reaction. Some positive Auer rods are found in M3, visible here in the middle cell and to the left

Fig. 83 a–g. AML, M3 subtype, response to treatment with all-trans retinoic acid (ATRA)

a Bone marrow smear in promyelocytic leukemia shows relatively mild atypias prior to therapy

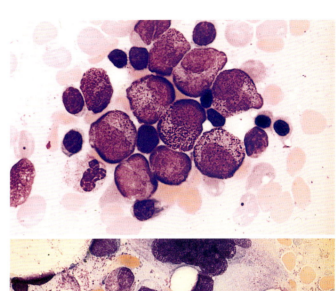

b Smear from same patient after 6 weeks' therapy shows definite maturation and "normalization" of the cells. The promyelocytes and myelocytes appear predominantly normal, and a few correspond to later maturation stages

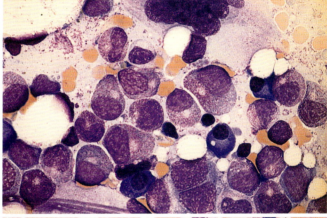

c After a total of 8 weeks' therapy, conspicuous bone marrow abnormalities have disappeared, and only subtle changes are noted in several mature forms

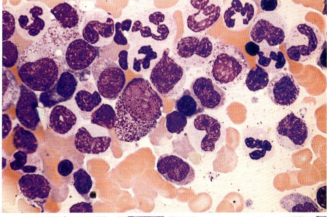

d Different case prior to therapy

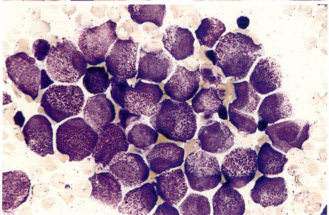

Fig. 83 e–g

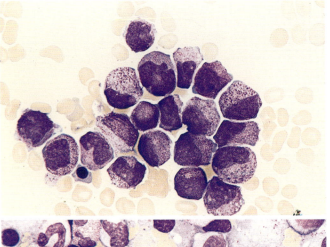

e Case in **d** after 4 week's therapy. Note that the granules generally are somewhat finer and the nuclei appear slightly more mature

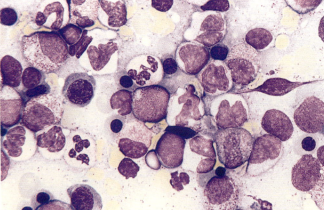

f After another 3 week's therapy, there is marked progression of maturation with segmented granulocytes

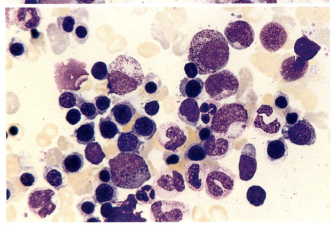

g After a total of 8 weeks' therapy the marrow appears morphologically normal, signifying a complete remission

Fig. 84 a – g. Other changes in response to ATRA therapy

a Another case of M3 prior to therapy. At *center* is a cell with Auer rods. At *left* is a basophilic granulocyte, and two others appear at *upper right* and *lower left*

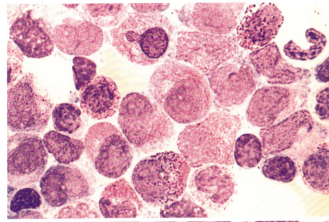

b After 4 week's therapy, definite signs of maturation are already seen. At *center* is a cell containing remnants of Auer rods

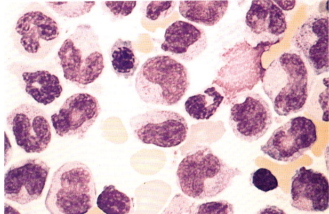

c Morphologic findings are normal after a total of 6 weeks' therapy. Extensive erythropoiesis and mature granulocytes are observed

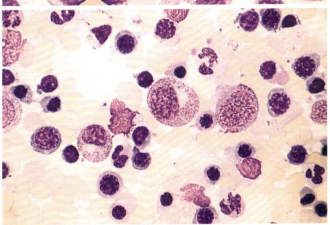

d Different case of M3 after just 3 weeks' treatment with ATRA. Segmented forms are already present, some still containing Auer rods (at *bottom* and *lower right*)

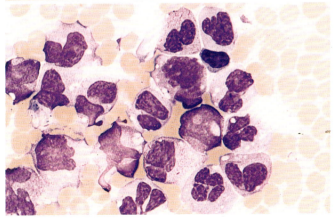

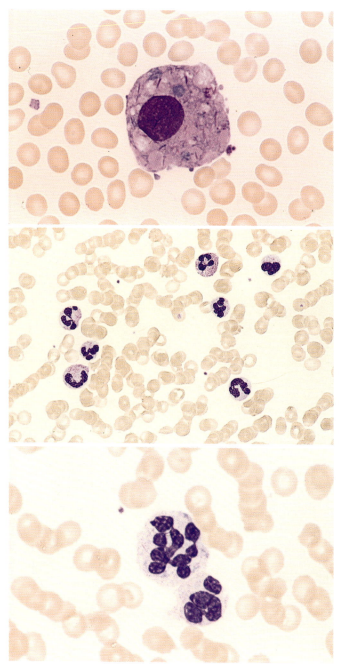

Fig. 84 e–g

e Same case as **d** shows macrophage with phagocytized cellular material, including Auer rods

f Blood smear in complete remission following ATRA therapy. The neutrophilic granulocytes appear essentially normal

g Hypersegmented neutrophil in the same patient

Fig. 85 a, b. Electron microscopic view of atypical promyelocytes in the M3 and M3 V subtypes of promyelocytic leukemia (Courtesy Prof. Dr. H. K. Müller-Hermelink, Würzburg)

a Atypical promyelocyte in M3. Note the large, irregular primary granules

b M3 V subtype. At *center* is a typical bilobed nucleus with a thin chromatin strand linking the two nuclear segments. At *right* is a large nucleolus. The cytoplasm contains small, sparse granules

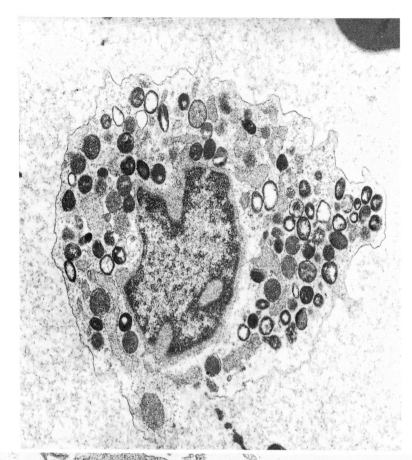

Fig. 85 a

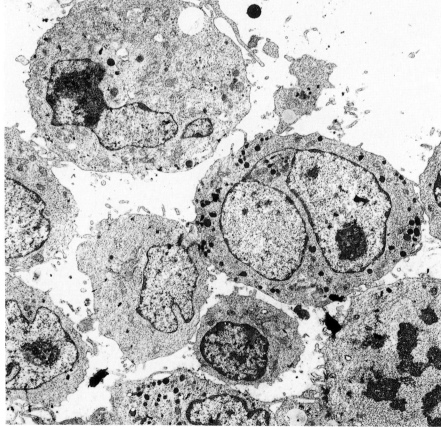

Fig. 85 b

Fig. 86. Schematic diagram and partial karyotype of the translocation t(15;17)(q22;q12), which is found in both the M3 and M3 V subtypes of promyelocytic leukemia. In the rare cases where cytogenetic analysis is unrewarding, the diagnosis can be established by molecular genetic detection of the PML/RARA translocation

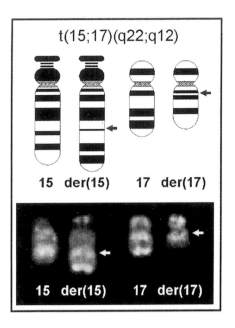

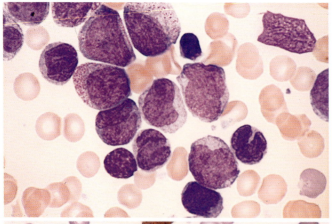

Fig. 87 a–g. Acute myelomonocytic leukemia, M4 subtype

a Bone marrow smear with undifferentiated blasts and precursors of the granulocytic and monocytic lines

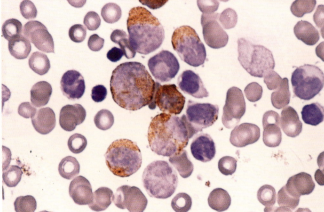

b Peroxidase reaction in the same patient shows peroxidase-positive blasts and later granulocytic precursors. Monocytic line is negative

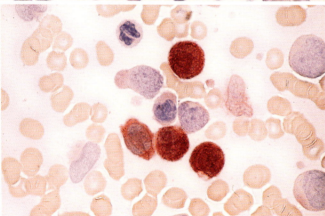

c Nonspecific esterase in the same patient shows strong, diffuse activity (brown) in four monocytes

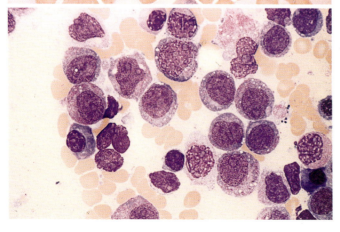

d Different patient. Blasts with grayish-blue cytoplasm (monocytic line). Several blasts contain coarse granules (granulocytic line)

Fig. 87 e–g

e CE reaction in the same case (**d**) shows strong activity in some cells (granulocytic line) and no activity in others

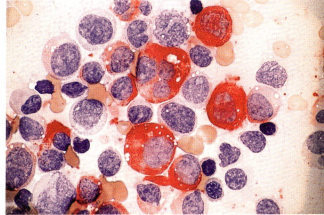

f Nonspecific esterase reaction in the same case shows strong, diffuse activity (grade 4) in most of the cells

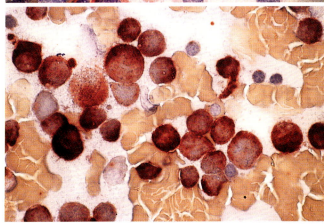

g Blood smear in M4 subtype demonstrates a large proportion of promonocytes and monocytes. There was just over 20 % granulocytopoiesis in the bone marrow, confirming the diagnosis of the M4 subtype

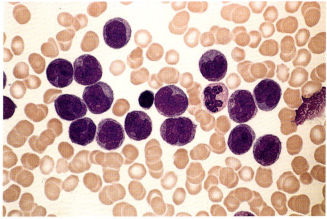

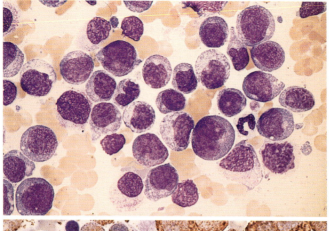

Fig. 88 a – g. Acute myelomonocytic leukemia, M4 subtype

a Pappenheim stain in bone marrow smear. Blasts and early precursors of granulocytopoiesis and monocytopoiesis are difficult to distinguish morphologically

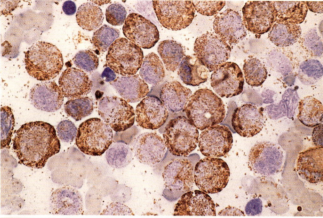

b Bone marrow from the same patient. Peroxidase reaction. Almost 100 % of the cells are peroxidase-positive

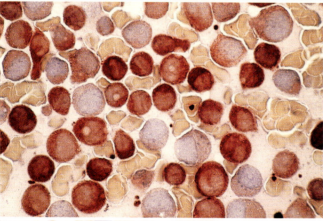

c Nonspecific esterase reaction in the same patient. Approximately 85 % of the cells are strongly and diffusely positive, confirming the diagnosis of M4. A large percentage of the leukemic cells have both monocytic and granulocytic properties

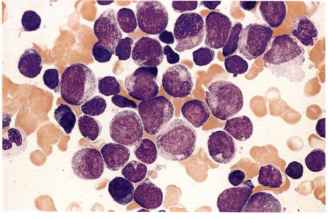

d Bone marrow from a different case of M4

Fig. 88 e – g

e Blood smear from the patient in **d**. At *center* is a segmented neutrophil with Auer rods. Below it are two monocytes with atypical nuclei

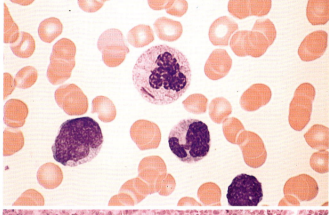

f Bone marrow histology in M4. Mega-karyocytes are increased, and some are dysplastic. HE stain

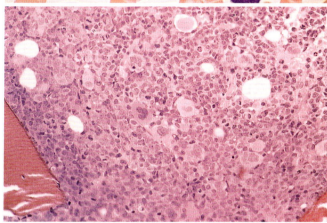

g Blood smear from the same patient shows greatly increased platelets and two monocytes

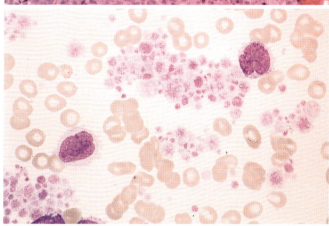

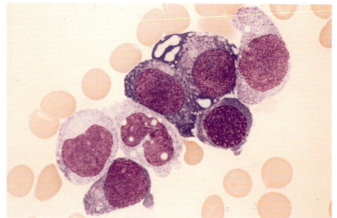

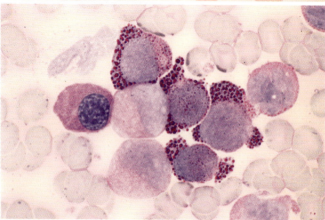

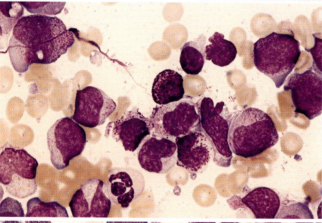

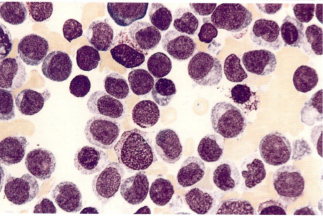

Fig. 89 a – d. Variants of the M4 subtype

a Severely dysplastic erythropoiesis. At *center* are three erythroblasts, two of which are very immature forms. The cytoplasm of the upper erythroblast is vacuolated

b PAS reaction in bone marrow from the same patient shows a strong, coarsely granular reaction in four atypical proerythroblasts and a diffuse reaction in an erythroblast at *left*. Three precursors of the white cell line show weak diffuse staining. There was less than 50 % erythropoiesis, excluding a diagnosis of erythroleukemia (M6 subtype)

c Bone marrow in M4 shows increased numbers of basophilic granulocytes. Three basophils surround the *center* of the field

d Increased basophilic granulocytes in the bone marrow from a different patient with M4. At *top and right* are two basophils with unusually fine granules. Toluidine blue stain confirms the metachromic reaction of the granules

Fig. 90 a – h. AML with abnormal eosinophils. M4Eo subtype

a This bone marrow smear contains precursors of granulocytopoiesis, monocytopoiesis, and blasts along with a high percentage of eosinophils, some of which (*left* and *right of center*) contain abnormal dark purple-violet granules. There are also mature eosinophils, some with very small granules

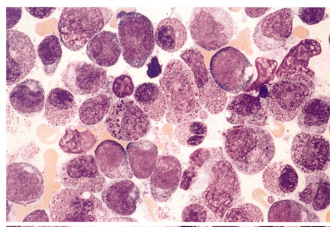

b Different case shows a striking abundance of abnormal eosinophils. These cells are easily mistaken for basophils with Pappenheim stain, but they do not show a metachromatic reaction with toluidine blue stain

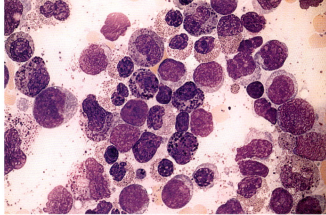

c Different case with many abnormal eosinophils. Note the pleomorphism of the abnormal granules

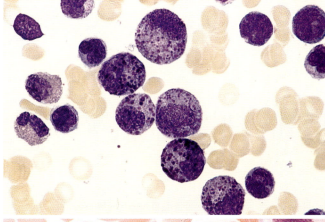

d Different case with two dysplastic eosinophils at the *center* of the field

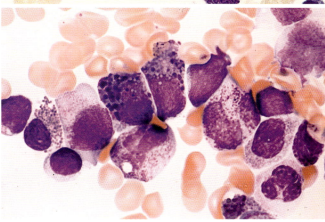

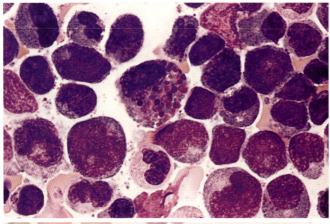

Fig. 90 e – h

e Severely dysplastic granules at *center*. The presence of this cell is sufficient to make a diagnosis

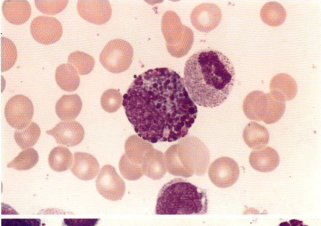

f Severely abnormal, immature eosinophil and an eosinophil containing very fine granules

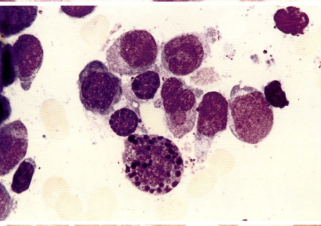

g Abnormal eosinophil (*bottom*) next to a group of monocytes

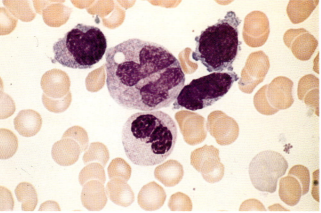

h Blood smear in M4Eo. At *top* are three very small monocytes and one monocyte with an abnormal nuclear structure. Below it is a pseudo-Pelger neutrophil form. Abnormal eosinophils are rarely found in blood films, and bone marrow examination is necessary to confirm the diagnosis

Fig. 91 a – f. Cytochemical findings in M4Eo

a The principal finding is the detection of CE in the granules of at least some of the abnormal eosinophils. This differentiates the abnormal eosinophils of M4Eo from reactive states and from eosinophils in other leukemias (e.g., M2 subtype of AML) in which eosinophils are increased. An exception is "pure" acute eosinophilic leukemia (see p. 253). This panel shows that a varying percentage of abnormal eosinophilic granules are CE-positive. At *upper left* is an eosinophilic myelocyte with large, 100 % positive granules

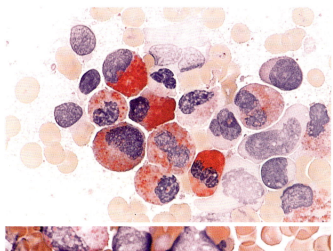

b From *top* to *bottom center* are three abnormal eosinophils that are CE-positive

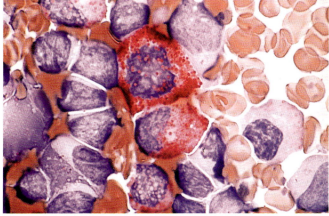

c Nonspecific esterase reaction in the bone marrow in M4Eo. The monocytes show the usual strong diffuse reaction. It is not uncommon, however, to find cases of M4Eo in which esterase activity is low compared with M4 and M5, without abnormal eosinophilia

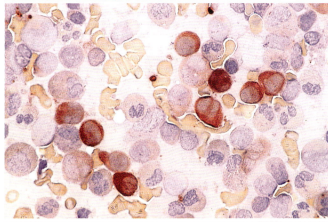

d PAS reaction. The abnormal granules may be PAS-positive. This finding is characteristic but not specific

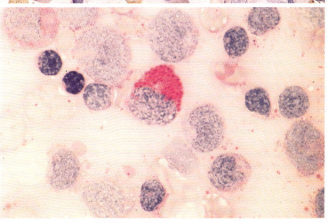

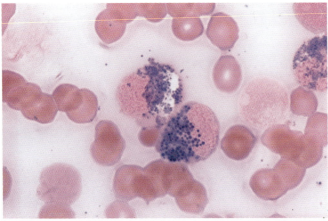

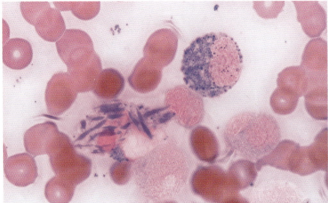

Fig. 91 e–f

e, f Adam's reaction for the detection of tryptophan. In the blood and bone marrow, this reaction is positive only in eosinophilic granules and so is the best technique for identifying eosinophils. Note that the abnormal granules and some Charcot-Leyden crystals, which form from eosinophilic granules (91f), are positive

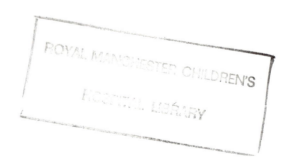

Fig. 92 a–g. Other findings in M4Eo

a, b In bone marrow with a high percentage of eosinophils, it is not unusual to find macrophages containing Charcot-Leyden crystals that have developed from eosinophilic granules. **a** Bone marrow smear in M4Eo. Two macrophages are laden with Charcot-Leyden crystals, which appear bright blue in this sample

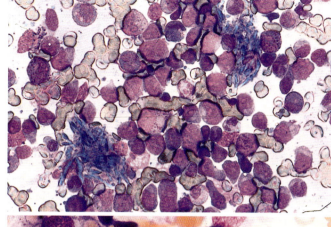

b Several pale Charcot-Leyden crystals in a slightly crushed macrophage, which also contains bluish material (phagocytized granules?)

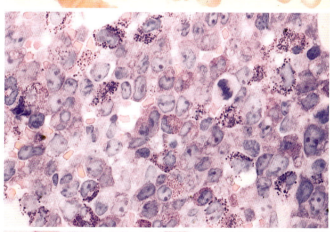

c Histologic section in M4Eo. Giemsa stain. The immature (bluish-violet) and mature (reddish) granules in the eosinophils are easily identified

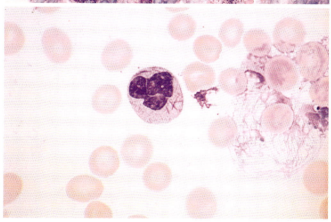

d Blood smear. Even in M4Eo, Auer rods are sometimes found in bone marrow cells and rarely in the peripheral blood

Fig. 92 e – g

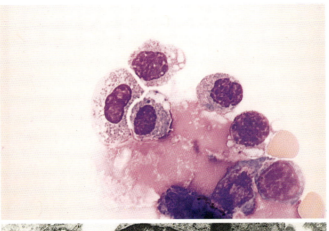

e Meningeal involvement may occur in M4Eo. In this case eosinophils were found in the CSF during a recurrence

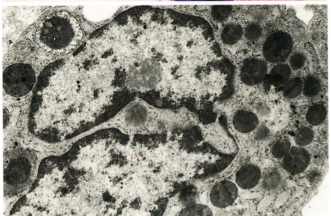

f Electron micrograph of an abnormal eosinophil. Predominantly eosinophilic progranules are visible in the cytoplasm. At *upper left* is a condensed vacuole, which develops into eosinophilic pro-granules. The crystalloid inclusions that are a typical feature of mature eosinophilic granules are poorly visualized. The small dark granules in the intergranular cytoplasm and in the pale rim of the condensed vacuole at *upper left* consist of glycogen

---

g Normal eosinophil for comparison. The granules contain typical crystalloid inclusions ▼

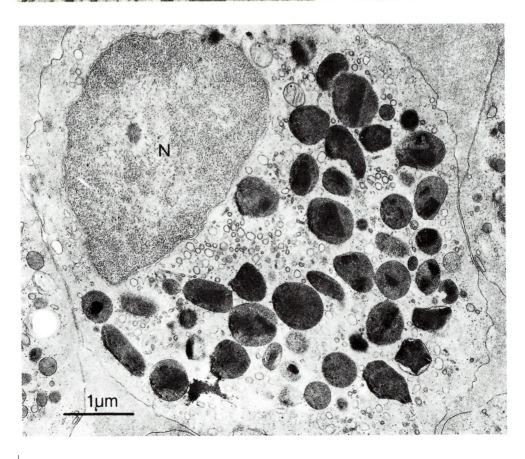

Fig. 93 a, b

a Schematic diagram and partial karyotype of the inversion inv(16)(p13;q22), which is found in acute myeloid leukemia of the M4Eo subtype. The arrows indicate the breakpoints

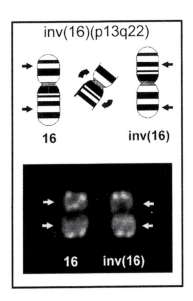

b FISH technique for detecting the inv(16) in interphase cells. Note the bright red eosinophilic granules in the cytoplasm and, above the nucleus, a signal (*blue-green dot* at *lower right*) from the normal chromosome 16 and a two-part signal (*two groups of small dots* at *left*) from the inverted chromosome 16. (From Haferlach et al. [1996] Blood. 87 : 2459 – 2463)

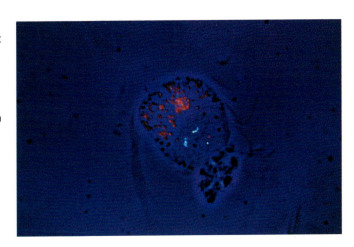

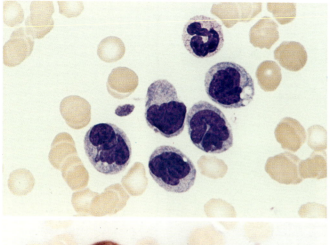

Fig. 94 a–h. Monocytic leukemia, M5b subtype. According to FAB criteria, at least 80 % of the nonerythroblastic bone marrow cells must be of monocytic lineage, and fewer than 80 % of these must be monoblasts

a Blood smear shows five somewhat atypical monocytes. At *top* is a neutrophil with a rod-shaped nucleus

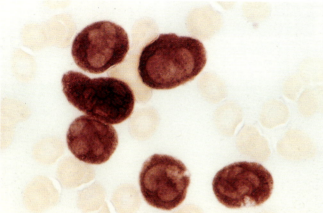

b Blood smear from the same patient. ANAE shows strong diffuse activity (grade 4) in all monocytic cells

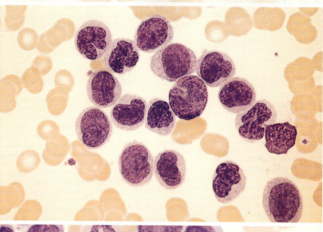

c Blood smear from a different patient with severe leukocytosis. Besides a monoblast at *top center*, the cells consist of monocytes and promonocytes

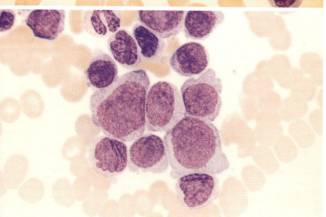

d Bone marrow from the patient in c. The proportion of monoblasts is larger but still less than 80 %

Fig. 94 e–h

e Blood smear from the same patient. ANAE demonstrates very strong diffuse reactivity (grade 4)

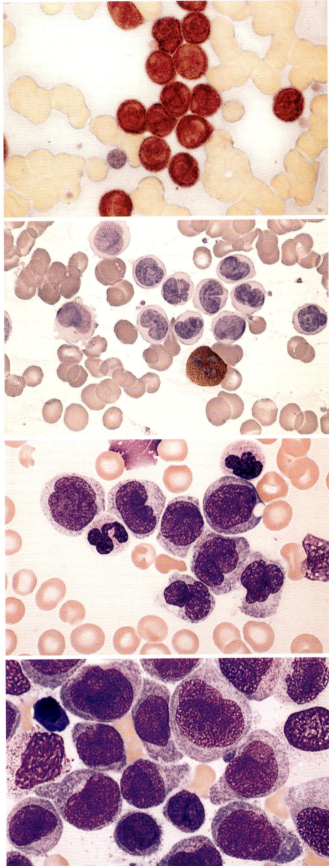

f Peroxidase reaction in the same patient shows a positive segmented neutrophil with negative monocytes and promonocytes

g Monocytes and promonocytes in the peripheral blood from a different patient

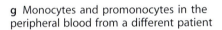

h Bone marrow smear from the patient in **g** shows a higher proportion of promonocytes and monoblasts than in the blood smear

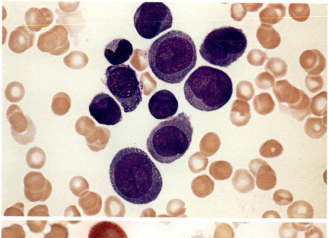

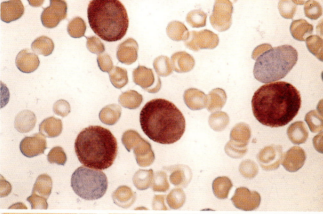

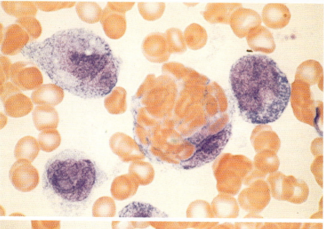

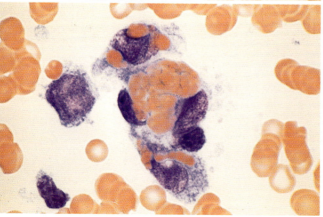

Fig. 95 a–d. Monocytic leukemia, M5b subtype

a Bone marrow smear from a different patient shows a large proportion of monoblasts. Borderline form with M5a

b ANAE in the same case shows strong diffuse activity in four cells

c, d Pronounced erythrophagocytosis in a case of M5b. The (8;16) translocation could not be detected

d

Fig. 96 a–h. Monoblastic leukemia, M5a subtype. Diagnostic criteria: at least 80 % of nonerythropoietic bone marrow cells must be of monocytic lineage, and at least 80 % of these must be monoblasts

a Bone marrow smear consists exclusively of monoblasts with round, frequently eccentric nuclei, distinct nucleoli, and abundant gray-blue cytoplasm

b Peripheral blood from the same patient also shows 100 % monoblasts, which appear slightly smaller and rounder

c Blood smear from the same patient. ANAE shows strong diffuse esterase activity in the cytoplasm of the blasts

d Peroxidase reaction in a bone marrow smear from the same patient. One residual granulocyte is positive, and all monoblasts are negative

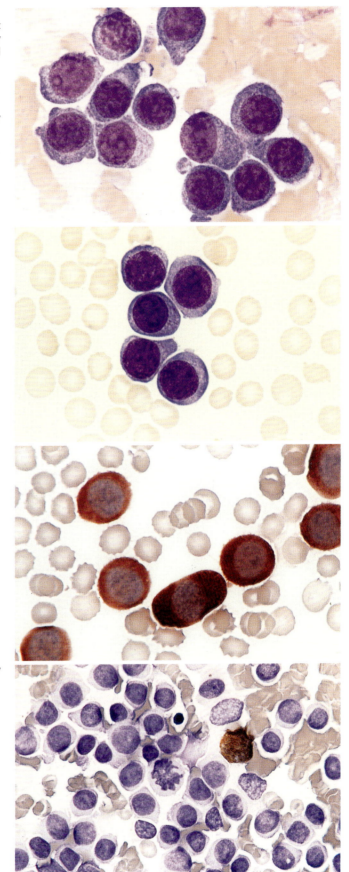

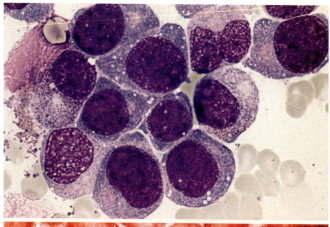

Fig. 96 e–h

e Bone marrow smear in a different case shows very immature-appearing monoblasts, which are sometimes interpreted as nonhematopoietic tumor cells

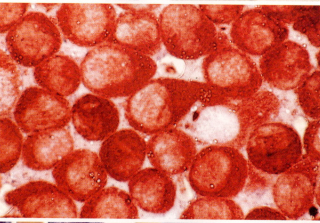

f Extremely strong ANAE activity in the bone marrow of the patient in **e**

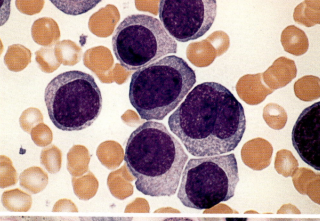

g Bone marrow smear from a different patient with M5a

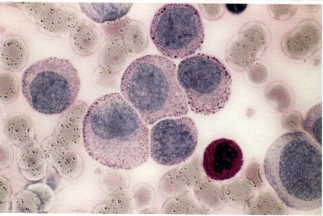

h Bone marrow smear from the patient in **g**. PAS reaction. A segmented neutrophil at *lower right* shows typical strong, diffuse reactivity. The monoblasts have a faint diffuse or finely granular reaction, which is condensed at the periphery of the cytoplasm to form coarse granules. This is a typical finding in the monocytic line

Fig. 97 a–h. Monoblastic leukemia, M5a subtype

a, b Different regions in the same bone marrow smear. In panel **a**, groups of monoblasts are seen to the *left of center* and on the *right*, along with abundant normal hematopoiesis. Panel **b** shows a different region with 100 % infiltration of the bone marrow by monoblasts

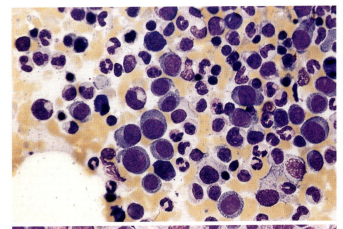

b

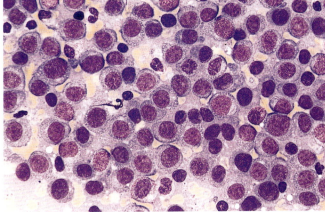

c–e Different regions of a histologic bone marrow section.

c Largely normal-appearing bone marrow with abundant megakaryocytes, erythropoiesis, and granulocytopoiesis

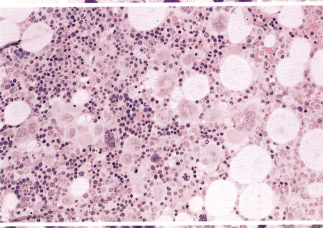

d Another site in the same specimen. A *line* from top center to lower left separates the monoblastic infiltrate at *lower right* from the area of normal hematopoiesis at *upper left*

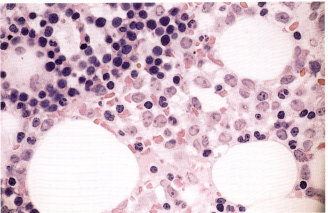

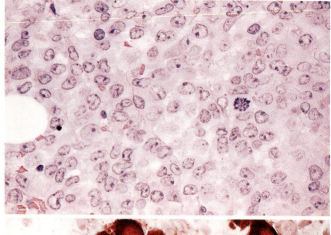

Fig. 97 e–h

e Another site showing 100 % monoblastic infiltration

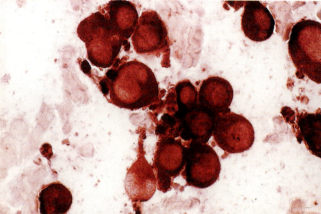

f ANAE reaction in a bone marrow smear from the patient in c–e shows extremely strong, diffuse reactivity in the monoblasts

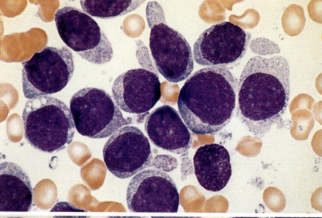

g Very immature monoblasts in another patient with M5a

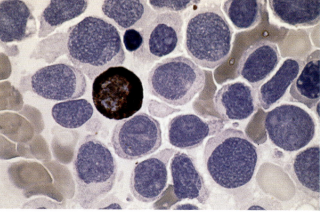

h Peroxidase reaction in a bone marrow smear from the patient in g. All the monoblasts are negative; only one normal residual granulocyte is positive

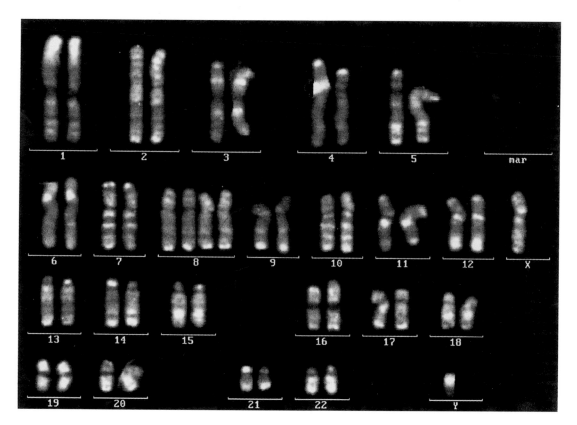

Fig. 98. Karyotype of AML, FAB type M5a, with the translocation t(11;16)(q23;p13) and tetrasomy 8 as a secondary aberration. Myelomonocytic and monocytic or monoblastic leukemias (FAB subtypes M4, M5b, or M5a) are mainly associated with translocations involving band q23 of chromosome 11. Besides t(11;16), the most important of these are t(9;11), t(11;14), and t(11;19). The translocation t(9;11) leads to the fusion gene AF9/MLL, which can be identified by molecular genetic analysis

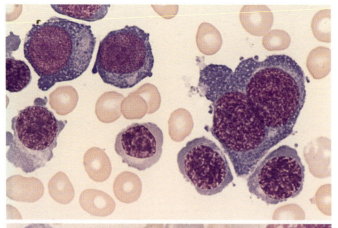

Fig. 99 a – h. Acute erythroleukemia subtype AML-M6. To meet the definition, erythroid progenitors must constitute at least 50 % of the marrow nucleated cells, and blasts must constitute at least 30 % of the nonerythroblastic cells (NEC). There are also "pure" erythroblastic leukemias (acute erythremia) with marked atypias of red cell precursors but very few myeloblasts. The proportion of red cell precursors may decline during the course of an erythroleukemia (e.g., after blood transfusion), resulting in an M1 or M2 type of pattern

a Megaloblastoid erythropoiesis. At *right* is a binucleated cell

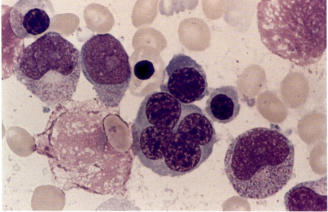

b At the *bottom of the field* is an erythroblast with four nuclei, and above it to the left is a myeloblast with an Auer rod

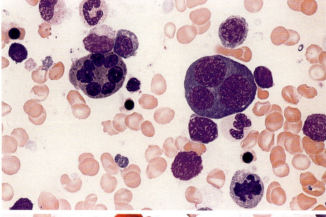

c At *left* is an erythroblast with seven nuclei and mature cytoplasm. At *right* is a trinucleated erythroblast with immature cytoplasm

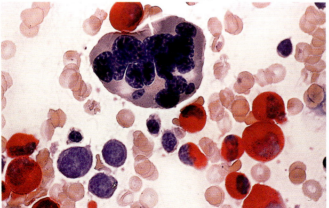

d CE reaction. At *top* is a multinucleated erythroblast with mature cytoplasm. A relatively large number of mature granulocytes are still seen

Fig. 99 e–h

e Marked megaloblastoid erythropoiesis in a case of M6

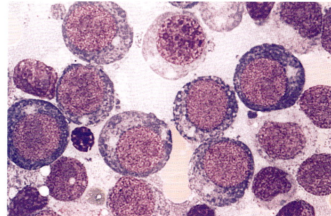

f Intense granular and diffuse PAS reaction in the bone marrow of the same patient. Such a strong PAS reaction is not seen in megaloblastic anemias caused by a vitamin B_{12} or folic acid deficiency

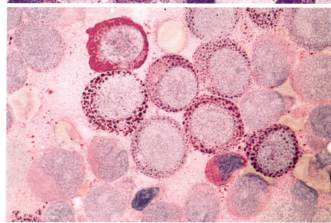

g Bone marrow from a different patient with M6 and mature erythropoiesis. The erythrocytes and some of the erythroblasts have cytoplasmic inclusions consisting of Pappenheimer bodies

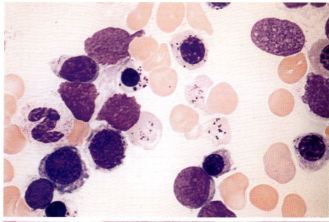

h Smear from the patient in **g** after iron staining. The inclusions in the erythrocytes (*center of field*) are positive. Ringed sideroblasts may be numerous in M6

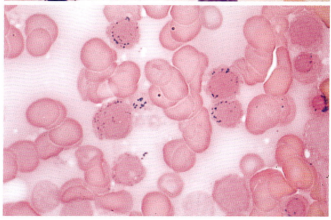

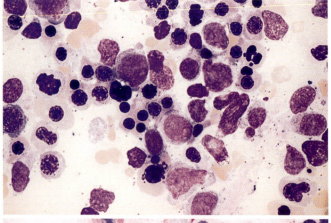

Fig. 100 a–h. **Acute erythroleukemia, subtype M6**

a Bone marrow from a patient with more mature but dysplastic erythropoiesis. Myeloblasts are visible above and below the *center* of the field

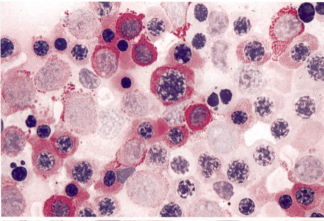

b PAS reaction in a bone marrow smear from the same patient demonstrates a very strong, predominantly diffuse reaction in the cytoplasm of the erythroblasts. Generally the reaction is clumped and granular in earlier precursors and diffuse in more mature forms

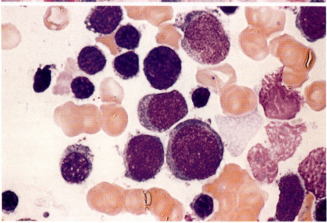

c Group of myeloblasts in another case of M6

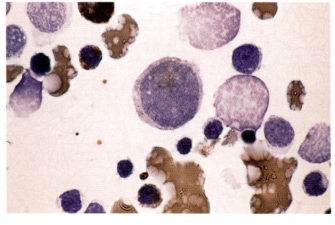

d Peroxidase-positive myeloblast in a smear from the patient in **c**

Fig. 100 e–h

e Focal acid phosphatase reaction in the erythroblasts of the same patient. This finding should not be mistaken for T-cell ALL

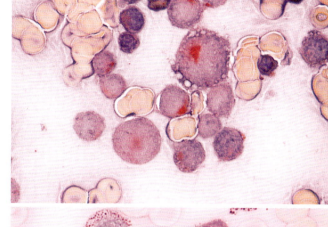

f PAS reaction in the bone marrow of the same patient

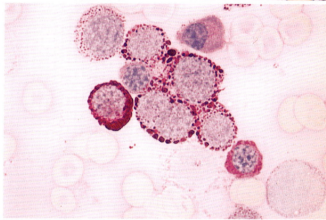

g Extremely immature form of M6. Some of the cells show vacuolated cytoplasm, and there is one abnormal mitosis

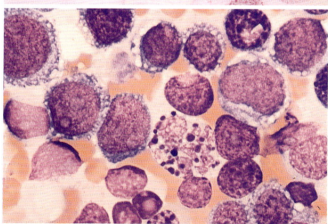

h PAS reaction in a smear from the same patient

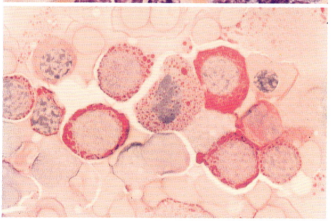

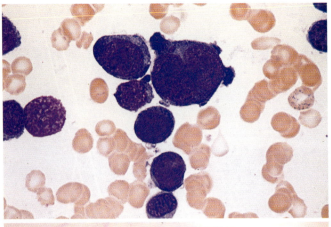

Fig. 101 a–h. Acute erythroleukemia, M6 subtype

a Extremely immature cells can be identified as erythroblasts only by the strong basophilia of their cytoplasm

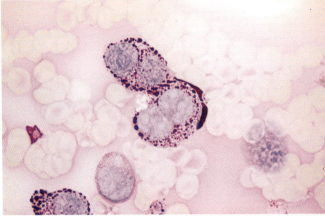

b PAS reaction as an additional criterion in the same patient. This is a case of "pure" erythremia, corresponding to the M6 V subtype

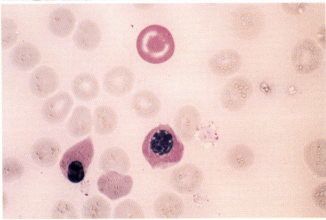

c Another case shows a markedly diffuse PAS reaction in an erythrocyte (target cell)

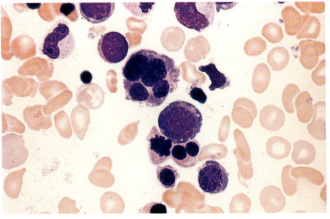

d Severely dysplastic erythropoiesis in another case of M6. Myeloblasts are visible at *left*

Fig. 101 e–h

e Bone marrow smear from the patient in **d**. ANAE reaction shows strong, diffuse activity in the cytoplasm of the blasts and more mature forms. This case is an M6 subtype involving the monocytic rather than granulocytic line

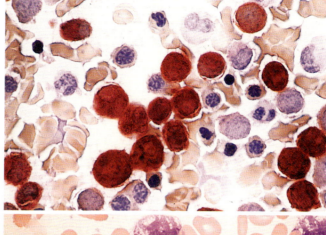

f Pappenheim stain in the same case shows a blast with a short Auer rod and, next to it, elliptical erythrocytes (acquired elliptocytosis)

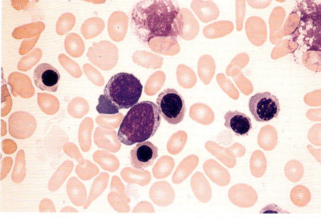

g, h Giant erythrocytes in another case of M6. Note the basophilic stippling and chromatin particles in **h**

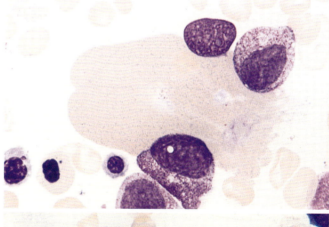

h

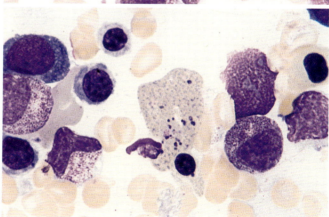

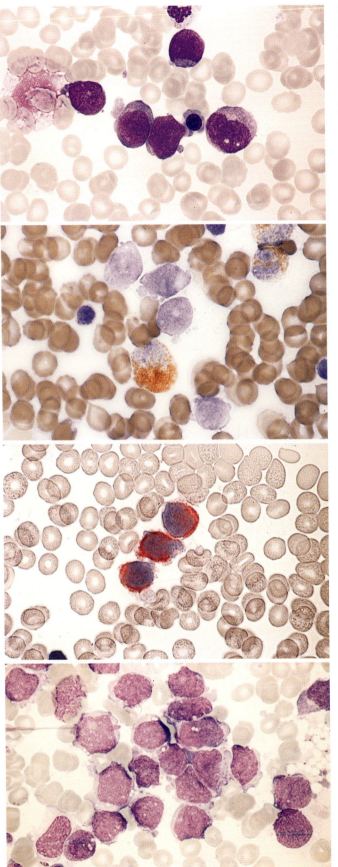

Fig. 102 a – g. Megakaryoblastic leukemia (M7). This last FAB-defined subtype of AML is more common in children than adults, with more than 15 % of cases diagnosed before 2 years of age. Only infants with the M7 subtype are found to have the (1;22) translocation as a specific chromosome abnormality. The definition requires 30 % megakaryoblasts in the bone marrow smear. Often these cells cannot be identified morphologically, and the diagnosis must be established by immunophenotyping (expression of the antigens CD41 and CD61). Bone marrow fibrosis often results in a dry tap; these cases require core biopsy and histologic evaluation

a Undifferentiated blasts with cytoplasmic budding (pseudopods)

b Smear from the same patient. Peroxidase reaction. The blasts are negative

c Immunocytochemical detection of CD41. APAAP technique. Blasts are positive (red)

d Undifferentiated blasts and cytoplasm fragments in bone marrow from a child. CD41 positive

Fig. 102 e–g

e ANAE reaction in the same patient shows a circumscribed, stippled pattern of activity

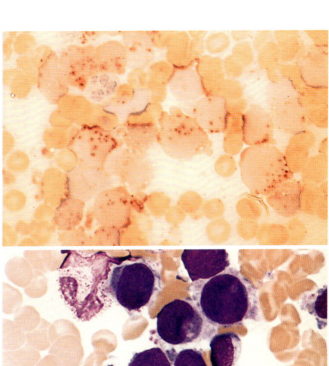

f, g Bone marrow smears from a different patient. The megakaryoblasts show relatively large nuclei, dense chromatin, and irregular cytoplasmic margins with detached flecks of cytoplasm. Cytoplasmic budding is particularly marked in **g**

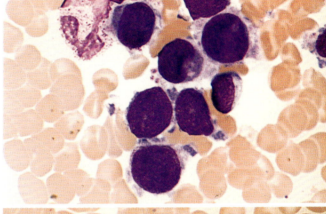

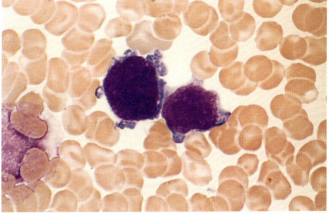

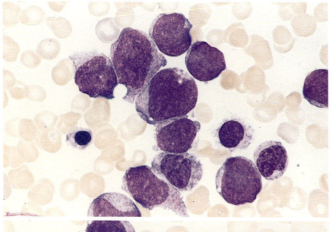

Fig. 103 a–c. Megakaryoblastic leukemia (M7)

a Different case showing large, pleomorphic blasts

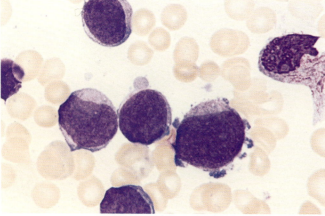

b Minimal cytoplasmic budding

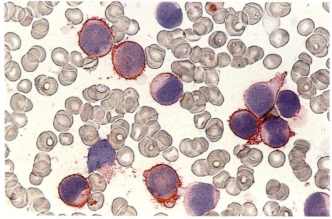

c APAAP technique. CD41 positive

Fig. 104 a – c. Transition from megakaryoblastic leukemia to a mixed megakaryoblastic-basophilic leukemia

a The blasts appear very immature, and a high percentage express CD34 in addition to CD41 and CD61

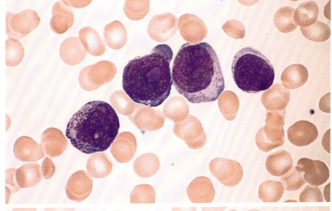

b Following a poor response to chemotherapy, the blasts contain dark-purple cytoplasmic granules that show metachromatic reactivity

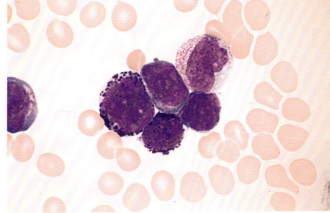

c Metachromatic reaction of the granules after toluidine blue staining. There has been a transformation from the megakaryoblast phenotype to basophilic precursors

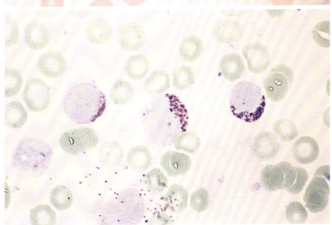

d, e Samples aspirated from the iliac crest in the area of a localized process

d Group of relatively large blasts show dense, homogenous-appearing nuclear chromatin and a wide, moderately basophilic cytoplasmic rim. CD61 and CD41 positive

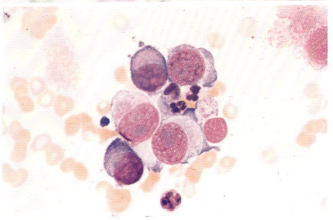

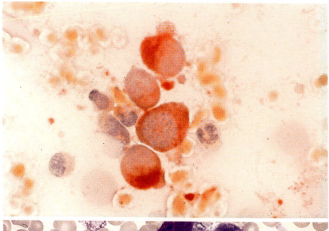

Fig. 104 e–f

e ANAE reaction. Cytoplasm shows intense enzymatic activity. Panels **d** and **e** illustrate a megakaryoblastoma

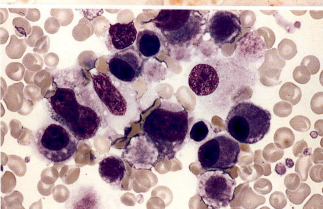

f Bone marrow smear from a small child with Down syndrome shows almost exclusive proliferation of megakaryoblasts and promegakaryocytes

Fig. 105. Partial karyotype of a (1;22) translocation from the bone marrow of an infant with megakaryoblastic leukemia. (Courtesy Prof. O. Haas, Vienna)

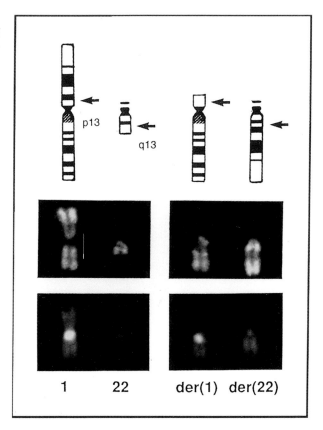

Fig. 106. Electron microscopic detection of platelet peroxidase in a megakaryoblast. The reaction is detectable in the nuclear membrane (*arrow*) and endoplasmic reticulum (*open arrow*) (*upper panel*). Typically the Golgi complex (*open arrows*) is peroxidase-negative while the nuclear membrane (*arrow*) shows definite peroxidase staining (*lower panel*). Mitochondria show nonspecific peroxidase staining. (Courtesy Dr. Heil, Hannover)

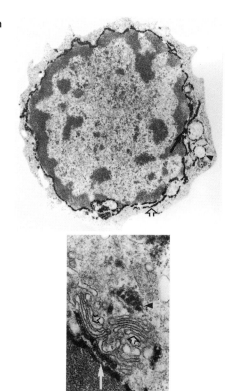

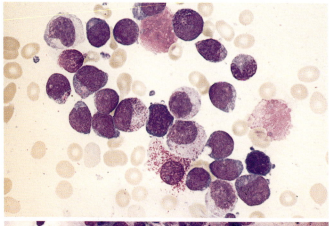

Fig. 107 and 108 Therapy-induced changes in acute leukemias (see also Figs. 83 and 84)

a AML, M2 subtype, prior to treatment

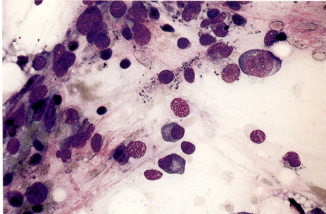

b Severe cytopenia following two cycles of chemotherapy

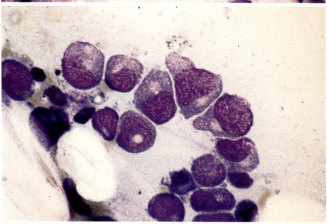

c Higher-power view of a small focus of granulocytopoietic regeneration with young promyelocytes. It can be difficult to distinguish between normal and leukemic precursors at this stage

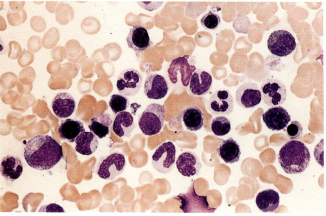

d Complete remission after an additional four weeks' therapy

Fig. 107 e–h

e Hypocellular bone marrow from a different patient following induction chemotherapy. Stromal cells, fat cells, plasma cells, and lymphocytes are found. Two mature granulocytes are seen at the *top*. This state may evolve toward remission or recurrence

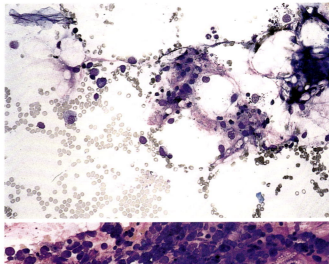

f Bone marrow findings in a different patient with AML-M5b, 18 days after induction chemotherapy with TAD (thioguainine, cytosine-arabinoside, daunorubicin). There is incipient regeneration of neutrophilic granulocytopoiesis

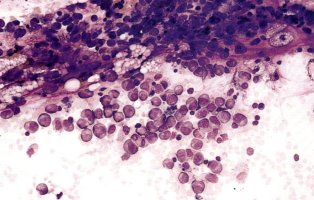

g Higher magnification of the same bone marrow demonstrates promyelocytes and myelocytes

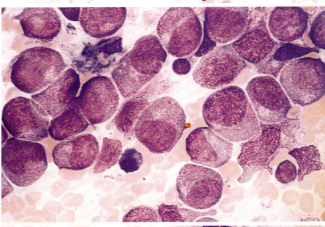

h Bone marrow smear with fat cells following chemotherapy

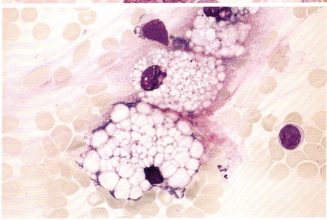

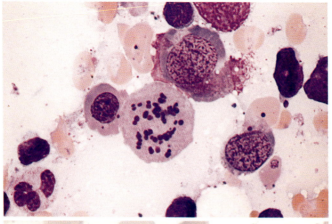

Fig. 108 a–d

a Bone marrow smear in ALL following combination chemotherapy that included vincristine demonstrates megaloblastic erythropoiesis and abnormal mitosis

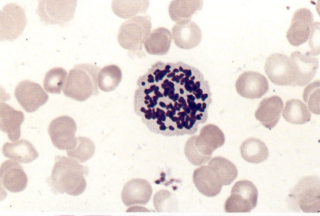

b Atypical chromosomes in a mitosis following cytosine-arabinoside therapy

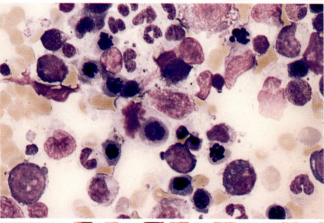

c Bone marrow smear in recurrent monoblastic leukemia (M5a) following vincristine therapy, with abundant arrested mitoses in erythroid precursors

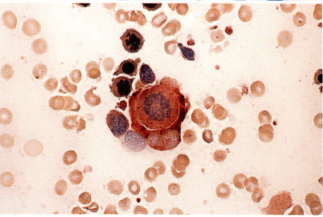

d ANAE reaction in the same patient. At *center* is a monoblast in mitosis (diffuse esterase activity) engulfed by the esterase-positive cytoplasm of a macrophage. At *left* are two arrested erythroblastic mitoses

Fig. 109 a – h. Secondary acute myeloid leukemias. Secondary AML may develop following chemotherapy with alkylating cytostatic drugs or with topoisomerase II inhibitors (particularly etoposide)

a Primary bone marrow findings in immunologically confirmed T-cell ALL. Complete remission was achieved initially

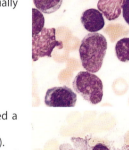

b Findings 12 months later suggested a "recurrence," which proved to be a secondary monocytic leukemia (M5b). Promonocytes and monocytes are found in the bone marrow

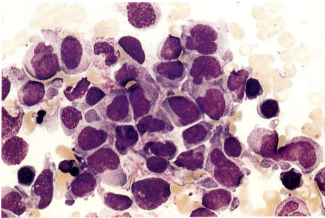

c Higher-power view of **b**

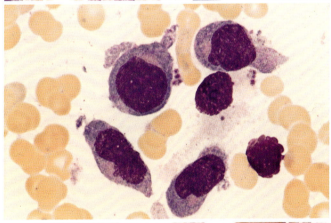

d Bone marrow smear in **c**, ANAE reaction

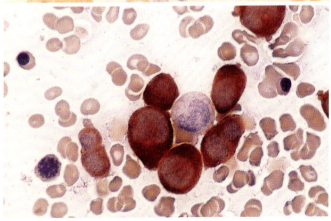

Fig. 109 e–h

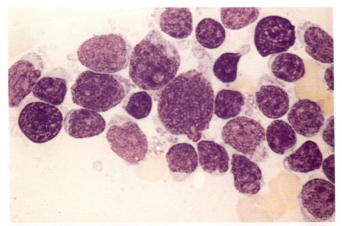

e Primary bone marrow findings in a patient with a long history of mantle cell lymphoma (MCL) in stage IV, which had been treated several times with chemotherapy including etoposide

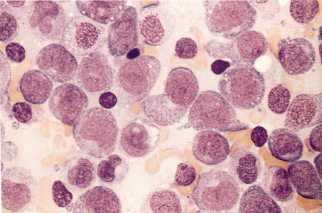

f Bone marrow findings on diagnosis of a secondary monoblastic leukemia (M5a). This field shows almost 100 % infiltration by monoblasts

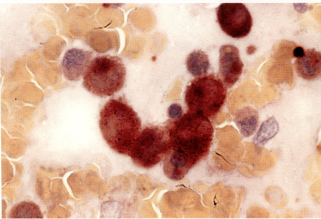

g ANAE reaction shows marked activity in the monoblasts

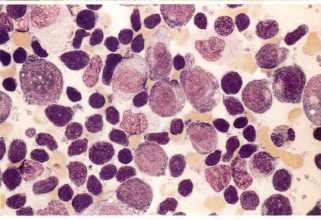

h View of a different site shows monoblasts interspersed with abundant lymphatic cells from the preexisting MCL. Concurrent cytogenetic studies identified a (11;16) translocation with an 11q23 breakpoint (characteristic of monocytic leukemia as well as secondary AML after topoisomerase II inhibitors) and also a t(11;14) with an 11q13 breakpoint (typical of MCL), confirming the coexistence of residual MCL cells and monoblastic leukemia

Fig. 110 a–f. Other secondary acute myeloid leukemias

a Monoblastic leukemia (M5a) with detection of the 11q23 aberration following chemotherapy for maxillary sinus carcinoma

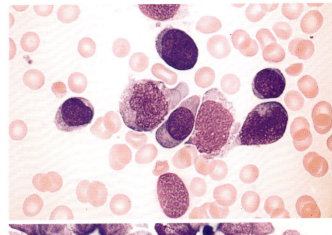

b, c Primary bone marrow findings in promyelocytic leukemia (M3). Faggot cell and hypergranular promyelocytes. Complete remission was achieved with combined ATRA and chemotherapy

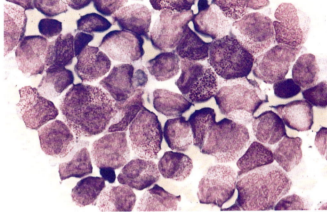

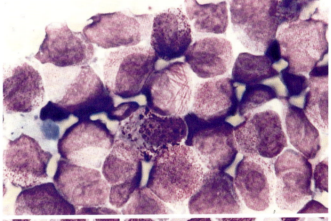

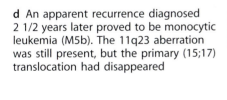

d An apparent recurrence diagnosed 2 1/2 years later proved to be monocytic leukemia (M5b). The 11q23 aberration was still present, but the primary (15;17) translocation had disappeared

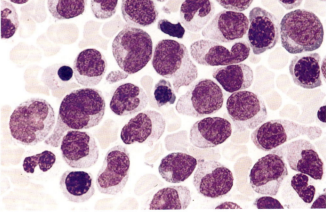

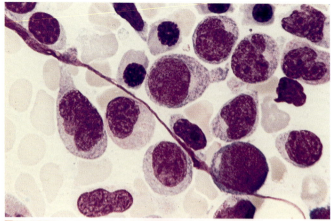

Fig. 110 e – f

e Higher-power view of d

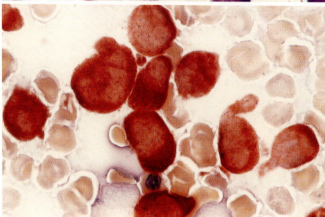

f ANAE reaction in the same smear

Fig. 111 a–e. Recurrence of AML with deficient granulocyte maturation

a Bone marrow at onset of the recurrence shows increased blasts

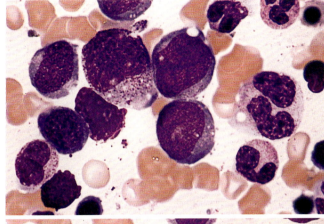

b Mature granulocytes are still relatively abundant but are accompanied by markedly dysplastic, polypoid forms

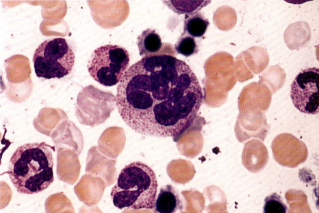

c, d Peroxidase reaction differentiates granulocytes that are still normal from the predominantly dysplastic granulocytes, which are peroxidase-negative

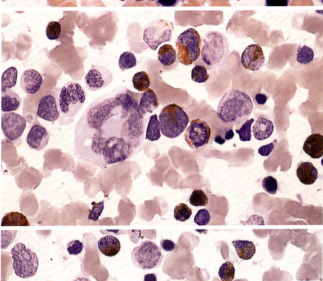

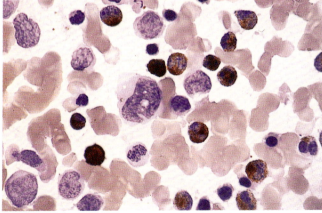

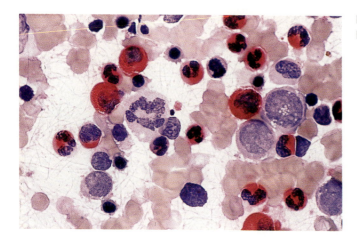

Fig. 111 e CE reaction shows the same pattern as peroxidase

Figs. 112–114. Rare acute myeloid leukemias

Fig. 112 a–h. Acute eosinophilic leukemia

a Blasts with reddish to purple granules and some large vacuoles that contain coarse inclusions

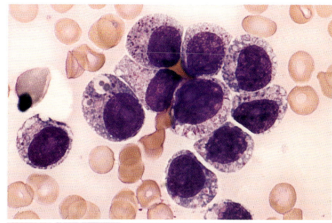

b Some of the granules are dark purple and highly variable in appearance

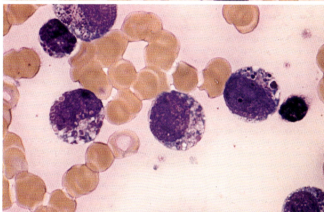

c Large vacuoles containing orange-colored granules

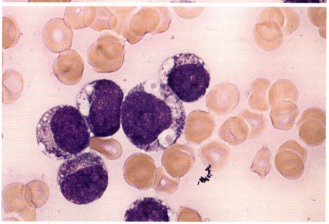

d, e Peroxidase reaction. Two neutrophilic precursors are seen at *top* and *center*. All other cells contain variable granules, some quite large and some with central pallor. These granules correspond to eosinophilic granules in precursors

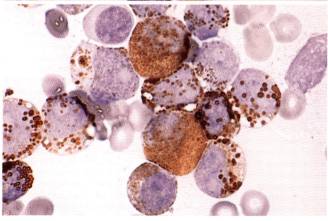

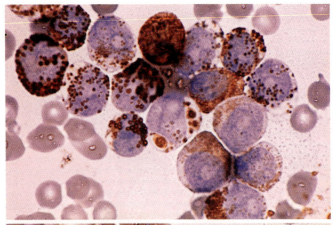

Fig. 112 e–h

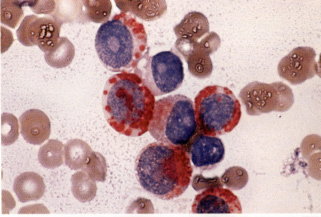

f, g CE reaction. The granules (red) are CE-positive and correspond in size and shape to those with peroxidase activity

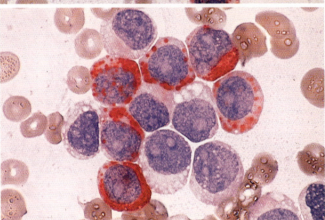

g

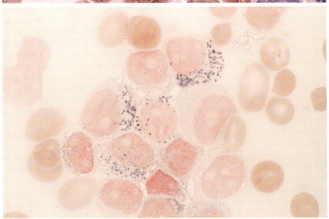

h The cells were identified as immature eosinophils by the positive Adam reaction of the granules (here grayish-blue) and by staining with luxol fast blue and the peroxidase modification for eosinophils. A specific chromosome aberration could not be identified in this patient, and molecular genetic analysis did not detect inversion 16 (CBFβ/MYH11)

Fig. 112 i, j Two additional cases of eosinophilic leukemia with a higher degree of maturation but also with atypical eosinophilic granulocytes containing very fine granules. Both patients were men, 20 and 63 years of age

i Clumped purple granules and pleomorphic nuclei in the 20-year-old man. As in the case above, the granules gave a positive Adam reaction. Cytogenetic analysis identified a t(10;11)(q11;p13–14) translocation. The Wilms tumor gene (wt1) was expressed, in contrast to hypereosinophilic syndrome

j The 63-year-old man had immature cells, also with Adam-positive granules. Some of the granules were CE- and peroxidase-positive. No chromosome abnormalities were found. The greater than 30 % proportion of blasts clearly identifies the disease as an acute leukemia

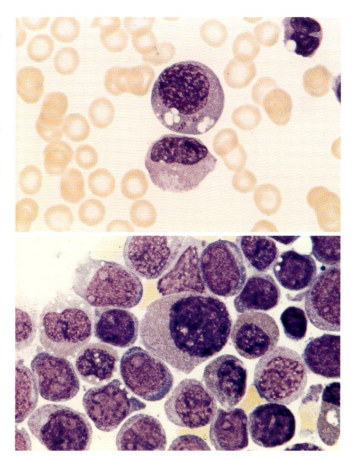

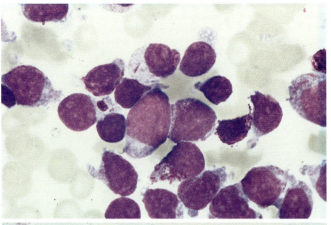

Fig. 113 a–f. Acute basophilic leukemia. These cases require differentiation from a basophilic phase of CML and from tissue mast cells leukemia

a, b Acute basophilic leukemia with a large proportion of blasts. Some cells contain abundant basophilic granules, and scattered inclusions like Auer rods are seen. Pappenheim stain (a), toluidine blue stain (b)

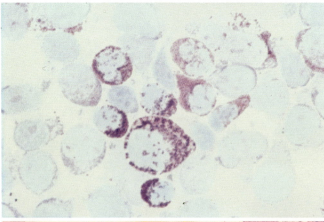

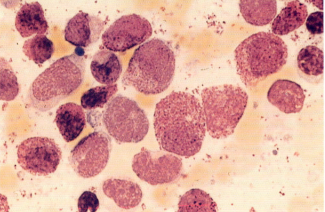

c Higher degree of maturation in a different patient

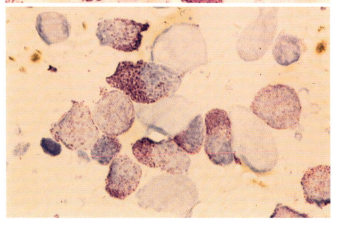

d Toluidine blue stain

Fig. 113 e–f

e Indistinct granules in a different patient

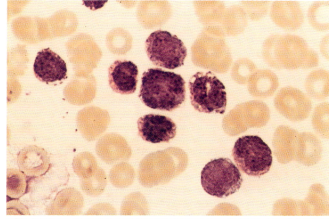

f Toluidine blue stain of a smear from the same patient shows a marked metachromatic reaction

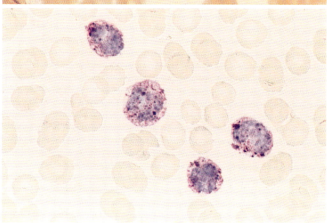

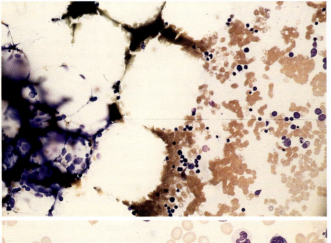

Fig. 114 a–d. Hypoplastic AML. Sample evaluation is feasible in these cases only if sufficient bone marrow fragments can be aspirated and mounted as smears. Otherwise the case should be evaluated by core biopsy and histologic examination. It can be very difficult to distinguish this variant of AML from aplastic anemias. Even histologic examination of the bone marrow can be misleading unless blasts are positively identified. The diagnosis relies on demonstrating a frequently circumscribed collection of blasts. Sporadic cases of acute lymphocytic leukemia may also start with an aplastic preliminary stage, and frequent follow-ups are necessary to establish a clear diagnosis

a Hypocellular bone marrow with increased fat cells

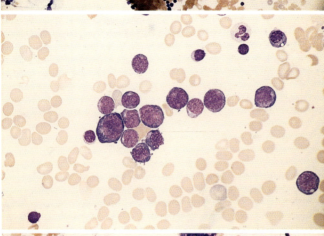

b Higher-power view of a more cellular site shows myeloblasts and erythroblasts (*left* and *bottom*)

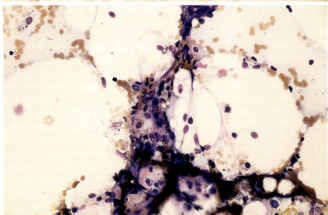

c Hypocellular bone marrow in a different patient

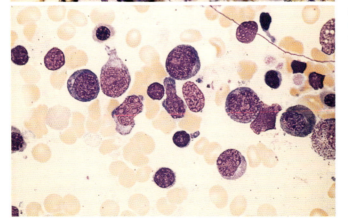

d Myeloblasts and isolated lymphocytes in an isolated hypercellular area of the same sample

Fig. 115 a – d. Acute lymphoblastic leukemia (ALL)

a Small blasts. These may closely resemble lymphocytes but are distinguished by their finer chromatin structure and the occasional presence of nucleoli

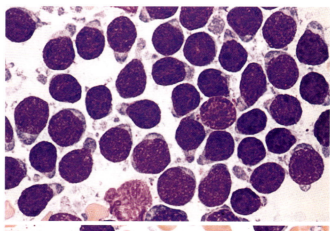

b Different case showing blasts of varying sizes, some with pleomorphic nuclei. Panels **a** and **b** illustrate B-lineage ALL

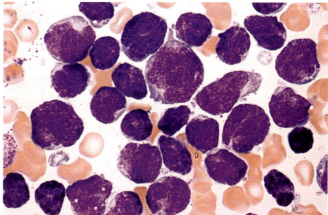

c Peroxidase reaction. All lymphoblasts are negative and are interspersed with residual cells of granulocytopoiesis, whose proportion is more clearly demonstrated by the peroxidase reaction

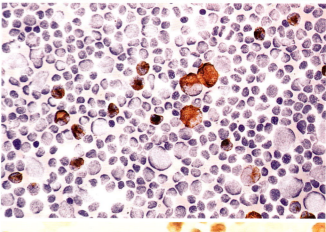

d Terminal deoxynucleotidyl transferase (TDT), detected by the immunoperoxidase reaction in the nuclei. TDT is not specific for lymphoblasts but is useful for differentiating forms of ALL from mature-cell lymphatic neoplasias and large-cell lymphomas. Today this reaction is usually performed in a fluorescence-activated cell sorter

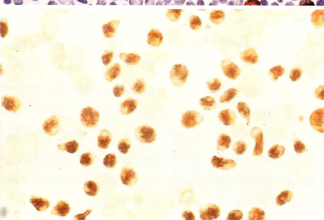

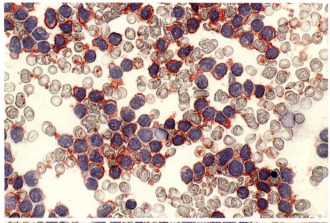

Fig. 116 a–g. B-lineage ALL

a The pan-B marker CD19 is very useful for the immunocytochemical detection of B-cell lineage. 100 % of the blasts in this sample are positive (red)

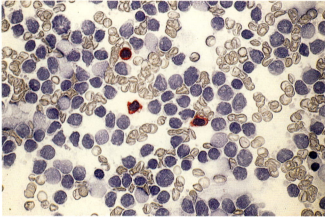

b Contrast with the T-lineage marker CD3: the blasts are negative, and interspersed mature T lymphocytes are positive (same case as **a**)

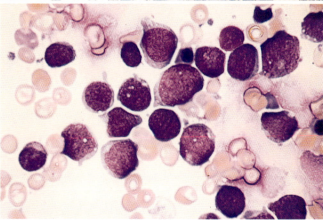

c Different case with lymphoblasts of varying size

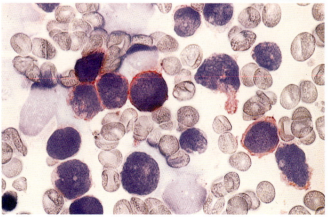

d Same case as **c**, demonstration of CD 19

Fig. 116 e–g

e Same case as **c** and **d**, demonstration of CD10. The detection of CD19 and CD10 correspond to C-ALL (BII)

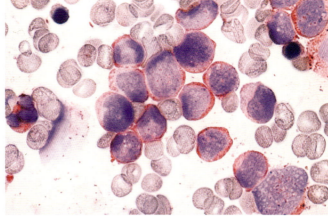

f PAS stain yields a granular reaction in a variable percentage of lymphoblasts, which show a coarse granular or flocculent reaction pattern

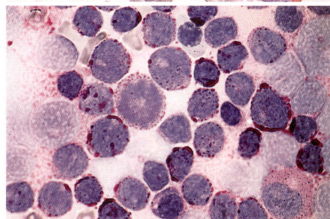

g Coarse granular and globular PAS reaction in a different case. The reaction pattern seen in **f** and **g**, when combined with a pale cytoplasmic background and negative peroxidase and ANAE, provides morphologic and cytochemical evidence of ALL

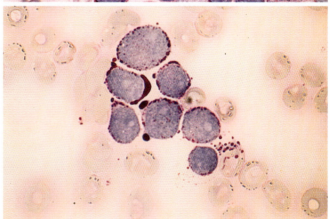

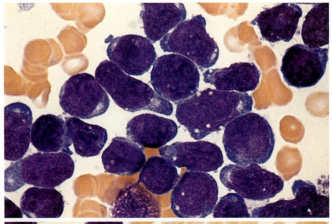

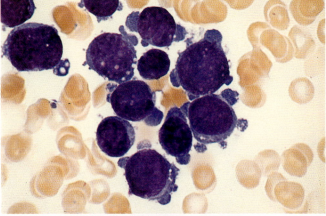

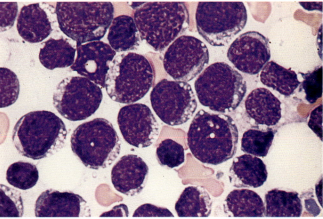

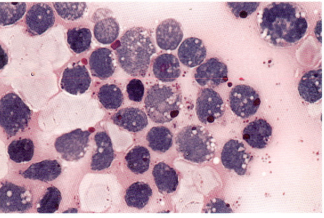

Fig. 117 a – g B-lineage ALL

a A range of morphologic features may be found in ALL. This sample shows relatively large blasts with an intensely basophilic cytoplasm

b Large blasts with marked cytoplasmic budding, at first suggesting megakaryo-blastic leukemia. Both **a** and **b** represent B-lineage ALL

c Vacuolation is not uncommon in ALL. Relatively large vacuoles are seen in this case

d Vacuoles in a different case. The coarse granular PAS reaction in the cytoplasm is not associated with the vacuoles

Fig. 117 e – g

e Large, partially confluent vacuoles in a different patient

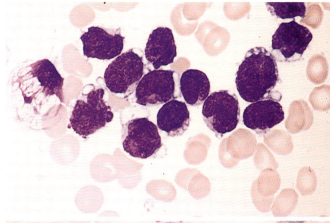

f PAS reaction in the same case (**e**) shows that the vacuoles are filled with glycogen

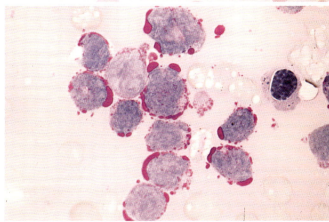

g Peroxidase reaction in the same case clearly demonstrates the vacuoles in the peroxidase-negative blasts

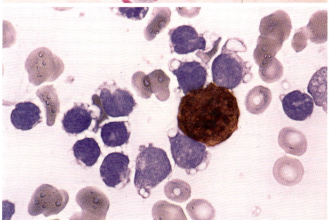

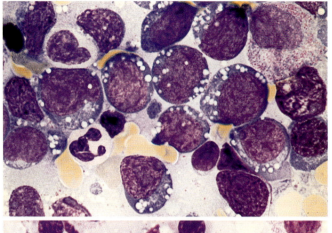

Fig. 118 a–d. Mature B-ALL (B IV) corresponding to the FAB subtype L3. This subtype of ALL is rare, but its recognition is important because the prognosis can significantly improve with specific therapy. Morphologic examination shows round, relatively uniform blasts of moderate size with intensely basophilic cytoplasm and sharply defined (fat-containing) vacuoles

a–c Various examples of this subtype of ALL

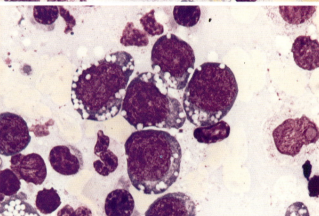

b

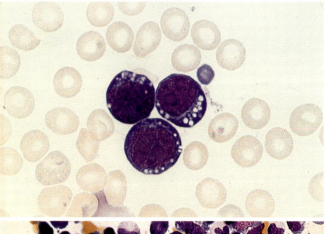

c

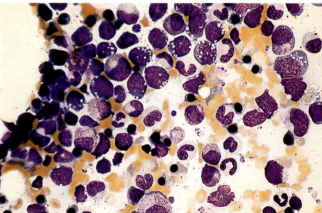

d Bone marrow smear in which infiltration is confined to the upper part of the field

Fig. 119 a – h. ALL with cytoplasmic granules. One morphologic subtype of ALL violates the dogma that cytoplasmic granules are suggestive of AML. This case is a B-lineage type of ALL with cytoplasmic granules that are peroxidase-negative and behave as lysosomes

a Blasts above the *center* of the field contain coarse purple granules. Several finer granules are visible below

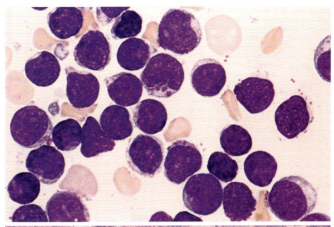

b PAS reaction. The abnormal granules stain pink, contrasting with the burgundy-red staining of the other glycogen granules

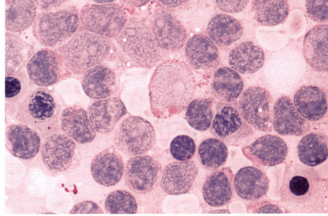

c ANAE reaction. The distinct, intensely reacting granules in the cytoplasm correspond to those seen in a and b

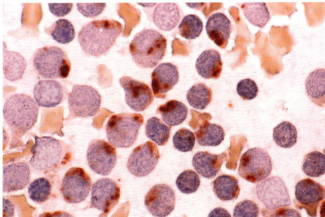

d Another case with very prominent dark-purple granules. They might be mistaken for basophilic granules but are distinguished by an absence of metachromasia

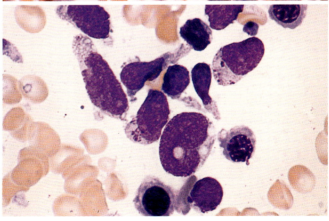

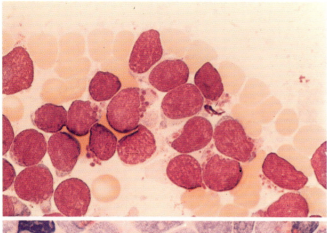

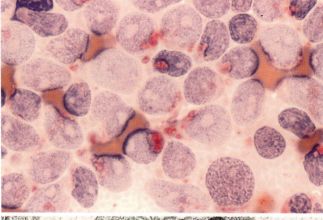

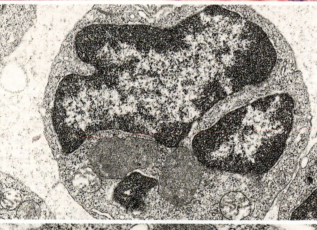

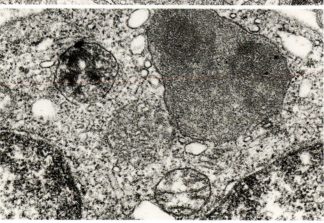

Fig. 119 e–h

e Relatively large, intensely staining granules in a different case

f Acid phosphatase reaction. Some of the granules are markedly positive

g, h Electron micrographs reveal large, membrane-bound inclusions in the cytoplasm with finely granular contents corresponding to the granules described above. (Courtesy of Prof. Dr. Müller-Hermelink, Würzburg)

h

Fig. 120 a, b. Chromosome abnormalities in ALL. The (9;22) translocation in ALL indicates a particularly unfavorable prognosis. This finding corresponds cytogenetically to that described in CML. In terms of molecular genetics, the minor breakpoint cluster region (m-bcr) is predominantly affected in ALL. a The (4;11) translocation, which also implies a poor prognosis. b The translocation t(8;14) (q24;q32), connected to Burkitt lymphoma and mature B-ALL (B IV)

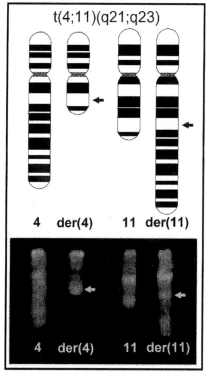

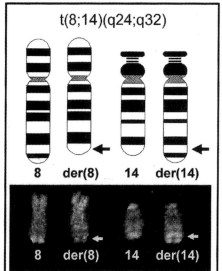

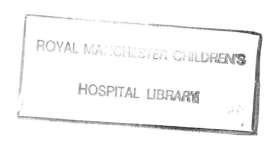

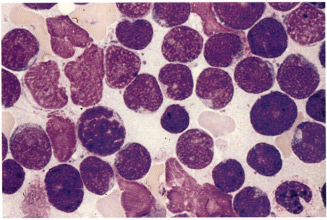

Fig. 121 a–f. T-lineage ALL. Usually the B-cell and T-cell forms of ALL are morphologically indistinguishable. The pronounced irregularity of the nuclear contour ("convoluted nucleus") and high rate of mitoses are more consistent with T-ALL

a Pappenheim stain in T-ALL

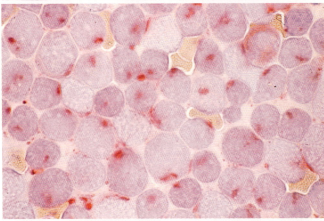

b The focal or paranuclear acid phosphatase reaction pattern shown here is typical of T-lineage ALL

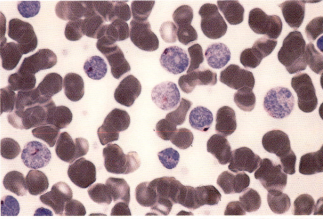

c Acid phosphatase reaction using a different technique (Sigma)

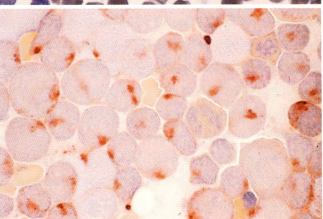

d The DAP IV reaction is a more specific but less sensitive method than acid phosphatase. It occurs at the same locations as the acid phosphatase reaction

Fig. 121 e–f

e A case of T-ALL with consistently round nuclei

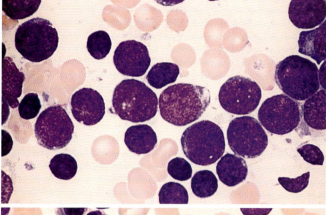

f Another case with some irregular nuclear contours

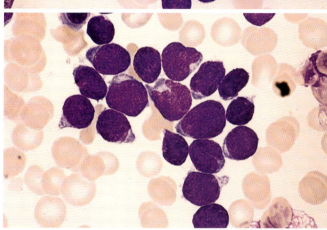

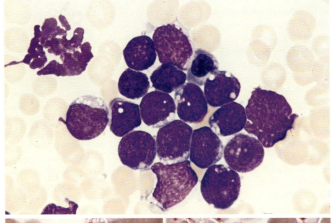

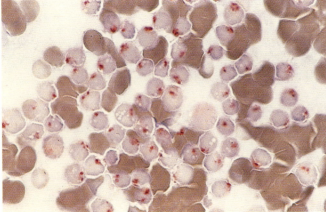

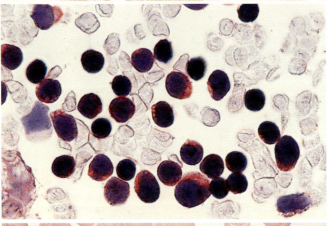

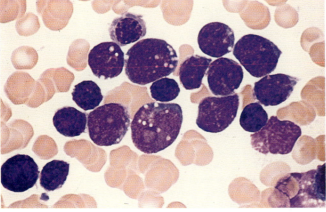

Fig. 122 a – d. T-lineage ALL

a Vacuolation of the cytoplasm may also be observed in T-ALL

b Acid phosphatase reaction at a typical location in the same case

c Detection of CD3 in the same case

d Basophilic cytoplasm and vacuoles in a different case

Fig. 123 a–h. Other morphologic variants of ALL

a "Hand-mirror" form with a handle-like extension of the cytoplasm. This morphologic subtype of ALL has no special significance but is shown to avoid confusion with monoblasts

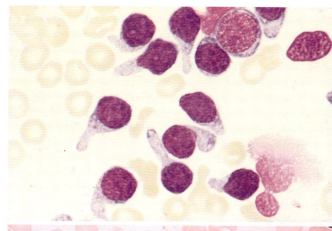

b Different case with fine granules and a hand-mirror configuration of the cytoplasm

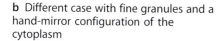

c Detection of CD19 in smears from the same patient

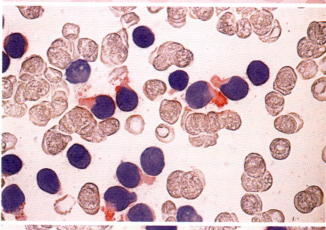

d Detection of CD10 in a smear from the same patient. Findings are consistent with C-ALL

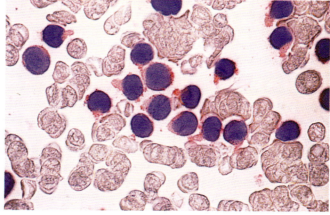

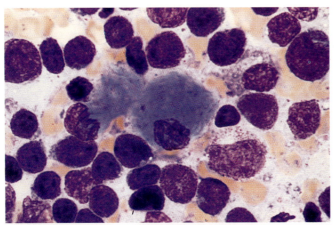

Fig. 123 e–h

e Very rarely, pseudo-Gaucher cells are also found in ALL. This case involves a T-ALL

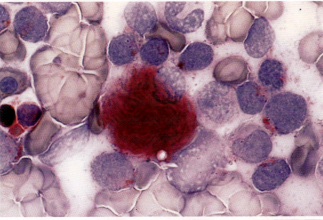

f Acid phosphatase reaction in the same case shows strong activity in the cytoplasm of a pseudo-Gaucher cell and a focal reaction in lymphoblasts

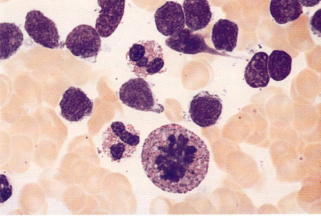

g Increase of eosinophilic granulocytes (two mature forms, one mitosis) in ALL

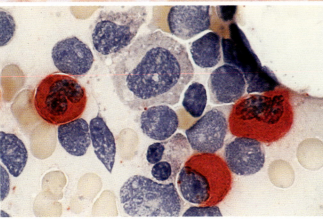

h CE reaction in the same case. The eosinophils are negative, and three neutrophils show a typical positive reaction. It is extremely rare to find increased eosinophils in ALL occurring in association with a (5;14) translocation

Fig. 124 a – g. Acute leukemias involving the lymphatic and granulocytic cell lines (hybrid, biphenotypic, bilinear, mixed lineage). At present there is no established definition for these acute leukemias. The European Group for the Immunological Characterization of Leukemias has proposed a point system to assist in classification [see Bene, MC et al (1995) Proposals for the immunological classification of acute leukemias. European Group for the Immunological Characterization of Leukemias (EGIL). Leukemia. 1995 Oct;9(10):1783 – 1786]. These types of leukemia most commonly occur in early T-ALL with myeloid markers. They also occur in true bilinear forms and occasionally in Philadelphia-positive forms of ALL, which also have a myeloid component

a Lymphatic blasts are interspersed with scattered mature lymphatic cells and large blasts with somewhat pleomorphic nuclei and lighter cytoplasm

b Higher-power view shows reddish granules in the cytoplasm of the larger blasts (lower right of center)

c A number of the large blasts are positive for peroxidase stain, confirming their granulocytic lineage

d The peripheral blood contains very small numbers of mature granulocytes with Auer rods

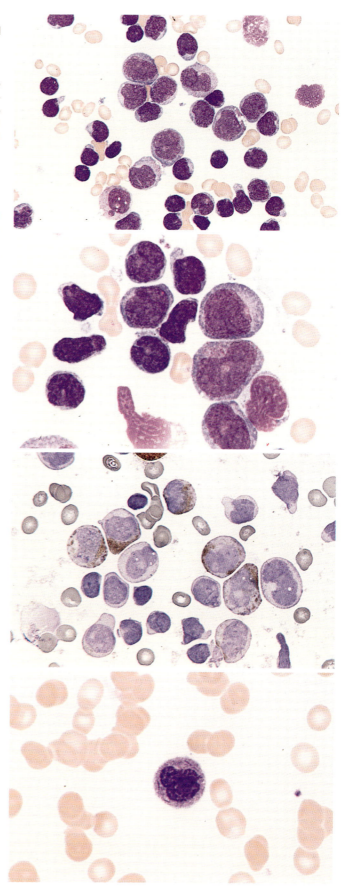

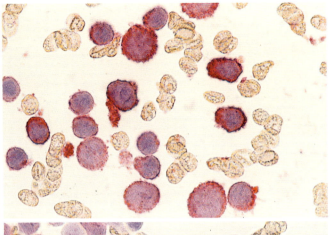

Fig. 124 e–g

e Almost all the blasts express CD13 on immunocytochemical analysis

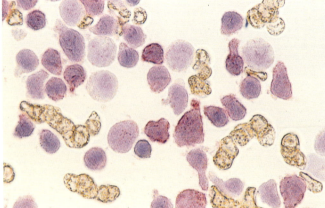

f More than 60 % of the small blasts are CD3–positive. Panels **a** through **f** illustrate the coexistence of T-ALL and AML

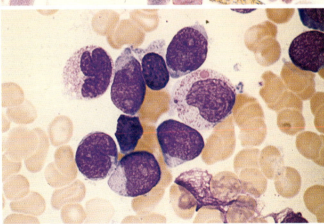

g In another case previously classified as T-ALL, we found myeloid precursors with atypias (*center right*, *upper left*), again demonstrating the involvement of granulocytopoiesis

Fig. 125 a–f. Originally diagnosed as AML, this case was identified by immunocytochemical analysis as bilinear AL with concomitant involvement of the T-ALL and myeloid lines.

a Peripheral blood reveals a blast with a round nucleus and mature granulocytes with Auer rods

b Higher-power view of a granulocyte with multiple Auer rods

c Low-power view of bone marrow shows a predominance of small blasts with round nuclei interspersed with large blasts showing pseudo-Chediak anomaly and splinter-like inclusions (arranged diagonally from *upper left* to *lower right*)

d Numerous fine Auer rods are seen at higher magnification

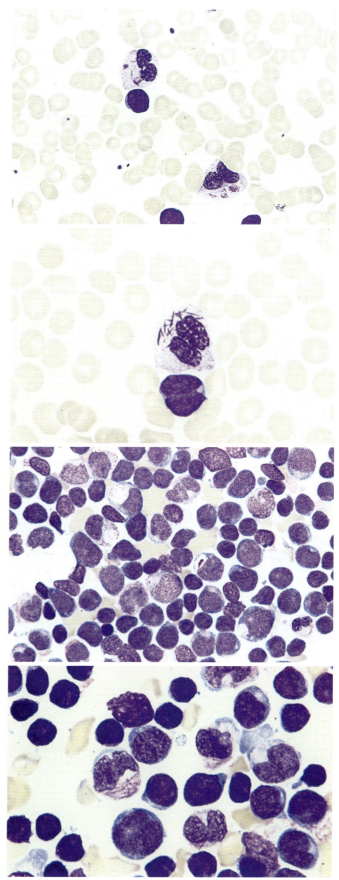

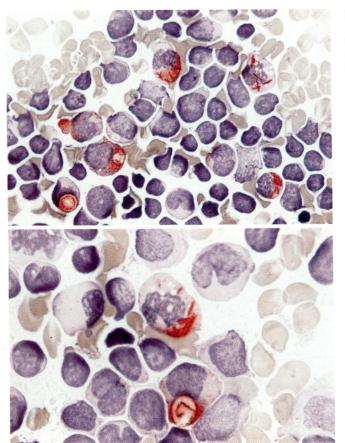

Fig. 125 e–f

e Low-power view of CE reaction. The Auer rods and positive inclusions are clearly demonstrated (red)

f Higher magnification demonstrates Auer rods and, below, inclusions with Auer rods

Fig. 126 a, b. In a case of Ph-positive ALL, severely dysplastic granulocytes are interspersed among the lymphoblasts, again confirming the involvement of granulocytopoiesis. The patient did not have prior therapy. Ph-positive cases of ALL are commonly associated with the coexpression of myeloid markers without detectable morphologic changes in granulocytopoiesis

a, b Marked dysplasia is evident in the maturation of granulocytopoietic precursors

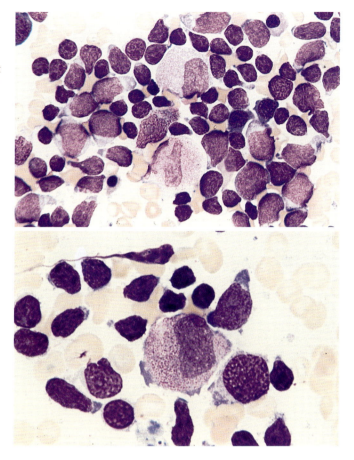

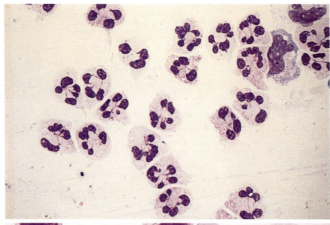

Fig. 127 a–f. CSF cytology in acute leukemias and malignant lymphomas. Samples were cytocentrifuged and Pappenheim-stained

a, b Inflammatory CSF findings for comparison

a CSF in purulent meningitis with neutrophilic leukocytes. A monocyte is visible at *upper right*

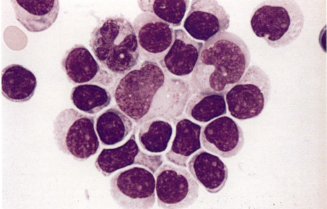

b CSF in viral meningitis. Lymphocyte changes in the CSF are similar to those seen when EDTA-treated blood is stored a long time before smears are prepared

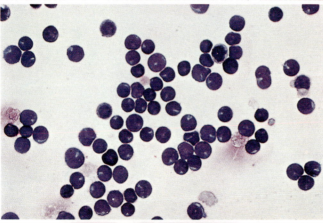

c CSF. Numerous typical lymphoblasts in leukemic meningitis

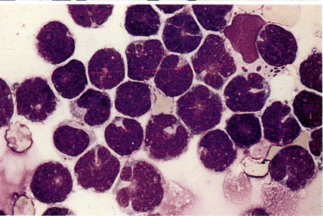

d CSF findings during lymphatic blast crisis in chronic myeloid leukemia

Fig. 127 e–f

e CSF findings in meningeal involvement by follicular lymphoma (cb/cc). Note the highly pleomorphic lymphatic cells and numerous mitoses

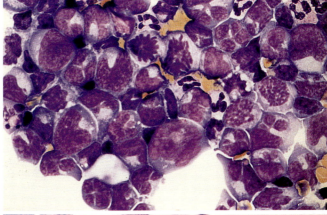

f CSF findings in meningeal involvement by monoblastic leukemia

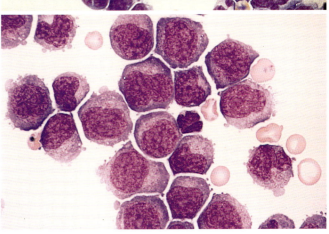

Neoplasias of Tissue Mast Cells (Malignant Mastocytoses)

We can distinguish mature-cell systemic mastocytoses with or without cutaneous involvement (urticaria pigmentosa) from immature-cell and leukemic forms (mast cell leukemias). As with normal mast cell, the tissue mast cells in mature-cell mastocytoses are identified by toluidine blue staining (to detect metachromasia) and by the CE reaction of the granules. As atypias become more pronounced, however, the metachromasia persists while the CE reaction weakens or becomes negative. By contrast, a positive tryptase reaction can be demonstrated both in mature-cell mastocytoses and in atypical immature-type tissue mast cells using immunocytochemical methods[1].

[1] Baghestanian M, Bankl Hc, Sillaber C, Beil WJ, Radaszkiewicz T, Fureder W, Preiser J, Vesely M, Schernthaner G, Lechner K, Valent P (1996) A case of malignant mastocytosis with circulating mast cell precursors: biologic and phenotypic characterization of the malignant clone. Leukemia 10:159–166

Fig. 128 a–d. Neoplasias of tissue mast cells (malignant mastocytoses). Tissue mast cells are positively identified by detecting a metachromatic reaction in the granules. Even with high grades of cellular atypia, it is usually possible to detect at least isolated metachromatic granules. Naphthol AS-D chloroacetate esterase (CE) is present in normal and reactive mast cells and in the mast cells of mature-cell (systemic) mastocytoses. As atypias increase, the enzyme disappears, and often it is no longer detectable when atypias are severe. Tryptase, however, can be detected even in immature malignant mastocytoses. Mature-cell systemic mastocytoses, which may or may not have cutaneous manifestations (urticaria pigmentosa), are distinguishable from immature-cell malignant mastocytoses and leukemic forms (tissue mast cell leukemia)

a Mature-cell mastocytosis in a bone marrow smear from a child. Pappenheim stain

b Toluidine blue stain in the same case shows pronounced metachromasia of the granules

c CE reaction demonstrates very high activity in the tissue mast cells

d Dense infiltration of a bone marrow fragment in the marrow smear of an adult with mature-cell systemic mastocytosis. Toluidine blue stain

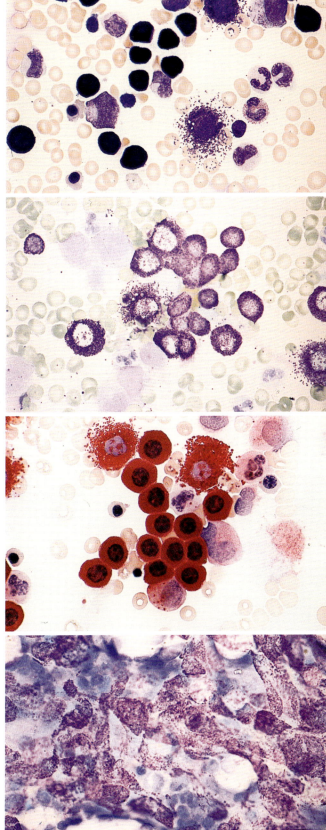

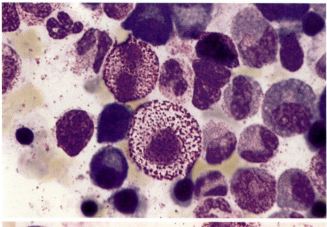

Fig. 129 a–h Malignant mastocytosis

a Immature-cell malignant mastocytosis with very coarse granules

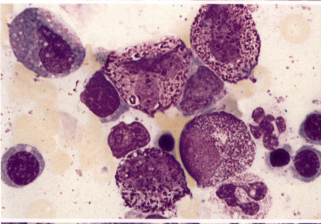

b Same case shows loosely arranged chromatin pattern in the enlarged and irregularly shaped nuclei. Granules are loosely distributed and markedly larger, and some are contained in vacuoles

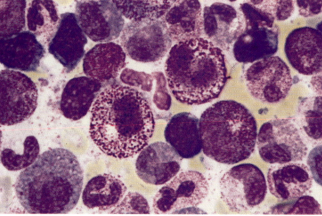

c View of a different site in the same sample

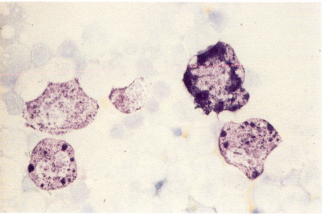

d Toluidine blue stain demonstrates masses of confluent granules

e Toluidine blue stain, higher-power view

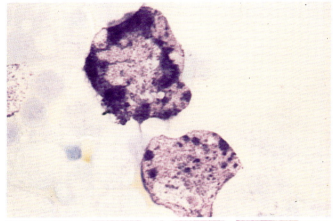

f Different case of malignant mastocytosis with very sparse granules, some localized to the perinuclear area

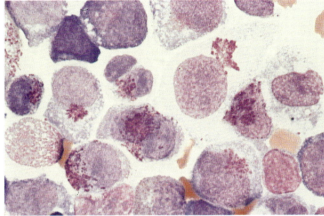

g Loosely scattered granules in the same case

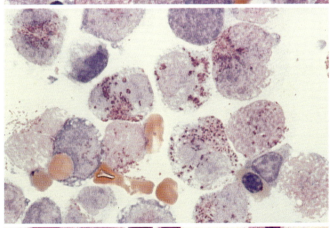

h Granules are visible only in some cells and appear indistinct

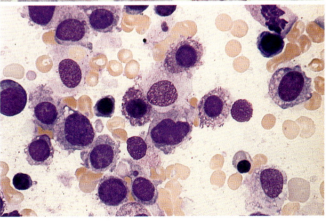

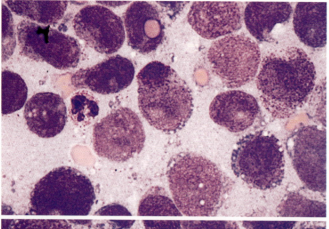

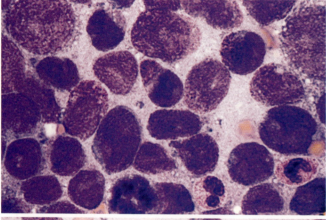

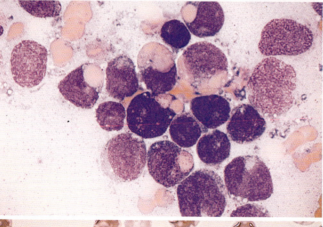

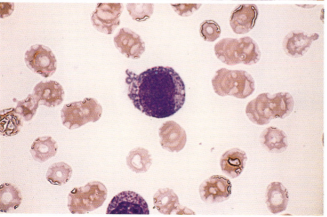

Fig. 130 a – e. Malignant mastocytosis with erythrophagocytosis

a Bone marrow smear shows very immature blasts that contain only a few metachromatic granules mostly localized to the perinuclear zone (*center*)

b Different site in the same bone marrow smear

c Same case, showing a high percentage of "mastoblasts" with erythrophagocytosis

d A mastoblast in the peripheral blood

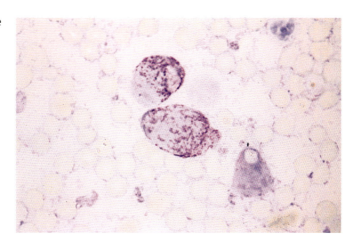

Fig. 130 e Toluidine blue stain of a bone marrow smear from the patient in **a–d**

C. Lymph Nodes and Spleen

An accurate diagnosis requires considerable experience in the interpretation of lymph node aspirates or touch preparations. Above all, the examiner must be familiar with the great morphologic diversity of reactive lymph node changes, and so particular attention is given to these changes in the present chapter. Four main types of cytologic pattern may be seen on the examination of smears prepared from lymph node aspirates (after Theml 1986):

1. A reactive cellular composition without specific cellular elements. Infections are usually causative, and reactive hyperplasia should be suspected.
2. A reactive cellular composition with specific elements, such as a preponderance of epitheloid cells (consistent with sarcoidosis) or Langhans cells (consistent with tuberculous lymphadenitis). Hodgkin cells and Sternberg cells should raise suspicion of Hodgkin disease.
3. A monotonic picture composed of lymphatic cellular elements. This should raise suspicion of non-Hodgkin lymphoma.
4. Cells extrinsic to the lymph nodes, consistent with a metastatic tumor.

Splenic aspiration has been used as a diagnostic procedure for more than half a century. Its importance has grown in recent decades owing to general improvements in cytologic methods and their expanded use. The procedure is best performed under direct laparoscopic vision or under ultrasound guidance when a percutaneous needle is used (see p. 5). In all cases it is preferable to use the Menghini needle or other thin-gauge needle in order to obtain material for both cytologic and histologic evaluation. The criteria for assessing the benignancy or malignancy of a cytologic smear are the same as in lymph node aspirates. Unfortunately, smear cytology is of little value in a number of conditions that are associated with splenomegaly (e.g., fibroadenia). The counting of splenograms is usually unrewarding.

In all diseases that are associated with lymph node enlargement, a serious effort should be made to supplement the cytologic examination with a histologic diagnosis.

Cytology of Lymph Node and Splenic Aspirates

The great majority of cells in aspirates or touch preparations of normal lymphatic tissue are small to medium-sized mature lymphocytes. These are largely identical to blood lymphocytes and are accompanied by smaller lymphatic cells or earlier precursors of lymphocytopoiesis, which are known collectively as large lymphoid cells. Usually the prevalence of these cells is 10 % or less. They consist of lymphoblasts, immunoblasts, and centroblasts. Small numbers of immature and mature plasma cells are also present. Tissue mast cells, granulocytes, histiocytes, and epitheloid cells are less commonly found. More common are heterogeneous groups called "reticulum cells." Below we shall describe cell types that display characteristic quantitative or qualitative changes during the course of reactive or autonomous lymph node disorders and are therefore helpful in making a diagnosis. Immunocytologic methods are particularly useful in differentiating normal cells of lymphocytopoiesis and their malignant equivalents.

The larger basophilic cells provide an important clue to the function and proliferative behavior of the lymphatic tissue, and they are readily distinguished from the mass of mature lymphocytes in the low-power microscopic field. However, they may show a range of morphologies that make it difficult to differentiate them according to type. The following three cell types are of primary interest:

The *immunoblast* (**Fig. 131 a, left**) can range from 25 to 30 µm in diameter according to its functional state. Normally its cytoplasmic rim is moderately wide and darkly basophilic, appearing broader and lighter when the cell is functionally stimulated. Often several vacuoles are present. The nucleus is usually centered and is round, oval, or slightly indented. It shows a fine reticular chromatin pattern that at times appears almost homogeneous. Usually there are well-defined, irregularly shaped nucleoli of a pale to dark blue color.

The second cell type is somewhat smaller than the immunoblast (approximately 20 μm in diameter). Its cytoplasmic rim is narrow and darkly basophilic. The centrally placed nucleus contrasts sharply with the cytoplasm owing to its pale color, which serves to distinguish the cell from the immunoblast, plasmablast, and lymphoblast. The nuclear chromatin pattern is relatively coarse and meshlike. One or more nucleoli may be visible and tend to be close to the nuclear membrane and of a pale color, especially in histologic sections. These cells (**Fig. 131 a, center**) are identical to the "*centroblasts*" described by Lennert.

Plasmablasts (**Fig. 131 a, right**) are usually somewhat smaller than immunoblasts. Their abundant cytoplasm stains a deep, dark blue. Perinuclear pallor is often found in the more mature forms. One or more cytoplasmic vacuoles are occasionally seen. The nucleus, which is concentrically placed in the younger "proplasmablasts" (= B immunoblast?), migrates closer to the cytoplasmic border as the cell matures, much as in mature plasma cells. The chromatin has a coarse trabecular structure and often appears stippled. Usually the nucleoli are poorly defined by panoptic staining. Plasma cells are described on p. 65, 66, tissue mast cells on p. 41, and epithelioid cells in **Figs. 136 a, d, 137 b, and 138**.

The *lymphoblast* (see **Fig. 131 b, c**) is 15 to 20 μm in diameter and has a relatively narrow and lightly basophilic cytoplasmic rim. The nucleus is centered, coarsely reticular, and contains a pale, medium-sized nucleolus.

The *histiocyte* is a relatively large cell (15–25 μm) whose morphology is frequently ill-defined. It is probably related to the monocyte. Its cytoplasmic rim is pale gray-blue to violet, depending on its functional state, and often contains fine reddish granules. The nuclear structure usually has a coarse, stringy appearance but may be relatively loose. One or more small, deep blue nucleoli are usually present. The cell is rich in enzymes, especially nonspecific esterase. Unlike the "lymphatic" reticulum cells, the histiocyte is peroxidase-positive.

Among the *reticulum cells* of the lymphatic tissue, the interdigitating and dendritic forms appear to play a special role. The *interdigitating reticulum cell* (see **Fig. 132**) is a specific cell of the thymus-dependent region of the lymph node (paracortical and interfollicular regions of the nodes and periarteriolar areas of the spleen). These cells have an irregularly shaped, often bi-

zarre nucleus with a relatively loose, delicate chromatin pattern and small, pale, indistinct nucleoli. The cytoplasm stains very weakly and tends to blend with its surroundings. These cells show an extremely weak acid phosphatase reaction and nonspecific esterase reaction on cytochemical staining (**Fig. 132 c, d**).

Dendritic reticulum cells occur exclusively in germinal centers, primary follicles, and occasionally in the outer follicular zone. Their cytoplasm stains very weakly with panoptic stain and contrasts poorly with its surroundings. The nucleus is oblong and sharply margined with loose, coarsely meshed chromatin and a pale blue nucleolus of moderate size. Cytochemical staining (**Fig 133 a, b**) elicits a weakly positive nonspecific esterase reaction and an apparently negative acid phosphatase reaction.

The remaining reticulum cells are at least partly derived from *histiocytes* and *macrophages*. It is by no means certain, however, that all storage cells are descendants of the monocyte-macrophage system, although this question is not critical to clinical evaluation.

The "*starry sky macrophages*" (**Fig. 134 a – c**) are unique among the macrophages in their morphologic and diagnostic importance. They are thought to be the result of an "ineffective germinal center proliferation" whose production is mediated by the effects of antigens, antibodies, or antigen-antibody complexes. These cells are easily recognized by their size and by the coarse particles (phagocytized nuclear debris) that they contain. They are strongly positive for acid phosphatase and nonspecific esterase (**Fig. 134 b, c**).

Splenic aspirates additionally contain cell forms that are not present in lymph node smears. *Serosa cells* are shed from the single layer of peritoneum that covers the spleen. Besides splenic aspirates, these cells are commonly found in the sediment of aspirated ascitic fluid. They are 20 to 40 μm in diameter and are often grouped in small clusters. Their borders are irregular, and their cytoplasm stains gray-blue to deep blue. The nucleus is often eccentrically positioned. The chromatin is relatively dense and coarse, and two or three bluish nucleoli are often present. Multinucleated forms sometimes occur.

Reactive Lymph Node Hyperplasia

This term may be applied collectively to all morphologic changes that affect lymph nodes, such as the nodes draining an area of infection or nodes responding to other kinds of *immunologic challenge*. While the morphologies of these changes are extremely varied, they are characterized very generally by an increase in the *large basophilic cell forms* described on p. 286. These cells also manifest significant qualitative changes. Typically they increase in size, their cytoplasmic rim widens and often becomes lighter and vacuolated, and the nuclear-cytoplasmic ratio increases. The nucleus enlarges to some degree, and its chromatin pattern appears less dense. Marked enlargement of the nucleoli is often a prominent feature. These changes can result in cells that resemble mononuclear Hodgkin cells (*"Hodgkin-like cells,"* see p. 297. As a rule, storage cells are also increased in size and number. Macrophages dotted with nuclear debris (*"starry sky macrophages,"* see pp. 292–294) are frequently seen as evidence of a follicular lymphatic hyperplasia. Besides the lymphatic cells, increased numbers of *tissue mast cells* and *granulocytes* are found in hyperplastic lymph nodes. The *eosinophils* are often very prominent, although their increase cannot be attributed to any specific pathogenic factors. A lymph node hyperplasia with a particularly marked increase in eosinophils is described as *hyperergic*. This term is appropriate in that the diffuse lymph node enlargement seen in these conditions is merely symptomatic of a severe disorder (probably allergic) that is associated with *hypereosinophilia* in the peripheral blood (see p. 105). These disorders probably belong to the large class of "undefined, abnormal immune reactions," whose best known representative is "immunoblastic lymphadenopathy."[1]

There are few diseases for which smear cytology can establish an etiology. The most important are *tuberculosis* (Langhans giant cells, epitheloid cells, liquefactions Fig. **137 a, b**), *sarcoidosis* (Boeck disease, epitheloid cells, isolated Langhans giant cells Fig. **138 a, b**), and *toxoplasmosis* (epitheloid-cell lymphadenitis of Piringer-Kuchinka, see **Fig. 136 a – d).**

In the examination of cervical lymph node aspirates, an enlarged *branchiogenic cyst* should be considered in the differential diagnosis. The morphologic features of these cysts are highly characteristic. They consist mainly of large epithelial cells with a small, dense, central nucleus and homogeneous cytoplasm. Abundant storage cells and necrotic material are usually seen as well.

---

[1] Lukes RJ, Tindle BH (1971) Immunoblastic lymphadenopathy. A hyperimmune entity resembling Hodgkin's disease. N Engl J Med 292:1–8.

Fig. 131 a – c. Lymph node cytology

a Immunoblast at *left*, two centroblasts at *center*, and a plasmablast at *right*

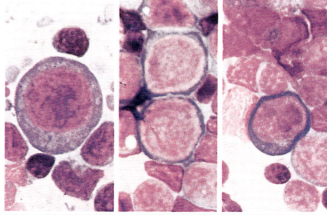

b Immunoblast at *center*, lymphoblast at *top center*

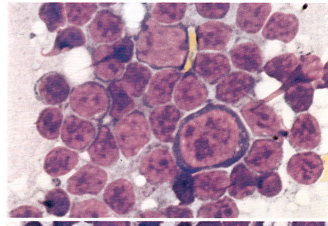

c Plasmablast at *upper left*, lymphoblast at *center*

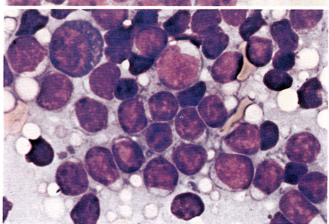

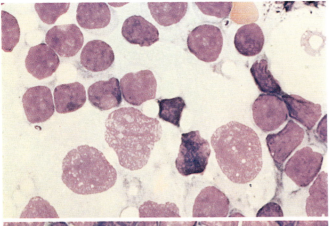

Fig. 132 a–d. Lymph node cytology, interdigitating reticulum cell

a, b Panoptic stain shows typical close relationship of lymphocytes to reticulum cells and their cytoplasmic extensions

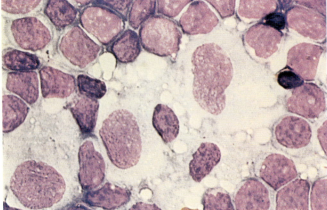

b

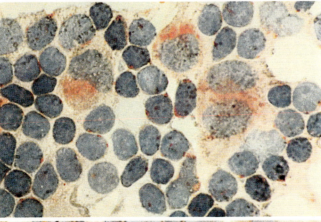

c Acid phosphatase reaction

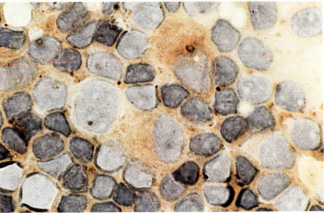

d Nonspecific esterase reaction. (Fig. 132 courtesy of Prof. E. Kaiserling, Tübingen)

Fig. 133 a, b. Lymph node cytology, dendritic reticulum cell

a Panoptic stain

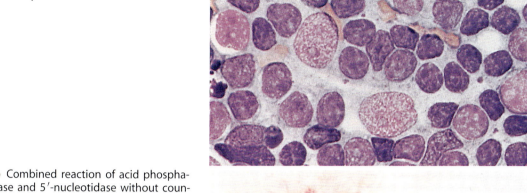

b Combined reaction of acid phosphatase and 5'-nucleotidase without counterstain. Pair of histiocytes at left and right (red reaction product); brown precipitate: dendritic reticulum cell with reaction product of 5'-nucleotidase

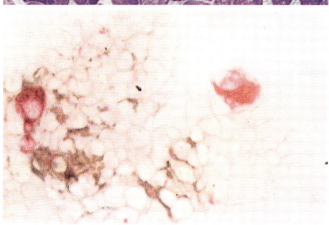

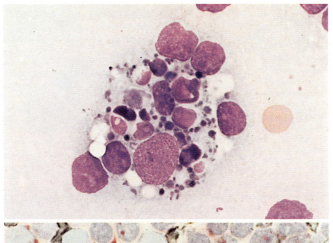

Fig. 134 a – d. Lymph node cytology, storage cells

a Starry sky macrophage (macrophage containing nuclear debris), panoptic stain

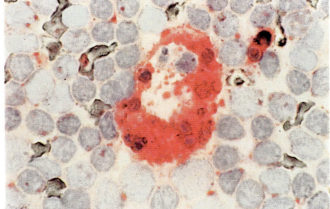

b Starry sky macrophage, acid phosphatase reaction

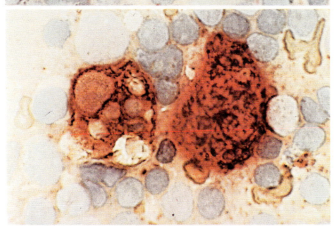

c Two starry sky macrophages, nonspecific esterase reaction. (Fig. 134 a – c courtesy of Prof. E. Kaiserling, Tübingen)

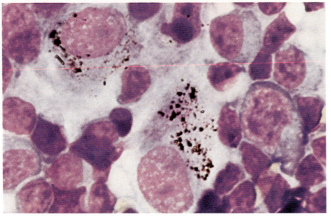

d Two storage cells containing anthracotic material (mediastinal lymph node). Immunoblast at *right*, above it two plasmablasts

Fig. 135 a – d. Lymph node hyperplasia

a Two immunoblasts and an eosinophil in lower half of field

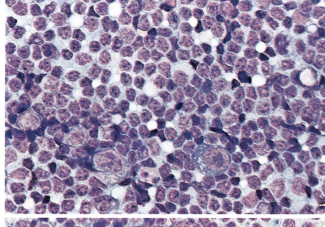

b Plasmablast at *top center*, several plasma cells at bottom, tissue basophil at *left*

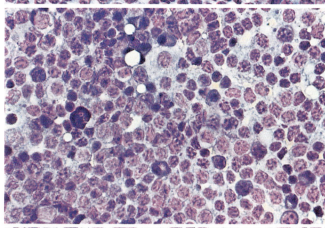

c Starry sky macrophage at *center*, several immunoblasts at *right*

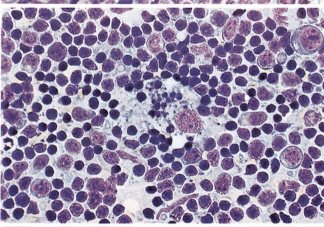

d Immunoblast at *upper left*, above it a centroblast, at *right* a reticulum cell

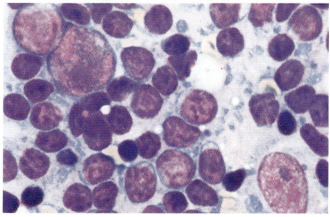

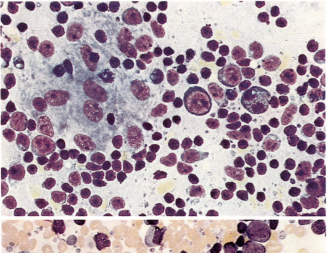

Fig. 136 a–d. Lymph node hyperplasia in toxoplasmosis

a Epitheloid cell lymphadenitis (Piringer-Kuchinka type). Epitheloid cell cluster at *left*, an immunoblast at *center*, to its right a binucleated plasma cell

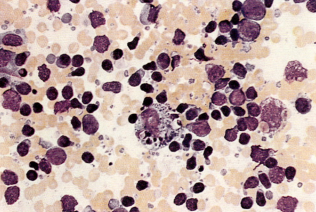

b Starry sky macrophage at *center*

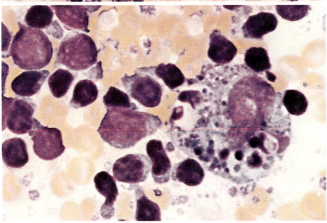

c Starry sky macrophage. Typical specimen with many coarse granular inclusions and cytoplasmic vacuoles

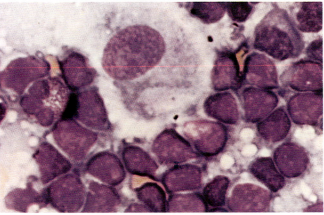

d Epitheloid cell shows typical fine but dense chromatin pattern with one or two blue, sharply defined nucleoli

Fig. 137 a, b. Tuberculous lymphadenitis

a Langhans giant cell

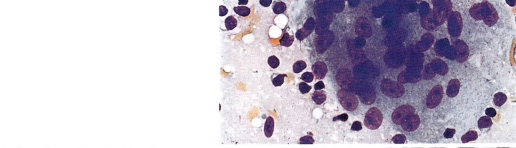

b Syncytium of epitheloid cells

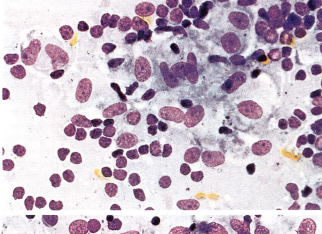

Fig. 138 a, b. Sarcoidosis (Boeck disease), lymph node

a Numerous epitheloid cells resembling a school of fish

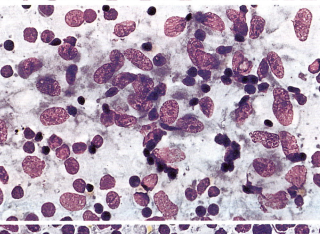

b Epitheloid cells in a "footprint" configuration

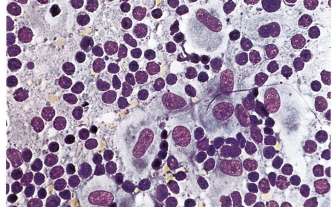

Infectious Mononucleosis

Infectious mononucleosis is caused by the Epstein-Barr virus. *Cytologically* it is the prototype of lymph node hyperplasias of viral etiology. The *clinical* picture may be dominated by lymph node enlargement and splenomegaly or by a pseudo-membranous, lacunar, or ulcerative sore throat. Fever may reach 39 °C and persists for several days or as long as 2 to 3 weeks. Often the fever precedes the onset of glandular swelling. The red blood count is usually normal, and mild anemia is rare. Generally there is a leukocytosis of 10,000 to 15,000/μL, which in rare cases exceeds 50,000/μL. Sporadic cases present with leukocytopenia; this finding plus the pharyngitis can mimic agranulocytosis. Thrombocytopenia is occasionally seen and may be so pronounced that a hemorrhagic diathesis results. The leukocyte distribution is characteristic. Examination of the blood smear shows a predominance of pleomorphic mononucleated cells (60 % – 90 %), which give the disease its name. Morphologically these cells may resemble young lymphocytes or lymphoblasts. Some appear as large blast-like cells with strongly basophilic cytoplasm. A significant increase in monocytes is not observed. Because similar cells can occur in other viral diseases, they have also been referred to as "virocytes" or lymphoid cells. The nuclei are pleomorphic, often kidney-shaped or irregular, and the nuclear chromatin forms a coarse meshwork of loosely arranged strands. One or more nucleoli are usually present. Azurophilic granules are found in some cells, which represent transformed T-lymphocytes. Bone marrow findings are generally non-specific, and thus the changes are typical of infection. The mononuclear elements of the bone marrow may be increased in a few cases, but never to a high degree.

By contrast, large numbers of typical cells are found in lymph node aspirates (**Fig. 139**). The picture is dominated by mononuclear cells very similar or identical to those in the peripheral blood. Once again, cytoplasmic vacuolation is a prominent feature. Particularly striking are the large basophilic cells whose "transformed" state is evidenced by their enlarged, blue-tinged nucleoli. The cytologic changes can even cause confusion with Hodgkin cells ("Hodgkin-like cells"). Isolated epitheloid cells are also found.

The diagnosis of infectious mononucleosis is established by detecting antibodies against the Epstein-Barr virus (EBV). While the rapid tests give a general impression as to whether infectious mononucleosis is present, their capabilities are otherwise limited.

Fig. 139 a–d. Infectious mononucleosis, lymph node

a Marked increase of immunoblasts, macrophage at *lower right*

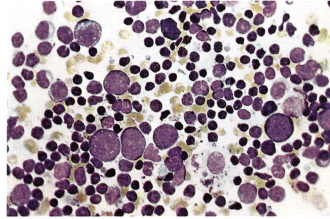

b At *center* an immunoblast, several plasma cells

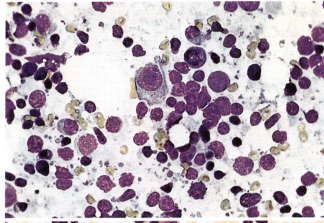

c Various immunoblasts, with several pleomorphic lymphoid cells in lower half of field

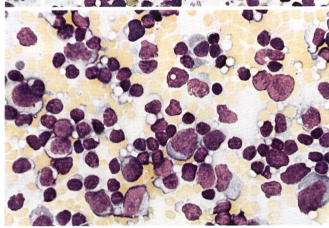

d Two strongly stimulated immunoblasts, Hodgkin-like cells

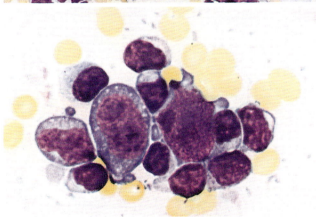

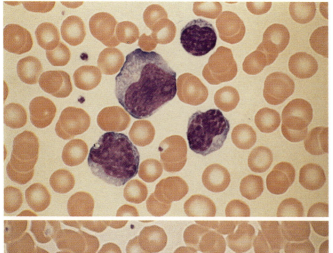

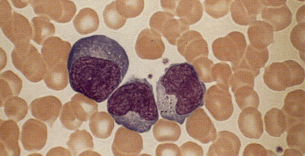

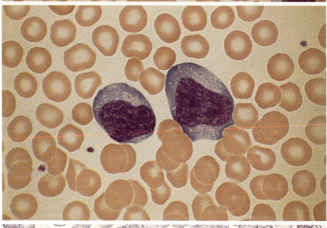

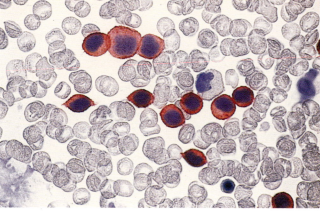

Fig. 140 a–d. Blood smears in infectious mononucleosis

a–c Typical pleomorphic lymphatic cells. Often these cells have irregular nuclear contours and basophilic cytoplasm, and some resemble blasts

b

c

d Detection of CD3, APAAP method. CD3 is detectable in the typical cells of infectious mononucleosis (*red*). These cells represent transformed T lymphocytes

Malignant Non-Hodgkin Lymphomas and Hodgkin Lymphoma

Whereas Hodgkin lymphoma represents a separate entity (with considerable variation in symptoms and prognosis), the malignant non-Hodgkin lymphomas constitute a *heterogeneous* group that are diverse not only in their manifestations, prognosis, and treatment but also in the changing classification schemes that are proposed. **Tables 16** and **18** review the diseases that are included in the class of malignant non-Hodgkin lymphomas. In the text we contrast the most commonly used nomenclatures so that clinicians who do not routinely see these disorders will be better able to cope with the bewildering variety of lymphomas.

The lesions may be broadly categorized as *B-cell or T-cell lymphomas* according to the lineage of the abnormal cells. B-cell lymphomas are more common in Europe and America, while T-cell lymphomas are predominant in Asia (**Table 17**). Lymphomas may be classified by morphologic and clinical criteria as *low-grade malignant* or *high-grade malignant*. Because this classification does not always reflect the true prognosis, it has been necessary to introduce a third subgroup called the *intermediate grade* because its prognosis is intermediate between the low- and high-grade forms.

Despite the fact that all lymphomas cannot be accurately classified by the examination of smears, there are a number of cytomorphologic criteria that allow at least a presumptive diagnosis to be made in most patients. These criteria are illustrated in the figures on the following pages.

Blood and Bone Marrow Involvement in Malignant Non-Hodgkin's Lymphoma (NHL) and Hodgkin's Disease

The present-day diagnosis and classification of malignant NHL is based on the histologic and immunologic examination of extirpated lymph nodes or other affected tissues. As in the acute leukemias, cytogenetic or molecular genetic findings are important or even critical adjuncts in making an accurate classification. Lymph node aspirates have a minor role in primary diagnosis except in cases where, for technical reasons, peripheral lymph nodes cannot be extirpated. On the other hand, diagnostic aspiration is an important adjunct in cases where abdominal or thoracic organs or intra-abdominal lymph nodes can be selectively aspirated under ultrasound or CT guidance. It additionally provides a helpful tool for rapid orientation and follow-up. The bone marrow is also affected in varying degrees, or substantial numbers of leukemic cells may be released into the peripheral blood. This section deals with the involvement of the blood and bone marrow in NHL. Further details may be found by consulting recent publications on the Kiel, Real or WHO classifications. Bone marrow involvement in Hodgkin disease is most readily detected by the histologic examination of biopsy samples and is rarely detectable in aspirate smears. The peripheral blood furnishes only indirect evidence in cases where lymphopenia or, rarely, eosinophilia is present. Our nomenclature is based upon the revised Kiel and Real classifications.

Suggested Further Reading

Schwarze EW (1986) Non-Hodgkin's Lymphoma. Cytology und Cytochemistry. G. Fischer, Stuttgart New York

Table 16. Low-grade non-Hodgkin lymphomas

B cell lineage
Chronic lymphocytic leukemia (B-CLL)
Lymphoplasmacytic immunocytoma (Waldenström macroglobulinemia)
Chronic lymphocytic leukemia/prolymphocytic leukemia (CLL/PLL)
(Atypical CLL)
Prolymphocytic leukemia (B-PLL)
Hairy cell leukemia (HCL)
Hairy cell leukemia variant (HCL-V)
Splenic lymphoma with villous lymphocytes (SLVL)
Follicular lymphoma (cb/cc = FL)
Mantle cell lymphoma (centrocytic lymphoma; MCL)

T cell lineage
Large granulated lymphocyte leukemia/lymphocytosis (LGL)
Prolymphocytic leukemia (T-PLL)
Sézary syndrome/mycosis fungoides (SS/MF)
Adult T-cell leukemia/lymphoma (ATLL)
Other peripheral T-cell lymphomas

Table 17. Immune markers in leukemic forms of low-grade non-Hodgkin lymphoma

Marker	B-CLL	B-PLL	HCL	FL	MCL	SLVL	T-CLL/LGL	SS	T-PLL	ATLL
S Ig	(+)	++	++	++	++	++	−	−	−	−	−
CD2	−	−	−	−	−	−	+	+	+	+	+
CD3	−	−	−	−	−	−	+	−	+	+	+
CD4	−	−	−	−	−	−	−	+	+/−	+
CD5	++	−	−	−	+	−	−	−	+	+	+
CD7	−	−	−	−	−	−	−	−	+/−	+	−/+
CD8	−	−	−	−	−	−	+	+/−	+/−	+/−	+/−
CD19/20/24	++	++	++	+	+	++	−	−	−	−	−
CD22	+/−	++	++	+	+	++	−	−	−	−	−
CD10	−	−	−	+/−	−	−	−	−	−	−	−
CD25	−	−	++	−	−	+/−	−	−	−	−	++
CD56	−	−	−	−	−	−	+	−	−	−	−
CD103	−	−	++	−	−	−	−	−	−	−	−
HL-DR	++	++	++	++	++	++	−	−	−	−	−

− = negative; (+) = weakly positive; + = positive; ++ = markedly positive; +++ = strongly positive; +/− = majority of cases positive; − /+ = majority of cases negative. CLL, chronic lymphocytic leukemia; PLL, prolymphocytic leukemia; HCL, hairy cell leukemia; FL, follicular lymphoma; MCL, mantle cell lymphoma; SLVL, splenic lymphoma with villous lymphocytes; LGL, large granulated lymphocyte leukemia; SS, Sézary syndrome; ATLL, adult T-cell leukemia/lymphoma

Low- and Intermediate-Grade Malignant Non-Hodgkin's Lymphomas (Tables 16 and 17)

Chronic Lymphocytic Leukemia (Chronic Lymphadenosis, CLL)

CLL is a chronic disease characterized by hematologic changes, multiple or generalized lymph node enlargement, splenomegaly, and frequent hepatomegaly. It predominantly affects older individuals. Peripheral blood examination usually reveals a leukocytosis with a strong preponderance of lymphocytes. Most of the cells appear morphologically as *small, mature lymphocytes* with a dense, coarse nuclear structure. Nucleoli are found only in a few "immature" cells. The cytoplasmic rim is narrow with a medium blue coloration. *Gumprecht shadows* or "smudge cells" (**Fig. 141 a–c**) is the term applied to crushed cells that, while often present in B-CLL, are not specific for that disease. A large percentage of the lymphocytes show marked, usually fine to moderate PAS granulations on cytochemical staining (**Fig. 141 f**). Small lymphocytes also predominate in the bone marrow (**Fig. 141 d**), lymph nodes, and spleen. Granulocytopoiesis, erythropoiesis, and thrombocytopoiesis are quantitatively depressed in the bone marrow, resulting in a progressive anemia, absolute granulocytopenia, and thrombocytopenia with their associated effects (which could also result from autoantibodies). The depletion of normal B-lineage cells from the bone marrow and lymph nodes almost always produces an increasing hypogammaglobulinemia that may culminate in an antibody deficiency syndrome.

The lymphocytes of CLL have B-cell properties (B-CLL) in the majority of cases seen in Europe and America. The existence of a T-CLL is controversial. The mature-cell type of T-cell leukemia or NK-cell leukemia is referred to as LGL (large granulated lymphocyte) leukemia or T-cell lymphocytosis. It is characterized by neutropenia and a chronic course. The abnormal cells have fine to medium-sized azurophilic granules in their cytoplasm and should be further identified by immunologic or molecular genetic criteria. T-cell leukemias (except for T-ALL) are classified mainly as T-cell prolymphocytic leukemias. The cells are frequently small and thus may be mistaken for the cells of B-CLL in improperly prepared smears. Most have nucleoli, however, and some have an irregular nuclear contour. A variant with a broader cytoplasmic rim and sharply defined vesicular nucleoli resembles B-cell prolymphocytic leukemia. Immunophenotyping is essential. The other leukemic forms of NHL are described in the figure legends.

Either of two staging systems may be used for evaluating the course of CLL and planning therapy:

1. Staging system of Rai et al.:

Stage 0: Blood lymphocytosis < 15,000/µL, bone marrow infiltration
Stage I: Stage 0 plus enlarged lymph nodes
Stage II: 0 with or without I, plus hepatomegaly and/or splenomegaly
Stage III: 0 with or without I and II, plus anemia (Hb < 11g%)
Stage IV: 0 with or without I–III, plus thrombocytopenia (<100,000/µL)

2. Staging system of Binet:
A. Lymphocytosis > 4000/µL,
   bone marrow infiltration > 40 %,
   hemoglobin > 10 g/dL,
   platelets > 100,000/µL,
   two lymph node regions involved (enlarged)
B. Same as stage A,
   plus enlargement of at least three
   lymph node regions
C. Same as A,
   plus anemia (Hb<10 g/dL) and/or
   thrombocytopenia <100,000/µL,
   with involvement of any number
   of lymph node regions

Immunocytoma (IC)

In the Kiel classification, this group of low-grade non-Hodgkin lymphomas includes lymphoplasmocytoid and lymphoplasmacytic immunocytoma. Cases that are CD5–positive on immunologic testing are presently classified as a form of B-CLL, whereas CD5-negative cases, often associated with an IgM type of monoclonal gammopathy and featuring lymphatic cells transitional with plasma cells, are classified as Waldenström disease. To date, no specific cytogenetic or molecular abnormalities have been described. The abnormal cell forms range from small lymphocytes to plasma cells. Bone marrow examination sometimes shows an increase in tissue mast cells (**Fig. 142 d, h**).

Prolymphocytic Leukemias

Prolymphocytic leukemias can be classified phenotypically as having a B-cell or T-cell lineage. B-cell prolymphocytic leukemia (B-PLL) is diagnosed if at least 55 % prolymphocytes are found on examination of the peripheral blood. These cells are larger than lymphocytes, have a broader cytoplasmic rim, and a round nucleus with a well-defined, vesicular nucleolus that is usually centered within the nucleus. Generally the leukocyte count is greatly elevated. Splenomegaly is present but there is little or no lymph node enlargement. Immunophenotypic analysis shows strong expression of the surface immunoglobulin (SJg). The B-cell markers CD19, CD20, CD24, and CD22 are markedly positive, FMC7 is positive, and CD5 is negative. No specific cytogenetic aberrations are known (**Fig. 150**).

T-cell prolymphocytic leukemia (T-PLL) is also associated with an elevated leukocyte count and splenomegaly. In contrast to B-PLL, however, lymph node enlargement is usually present and is sometimes accompanied by cutaneous infiltrates and effusions. The cells resemble those of B-PLL in approximately 50 % of cases but usually show an irregular nuclear contour. In other cases the cells are smaller and have a narrower and markedly basophilic cytoplasmic rim. In approximately one-third of cases the nucleoli are difficult to detect with light microscopy but are clearly defined by electron microscopy. At one time such cases were frequently diagnosed as T-CLL, and indeed there are sporadic cases that do not display the features of LGL leukemia and must be classified as T-CLL. The T-cell markers CD2, CD3, CD5, and CD7 are positive on immunophenotypic analysis. CD4 and the T-cell receptor are positive in more than 50 % of cases, and CD8 is rarely detectable.

Cytogenetic analysis frequently demonstrates an inv(14) or trisomy 8q (**Figs. 157, 158**).

Mantle Cell Lymphoma (MCL)

This lymphomatous disease was previously recognized by the Kiel group as a separate entity ("centrocytic lymphoma") because of its poor prognosis, but the entity was accepted internationally only after the cytogenetic detection of the (11;14) translocation (**Fig. 151 f**). The abnormal cells are derived from the mantle zone of the lymphoid follicle and require differentiation from true follicular cells (from the center of the follicle). They may equal or greatly surpass lymphocytes in size. The smaller cells usually have an irregular nuclear contour but are sometimes difficult to distinguish from the cells of CLL; even the immunologic detection of CD5 and standard B-cell markers cannot provide reliable differentiation. These cases are diagnosed by using cytogenetic analysis or the FISH technique to detect the (11;14) translocation. The variant with larger and sometimes anaplastic cells is identified by a conspicuous pleomorphism of nuclear contours and a very coarse ("rocky") chromatin pattern (**Fig. 151**).

Centroblastic-Centrocytic Lymphoma (Low-Grade Follicular Lymphoma)

The cells of centroblastic-centrocytic lymphoma are derived from the center of the follicle. Mature lymphatic forms predominate, and blasts are rarely observed in blood and bone marrow smears. Deep nuclear clefts are typically found in the more mature forms and may almost completely divide the nucleus ("cleaved cell," **Fig. 152 e**). Additionally there are cells with round nuclei and isolated blasts. Cytogenetic analysis reveals a t(14;18) in approximately 70 % of cases, and molecular analysis shows the hyperexpression of bcl-2. The t(14;18) can be detected with high sensitivity by FISH and PCR and therefore makes a useful differentiating criterion. On immunophenotyping, the cells of low-grade follicular lymphoma may express CD10 in addition to standard B-cell markers. CD5 is negative.

Hairy Cell Leukemia (HCL)

Hairy cell leukemia is always associated with splenomegaly, which tends to progress slowly during the course of the disease. Lymph node enlargement is usually absent. Most cases present hematologically with leukopenia, neutropenia, and typically with monocytopenia. Lymphocytes and only small numbers of hairy cells are found in blood films (**Fig. 144 a**). The hairy cells are roughly the size of lymphocytes or slightly larger. The grayish-blue cytoplasm appears finely honeycombed and has irregular borders with typical hairlike projections that give this disease its name. Other cells may present denser, pseudopod-like cytoplasmic extensions. Azurophilic granules are occasionally present in the cytoplasm. The nucleus is usually oval, and its chromatin is finer than in lymphocytes (**Figs. 144– 146**). A single, small nucleolus is rarely present. Cytochemical staining demonstrates a strong acid phosphatase activity that is not inhibited by tartrate (see method on p. 14). This is due to the presence of isoenzyme 5 in the hairy cells (**Fig. 147 a–d**). When these cells are seen in the bone marrow, which may be difficult or impossible to aspirate (dry tap), they are frequently arranged in clusters. If a dry tap is obtained, a core biopsy is necessary for a definitive diagnosis (**Fig. 146 c – e**). The hairy cells are a special variant of the B-lymphocyte line that have a typical immunophenotype. They express the standard B-cell markers in addition to CD11c and CD103. Besides typical hairy cell leukemia, there is a variant (HCL-V) characterized by elevated white cell counts in the peripheral blood. In contrast to typical HCL, a decrease in monocytes is usually not observed. Most of the cells have a broader and more basophilic cytoplasm than the typical hairy cells. Their denser nuclear chromatin and distinct nucleoli create a picture that resembles the nuclei in B-PLL. Tartrate-resistance acid phosphatase is usually absent (**Fig. 148**).

Table 18. High-grade non-Hodgkin lymphoma according to the Revised European American Lymphoma (REAL) classification

B-cell type	Diffuse, large cell (Centroblastic) (Immunoblastic) Burkitt Burkitt-like Primary mediastinal, large-cell, B-cell lymphoma[a] Anaplastic B-cell lymphoma
T-cell type	Peripheral T-cell lymphoma, unspecified Anaplastic, large-cell, T-cell lymphoma

[a] In accordance with the recommendation of the WHO, in diffuse, large-cell, B-cell lymphomas, an additional distinction is drawn between an intravascular and a primary effusion lymphoma (in the HIV infected).

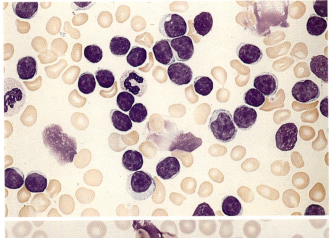

Figs. 141–152. Low-grade and intermediate non-Hodgkin lymphomas

Fig. 141 a–f. Chronic lymphocytic leukemia of B lineage (B-CLL)

a–c Peripheral blood smears show predominantly mature lymphocytes, some with a clumped chromatin pattern (**c**). Occasional crushed nuclei (Gumprecht nuclear shadows) are seen

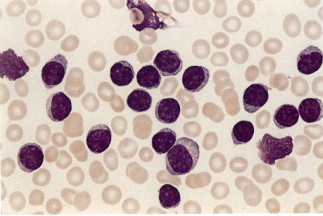

b

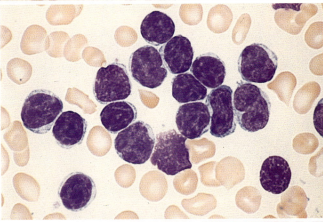

c

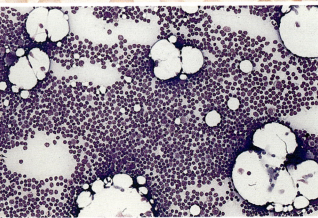

d Bone marrow smear in B-CLL, with diffuse infiltration of the bone marrow

Fig. 141 e–f

e Bone marrow smear from the same patient. Immunocytochemical detection of CD5. All the lymphocytes are positive (*red*) – a characteristic feature of B-CLL. Standard B-lineage markers are also found

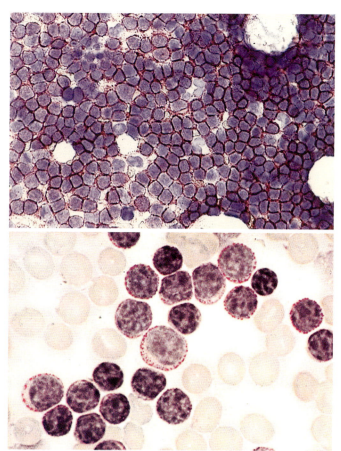

f Peripheral blood, PAS reaction. Numerous cells show a strong, finely granular PAS reaction

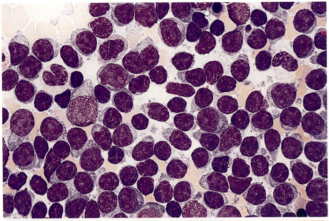

Fig. 142 a–h

a Cellular pleomorphism is greater than in Fig. 141, and there are scattered younger forms with well-defined nucleoli. This is an atypical form of CLL (formerly classified as immunocytoma)

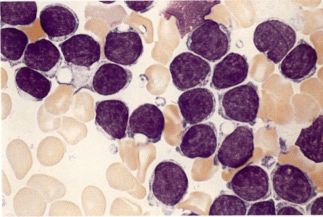

b Different case with vacuoles in the cytoplasm

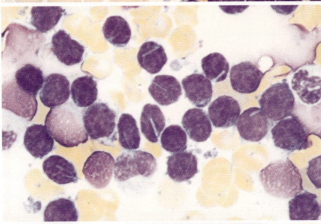

c Different case with rod-shaped crystalline inclusions in the cytoplasm

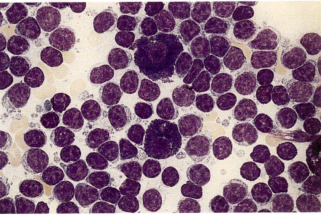

d Two mature tissue mast cells surrounded by lymphocytes, which often have a somewhat broader and more basophilic cytoplasm. Similar findings are seen in Waldenström disease

Fig. 142 e – h

e, f Filiform, spaghetti-like inclusions in the cytoplasm

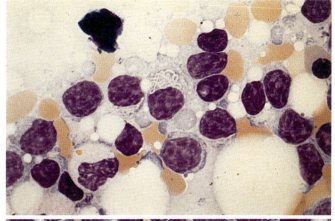

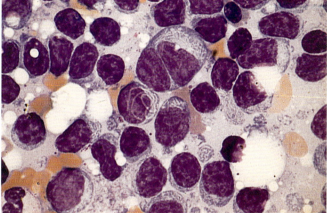

g Different case with markedly broader and more basophilic cytoplasm suggestive of immunocytoma (marginal cell lymphoma?)

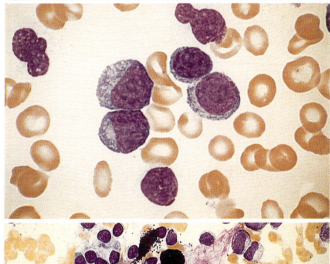

h Bone marrow smear showing granuloma-like infiltration and five tissue mast cells. Sample from a patient with Waldenström disease

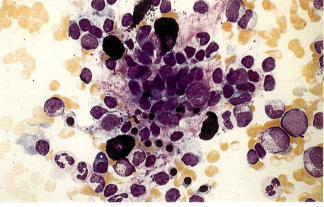

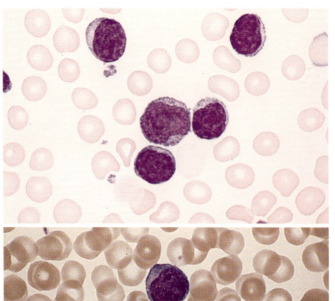

Fig. 143 a – d. Transitional form of CLL/PLL or atypical CLL

a Besides small lymphocytes, there are more than 10 % prolymphocytes with distinct nucleoli

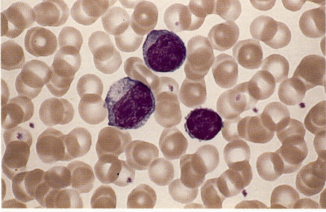

b Larger cells with broader, basophilic cytoplasm

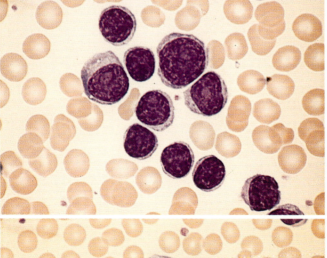

c Different case with small lymphocytes and larger lymphocytes containing a distinct nucleolus (prolymphocytes)

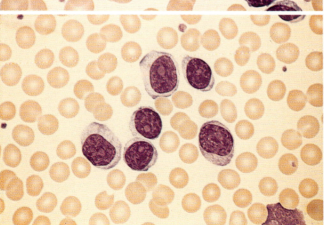

d Different site in smear **c**. Here all the cells have nucleoli, showing that the distribution of cells in a smear can be very heterogeneous

Fig. 144 a – g. Hairy cell leukemia (HCL)

a Typical hairy cell, shown with a normal lymphocyte for comparison

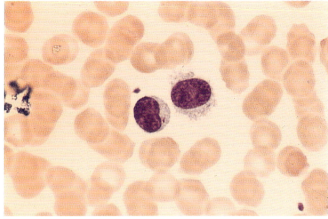

b Hairy cell with abundant, agranular, very "hairy" cytoplasm

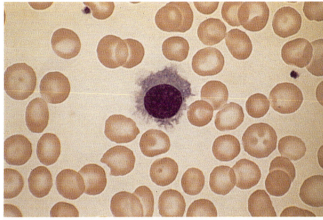

c More hairy cells with abundant cytoplasm, which has a shredded appearance

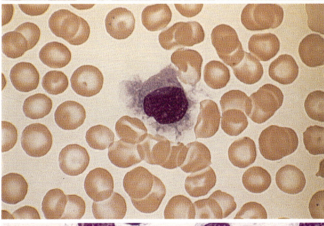

d Exceptionally cellular bone marrow smear in HCL. The nuclear indentation at *center* is not unusual. The cytoplasm shows a fine honeycomb structure

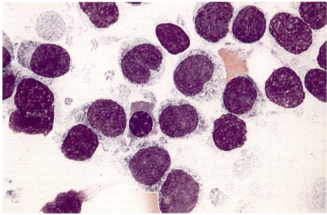

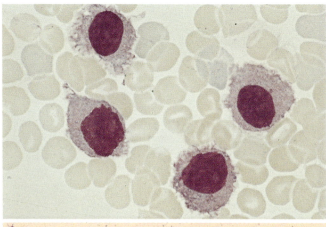

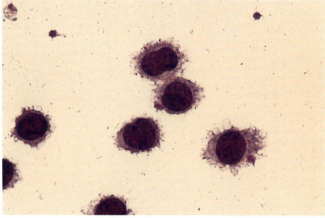

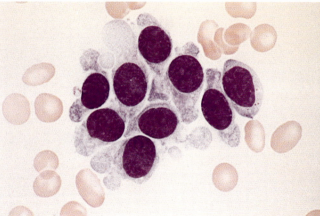

Fig. 144 e–g

e Large-cell type of HCL with abundant cytoplasm

f Very conspicuous "hairs" are seen in the leukocyte concentrate from a different case

g Different case with a broad, smooth cytoplasmic rim

Fig. 145 a, b. Hairy cell leukemia. The cytoplasm contains pale, streaklike, relatively well-defined structures corresponding to the ribosome-lamellar complex (RLC) seen on electron microscopy (*upper left* in **b**)

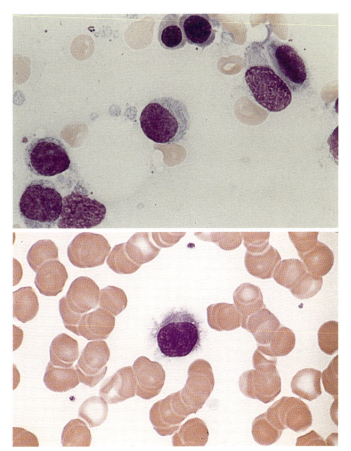

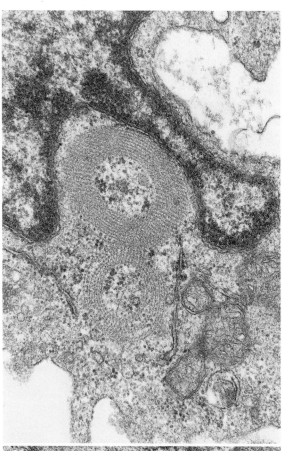

Fig. 145 c, d. Electron microscopic appearance of the RLC, whose light microscopic equivalent is shown in a and b.

c RLC in cross section

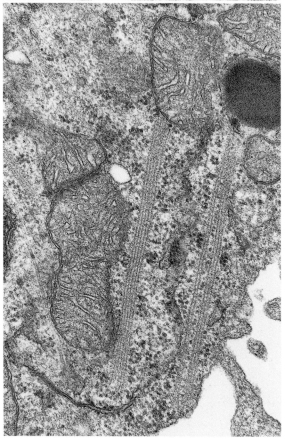

d RLC in longitudinal section. The parallel structures are each composed of five lines. (**Fig. 145 c, d** courtesy of Prof. F. Gudat, Institute of Pathology, Basel)

Fig. 146 a – d. Hairy cell leukemia

a Unusual nuclear form ("flower cell") not normally seen in HCL. Typical hairy cells were found elsewhere in the sample

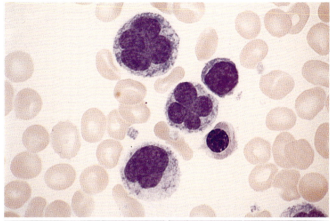

b Bone marrow smear in HCL shows loosely arranged nuclei of hairy cells and interspersed tissue mast cells (violet "blotches")

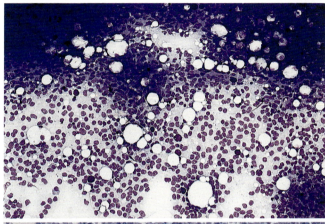

c Bone marrow section, Giemsa stain. The loose arrangement of the hairy cells contrasts with the dense arrangement seen in B-CLL

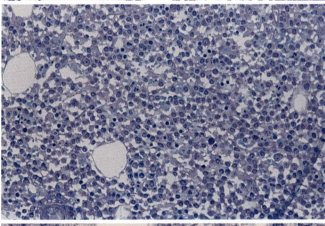

d Higher-power view of an isolated hairy cell at the *center* of the field. Below it is a tissue mast cell

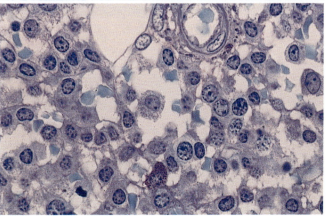

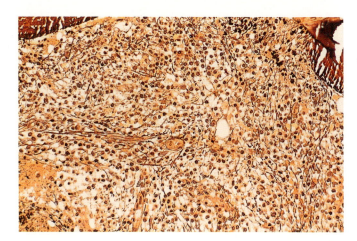

Fig. 146 e. Appearance of reticular fibers in histologic section. Note how the hairy cells are trapped in the reticular fiber meshwork. This explains the generally poor aspirability of the bone marrow (dry tap)

Fig. 147 a–g. Cytochemistry and immunocytochemistry of HCL

a Tartrate-resistant acid phosphatase (TRAP) activity in three hairy cells

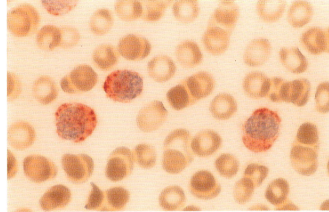

b Different smear shows varying degrees of positive TRAP staining

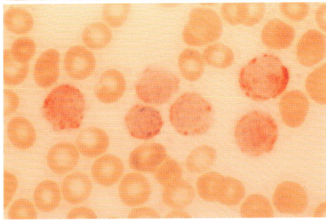

c TRAP in bone marrow from a different patient. Neutrophils and lymphocytes are negative

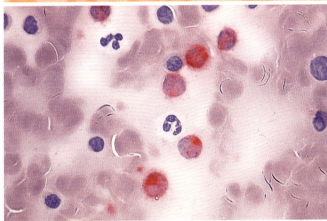

d TRAP demonstrated by a different technique (Sigma)

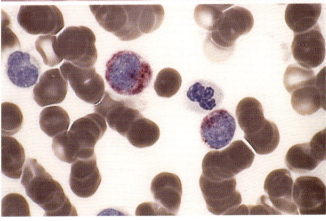

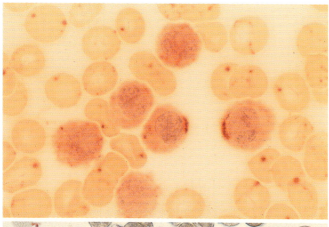

Fig. 147 e–g.

e Esterase reaction (pH 7.4) shows weakly diffuse and polar-cap patterns of activity

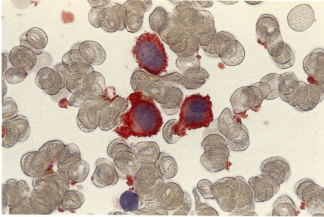

f Immunocytochemical detection of CD11c

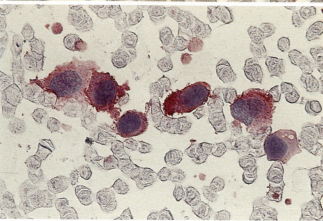

g Immunocytochemical detection of CD103. APAAP technique

Fig. 148a – d. Variant of hairy cell leukemia (HCL-V). This is another B-lineage
form, usually associated with marked
leukocytosis. The nuclear structure resembles that of prolymphocytes with
nucleoli, but the cytoplasm is somewhat
less "hairy" than in typical HCL

a, b Typical cells of HCL-V with small,
distinct nucleoli

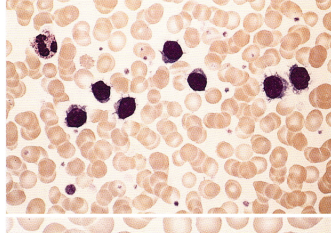

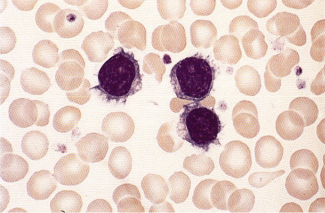

c A lymphocyte with granules appears
among the abnormal cells

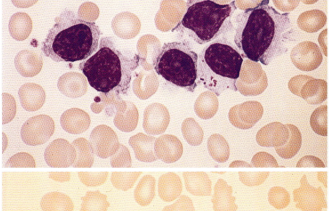

d Different case of HCL-V

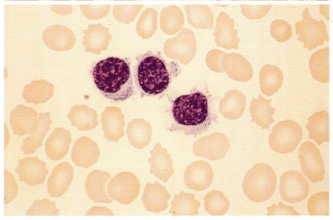

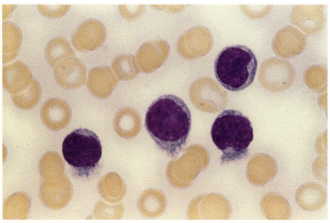

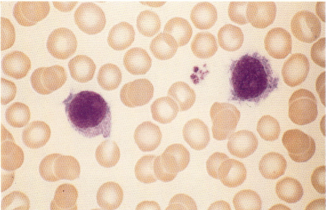

Fig. 149 a, b. Splenic lymphoma with villous lymphocytes (SLVL). The cells in the blood smear are more variegated than in HCL. The nuclei usually have a distinct nucleolus and sometimes resemble the nuclei of B-cell prolymphocytic leukemia. The cytoplasm shows variable basophilia. Cytoplasmic irregularities ("hairs") at one pole of the cell are characteristic. SLVL probably belongs to the class of marginal cell lymphomas

Panels **a** and **b** show typical samples of peripheral blood

Fig. 150 a–e. B-cell prolymphocytic leukemia. The cells are larger than lymphocytes and have round nuclei with distinct, usually sharply circumscribed nucleoli

a Typical prolymphocytes with well-defined nucleoli

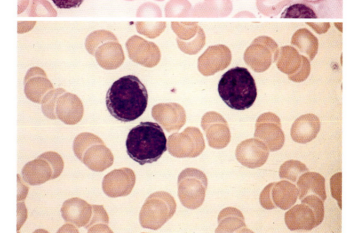

b Peripheral blood in a different case

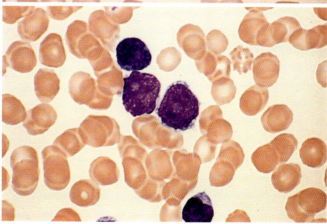

c Different case showing two typical prolymphocytes and one lymphocyte

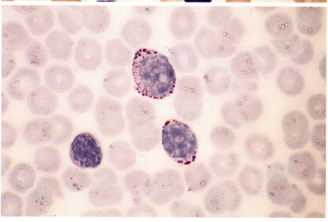

d PAS reaction shows relatively coarse granules in the cytoplasm, similar to those in ALL. Therefore this reaction is not useful for distinguishing B-PLL from ALL

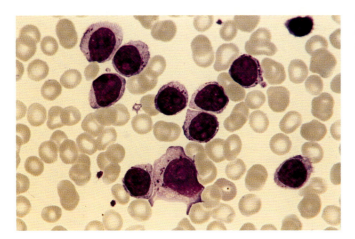

Fig. 150 e. Extremely unusual case with coarse azurophilic granules in the cytoplasm. Definite B-cell markers could be detected immunologically

Fig. 151 a–e. Mantle cell lymphoma. Called centrocytic lymphoma in the Kiel classification, this disease has a poor prognosis. It differs from the follicular lymphomas and other low-grade lymphomas by the (11;14) translocation and can also be identified by molecular genetic testing. CD5 is detected on immunocytochemical analysis; this can make mantle cell lymphoma difficult to distinguish from B-CLL, especially when the cells are very small. Morphologically, the cells often have somewhat irregular nuclei, dense chromatin, and scant cytoplasm. Less mature forms with distinct nucleoli are sometimes difficult to distinguish from blasts. There are also highly pleomorphic forms with clefted, "rocky"-appearing nuclear chromatin

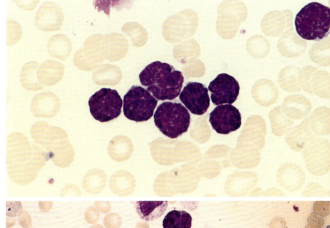

a Very small cell type with an irregular nuclear contour

b Bone marrow smear in a different case

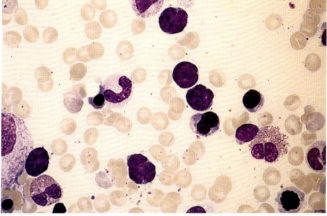

c Bone marrow from another case shows multiple nuclear indentations

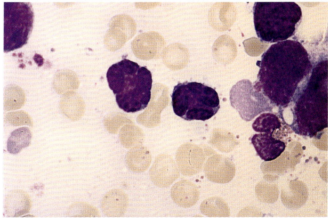

d Bone marrow from another case shows a high degree of nuclear pleomorphism

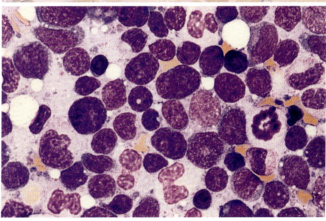

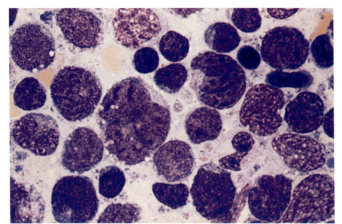

Fig. 151 e–f

e Higher-power view of the case in **d** shows relatively large cells with a clefted chromatin pattern

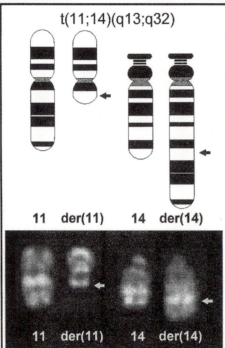

t(11;14)(q13;q32)

11   der(11)   14   der(14)

11   der(11)   14   der(14)

f Schematic diagram and partial karyotype of the translocation t(11;14)(q13;q32), which is found in mantle cell lymphoma. The *arrows* indicate the breakpoints

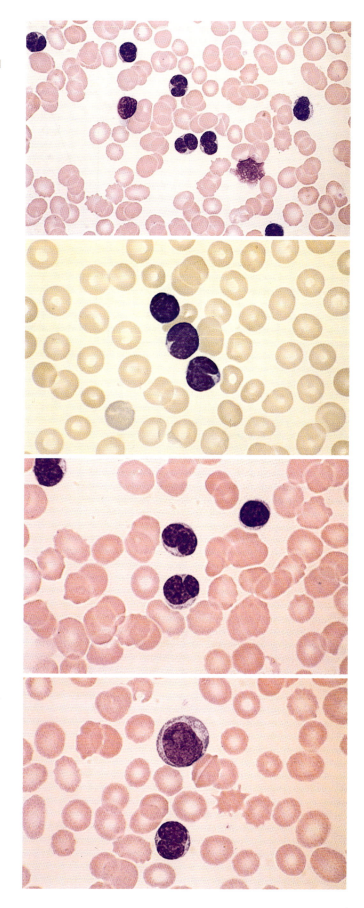

Fig. 152 a–e. Low-grade follicular lymphoma (cb/cc)

a–c Typical cases with singly notched nuclei and small cells

d A centroblast. Centroblasts are an extremely rare finding in blood smears

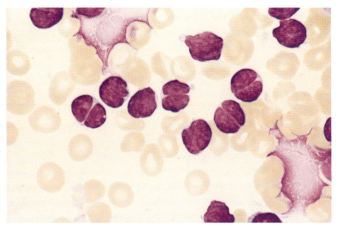

Fig. 152 e–f

e Deeply clefted nuclei in follicular lymphoma

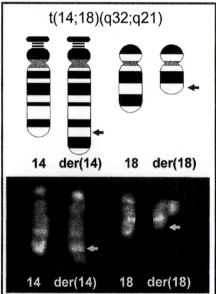

t(14;18)(q32;q21)

14   der(14)   18   der(18)

14   der(14)   18   der(18)

f Schematic diagram and partial karyotype of the translocation t(14;18)(q32;q21), which is found in centroblastic-centrocytic and centroblastic lymphomas. *Arrows* indicate the breakpoints

Sézary Syndrome

Sézary syndrome is a cutaneous T-cell lymphoma that is closely related to mycosis fungoides. It presents clinically with diffuse erythroderma, and typical histologic skin changes are observed. Highly characteristic T lymphocytes called Sézary cells are found in the peripheral blood. These cells range from the size of lymphocytes to the approximate size of monocytes. They have scant, lightly basophilic cytoplasm, and the typically oval nucleus shows a pathognomonic morphology. When seen in blood smears, the nucleus appears permeated by fine furrows caused by highly convoluted nuclear folding, which creates a "cerebriform" pattern on electron microscopy. Usually there are no detectable nucleoli. The nuclear contour may be smooth or slightly irregular, and deep indentations are rare. On immunophenotyping, the cells predominantly express CD4 along with CD3, and they rarely express CD8. Cytochemical stains are relatively nonspecific, demonstrating a dotlike esterase reaction and weak acid phosphatase activity.

A rare variant, which some also consider a variant of T-cell prolymphocytic leukemia, is Sézary cell leukemia. Peripheral blood examination shows an increased cell count with an overwhelming predominance of relatively small Sézary cells.

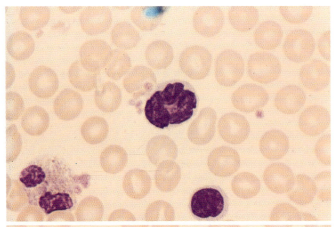

Figs. 153–158. Low-grade lymphomas of T-cell lineage

Fig. 153 a–f. Sézary syndrome. Lymphatic cells in the peripheral blood have distinctively furrowed, convoluted nuclei, which sometimes are indented. Electron microscopy shows cerebriform nuclear folding

a Very deep nuclear indentation in Sézary syndrome

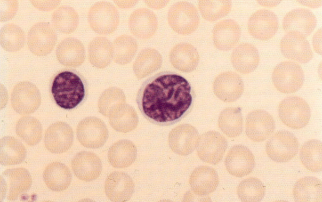

b, c Two different cases with nuclear furrowing

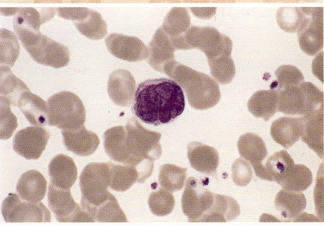

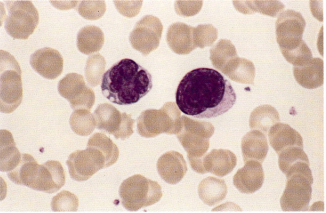

d Pleomorphic nucleus at *left*, large Sézary cell at *right*

Fig. 153 a – f

e Leukocyte concentrate demonstrates many small Sézary cells and one larger cell

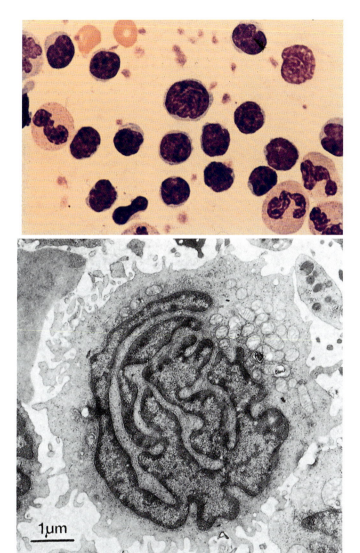

f Electron micrograph of a Sézary cell shows the typical bizarre, cerebriform folding of the nucleus

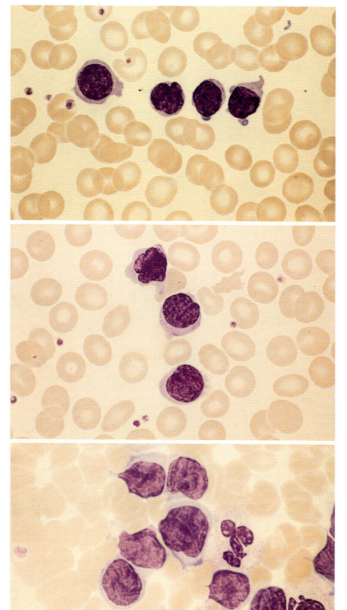

Fig. 154 a–f. Sézary cell leukemia. These patients generally do not have erythroderma as in Sézary syndrome, but there is pronounced leukocytosis. It has been postulated that Sézary cell leukemia may be a variant of T-cell prolymphocytic leukemia

a–d Peripheral blood examination shows leukocytosis with many small Sézary cell displaying a typical nuclear structure

Fig. 154 e – f

e Immunocytochemical detection of CD3

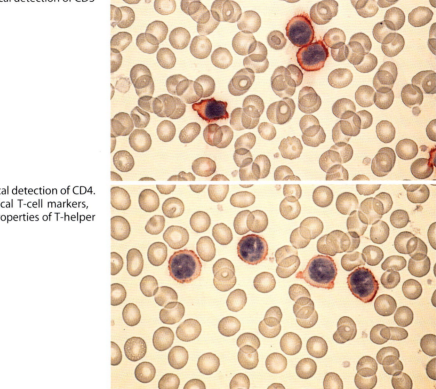

f Immunocytochemical detection of CD4. The cells express typical T-cell markers, and some have the properties of T-helper cells

Large Granulated Lymphocyte (LGL) Leukemia

Another form of mature-cell T- or NK-cell leukemia is *LGL leukemia* (large granulated lymphocyte leukemia), which is very rare. Two distinct immunologic forms have been identified. The first is the T-cell type, characterized by an indolent course, increased T cells in the peripheral blood, and neutropenia. Immunologic studies demonstrate CD2, CD3, CD8, and CD16. CD 57 may be positive or negative, and the T-cell receptor α/β is positive. The second is the NK-cell type, which takes an aggressive clinical course. CD2 is positive, CD3 is negative, CD16 is positive, and CD56 and CD57 may be positive or negative. The T-cell receptor α/β is negative. Peripheral blood examination in both variants shows mature lymphatic cells with azurophilic granules, some of which are very fine and difficult to identify (**Fig. 155**).

Fig. 155 a–d. LGL leukemia

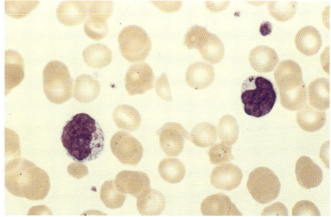

b–d These cells contain distinct azurophilic granules, some of which are very
fine. If possible, a molecular genetic study
should be performed to establish the
diagnosis

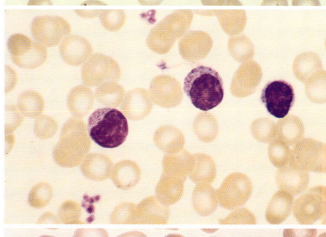

c

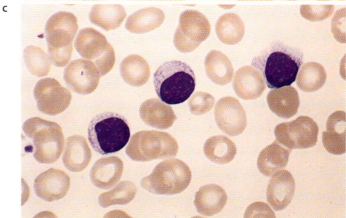

d

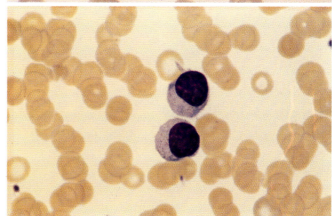

Adult T-Cell Leukemia/Lymphoma (ATLL)

Adult T-cell leukemia/lymphoma (ATLL) occurs in an endemic form in southwestern Japan and the Caribbean. Its etiology is based on infection with the human T-cell leukemia virus (HTLV-1). Sporadic cases have also been reported in Europe and other regions (**Fig. 156 a, b**).

Fig. 156 a – e

a, b Adult T-cell leukemia/lymphoma
(ATLL). The pleomorphic, flower-like
nuclei ("flower cells") are characteristic.
(Courtesy Prof. D. Catovsky, London)

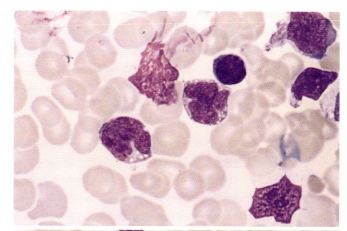

b

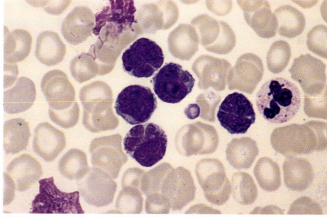

c – e Morphologically similar T-cell leu-
kemia, which was observed in Germany.
There was no evidence of infection with
HTLV-I

c, d Peripheral blood, Pappenheim stain

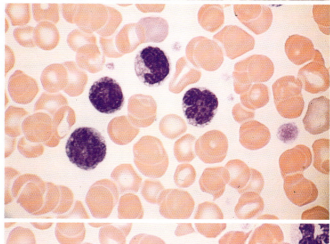

d

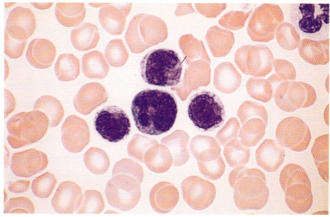

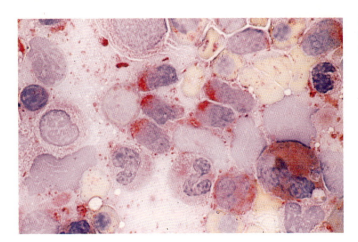

Fig. 156 e. Bone marrow smear. Acid phosphatase reaction shows definite perinuclear activity

Fig. 157 a – h. T-cell prolymphocytic leukemia (T-PLL). In contrast to B-PLL, the nuclei are usually irregular and the nucleoli are not as distinct. Cytochemical staining shows a pronounced acid esterase reaction (ANAE)

a Pleomorphic nuclei with indistinct nucleoli

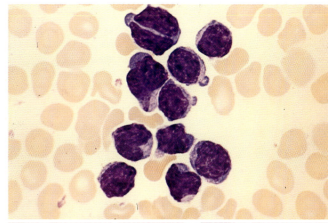

b Characteristic dotlike ANAE staining pattern

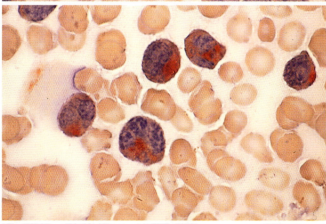

c The cells are very strongly positive for another cytochemical T-cell marker, DAP IV

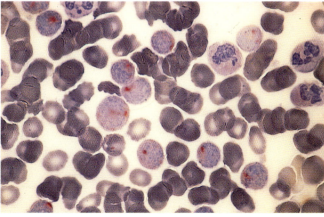

d Acid phosphatase reaction similar to that found in T-ALL

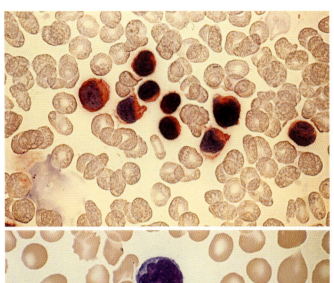

Fig. 157 e–h. T-PLL

e Immunocytochemical detection of CD3

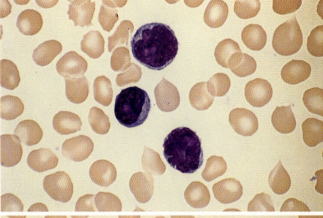

f Different case of T-PLL with distinct nucleoli and irregular nuclear contours

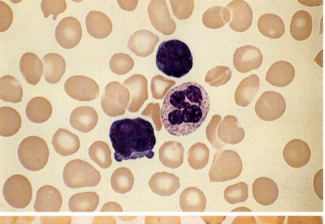

g Two prolymphocytes in the peripheral blood

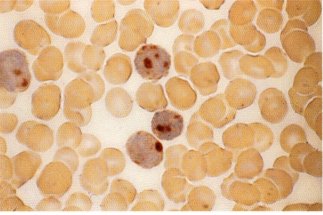

h Very strong ANAE activity in the same case

Fig. 158 a–f. T-prolymphocytic leukemia (T-PLL)

a Round nuclei and distinct nucleoli in T-PLL

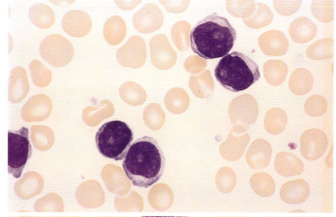

b Different case, apt to be mistaken for B-PLL

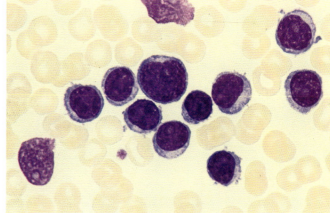

c Same case shows a typical dotlike reaction pattern of ANAE

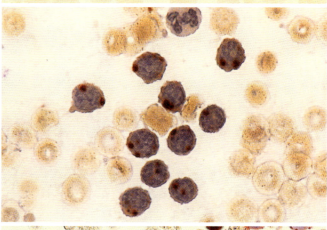

d Immunocytochemical detection of CD3

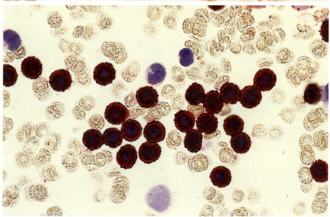

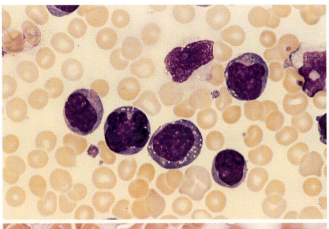

Fig. 158 e–f

e, f Large-cell T-PLL with strongly basophilic cytoplasm

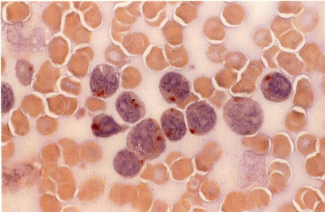

f Dotlike ANAE staining pattern

Fig. 159 a – k. High-grade non-Hodgkin lymphomas (NHL)

a Lymph node touch preparation in high-grade Burkitt-type B-cell lymphoma with "starry sky macrophages" among the lymphoblasts

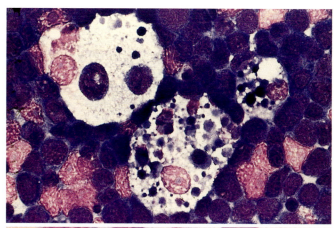

b – g Centroblastic NHL (large-cell, diffuse) with a fine chromatin pattern and pale nucleoli. The cells may also show greater pleomorphism

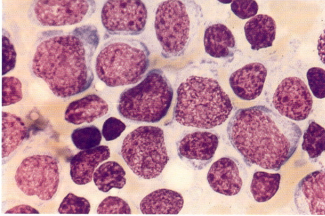

c

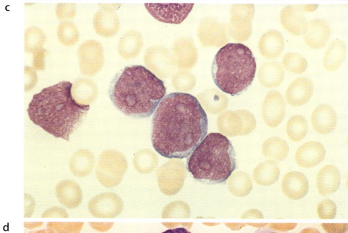

d

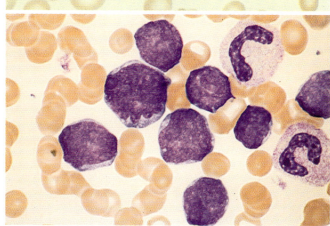

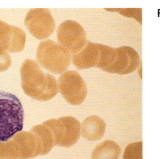

Fig. 159 e – g

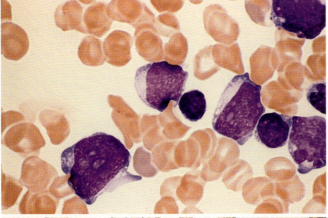

f

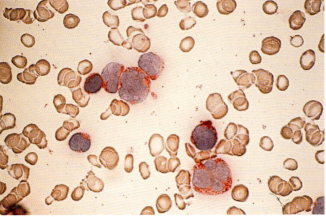

g Detection of CD10. This marker, originally used in diagnosing C-ALL, is also expressed in centroblastic lymphomas

Fig. 159 h – k

h – k Unusually large-cell form of high-grade T-cell lymphoma

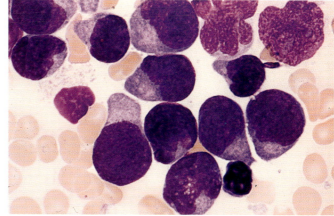

i These cells have large nuclei, usually indented and occasionally lobulated, and a strongly basophilic cytoplasm

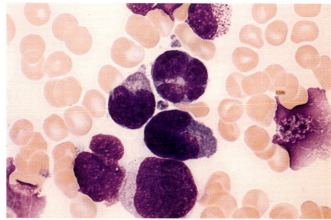

j Extremely strong acid phosphatase activity localized to the paranuclear area

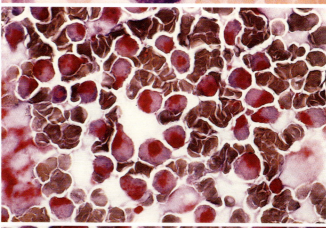

k Higher-power view of **j**

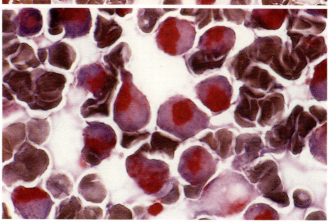

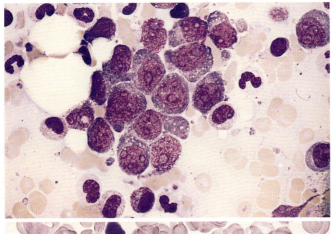

Fig. 160 a – f. High-grade non-Hodgkin lymphoma

a Large-cell high-grade B-cell lymphoma with intensely basophilic cytoplasm and distinct nucleoli

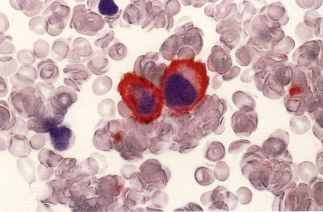

b Immunocytochemical detection of the B-cell marker CD19 in the same case

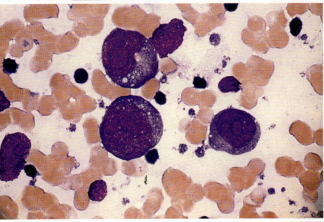

c Large-cell anaplastic B-cell lymphoma with large nucleoli

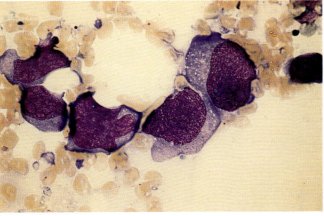

d Different large-cell lymphoma with expression of CD30 (Ki-1 lymphoma)

Fig. 160 e – h

e Same patient as in **d**

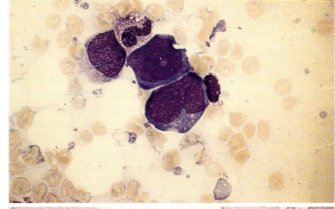

f Immunocytochemical detection of CD30

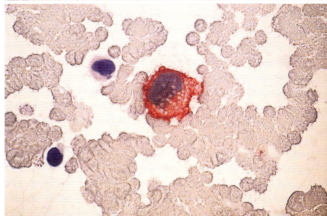

g, h Richter syndrome
Characterized by the presence of large blasts with large nucleoli in a patient with preexisting B-CLL. In some cases the blasts belong to the same clone as the preexisting CLL. In bone marrow smears, large blasts with copious cytoplasm and distinct nucleoli are interspersed among the small lymphocytes

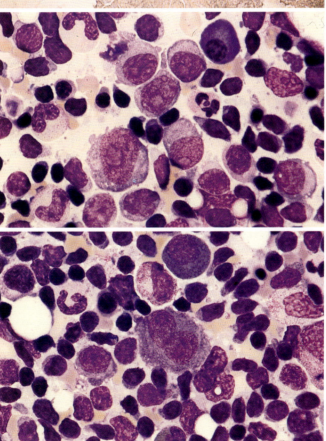

Plasmacytoma
(Multiple Myeloma, Kahler Disease)

Plasmacytoma is characterized by a proliferation of abnormal plasma cells. It may take the form of a solitary tumor or multiple tumors (multiple myeloma), or the changes may permeate the bone marrow diffusely. The most common form is *multiple myeloma,* characterized by multiple, sharply circumscribed osteolytic foci that are conspicuous on radiographs. The *diffuse form* of the disease presents radiographically as a generalized decalcification and rarefaction of the bony structure, resembling osteoporosis. *Solitary plasmacytomas* may become generalized in the course of the disease, just as initially diffuse lesions can in time produce multiple plasma cell tumors. Since plasma cells are descendants of B lymphocytes, which are ubiquitous, plasmacytomas are not confined to the bone marrow (extramedullary plasmacytoma). It is relatively uncommon for large numbers of plasma cells to enter the peripheral blood. This condition is called *plasma cell leukemia.*

Because plasma cells manufacture immunoglobulins, qualitative and quantitative protein abnormalities are a consistent feature of plasmacytomas. Generally there is a pronounced increase in immunoglobulins, whose homogeneity on immunoelectrophoresis ("monoclonal paraproteinemia," "monoclonal gammopathy") reflects the monoclonality of the malignant plasma cell population, demonstrable by immunocytologic analysis. Several immunologic classes of plasmacytoma are currently recognized: IgA, IgG, IgD, and IgE. IgM paraproteinemia, by contrast, is seen chiefly in immunocytomas (Waldenström's macroglobulinemia). If the structure of the immunoglobulins in the plasma cells is rudimentary, a *Bence Jones myeloma* (light-chain plasmacytoma) is said to be present, and the patient will manifest a characteristic Bence Jones proteinuria. The different variants of plasmacytomas cannot be distinguished morphologically. The *clinical picture* of plasmacytoma is marked by the proliferation of plasma cells and by the diverse effects of abnormal protein formation.

The *morphologic features* of plasmacytoma are characteristic and are easily recognized in fully developed cases. There are sheets or islands of plasma cells that usually show the characteristics of mature plasma cells ("mature-cell" or "plasmacytic" myeloma) but may show considerable pleomorphism (**Figs. 161–169**) or may even lose their plasma cell characteristics ("immature-cell" or "plasmablastic" myeloma; see **Fig. 162**; the reference to plasma cell precursors may be a misnomer, as it is more reasonable to assume a higher grade of malignant transformation based on immunologic findings). The cytoplasm of the myeloma cells may contain reddish-violet granules, called *Russell bodies* (dilated, immunoglobulin-filled ergastoplasm sacs, see **Fig. 163 f, g**), or vacuoles (Russell bodies dislodged by the staining process), which may culminate in the formation of morula cells. Some plasma cells take a reddish-violet cytoplasmic stain, which has earned them the name "flaming plasma cells" (see **Fig. 161 f**) and is seen in IgA myelomas.

Cytochemical staining typically demonstrates very strong acid phosphatase activity and often shows nonspecific esterase activity (see **Fig. 164 d–g**), but this is rarely necessary to establish a diagnosis. Differential diagnosis may prove difficult in early stages when the plasma cell increase does not yet permit a definitive diagnosis to be made. The picture is further complicated by the substantial plasma cell increases that can arise in the course of severe, prolonged infections and neoplastic diseases (see also **Table 7**). When doubt exists, the immunocytologic differentiation of monoclonal and polyclonal plasma cell populations can be helpful. The neoplastic plasma cells usually do not express CD19, but the majority express CD38 and CD56.

As the plasma cell population expands, the *cells of normal hematopoiesis* become less and less prominent, and the blood picture may ultimately become pancytopenic. The rare plasma cell leukemias have a particularly poor prognosis.

Fig. 161 a–g. Multiple myeloma (plasmacytoma)

a, b Rouleaux formation of erythrocytes in the blood smear, caused by the increased amount of abnormal immunoglobulin in the plasma. A small plasma cell is seen in **b**

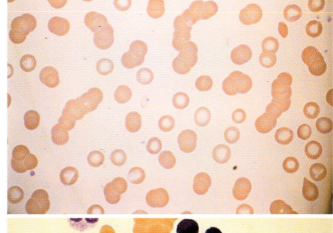

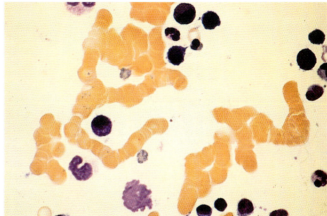

c Moderately pleomorphic plasma cells with nucleoli, and one binucleated form

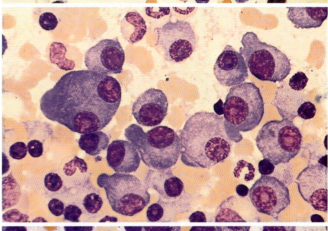

d These plasma cells appear fairly mature but contain distinct nucleoli

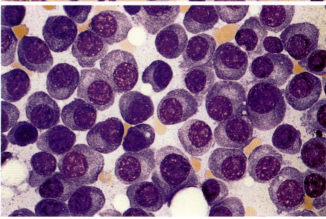

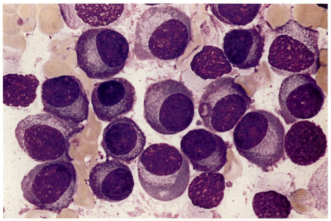

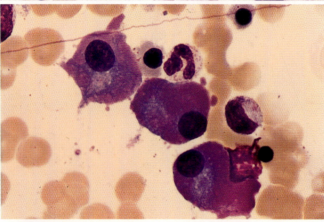

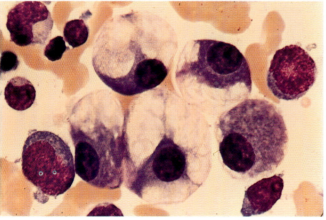

Fig. 161 e–g

e Mature-cell plasmacytoma in a different case

f "Flaming" myeloma cells with red-staining, homogeneous-appearing cytoplasm. This type of myeloma cell is seen mainly in IgA gammopathy

g Giant vacuoles in myeloma cells

**Fig. 162 a–f. Multiple myeloma
(plasmacytoma)**

a Plasmablastic type of multiple
myeloma

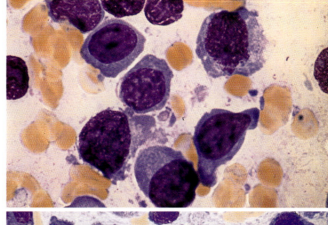

b Distinct nucleoli

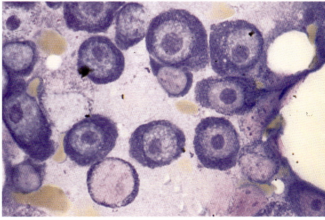

c The large nucleoli are clearly demonstrated by specific nucleolar staining

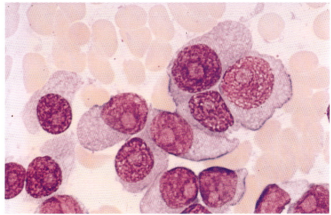

d Extremely immature plasmacytoma

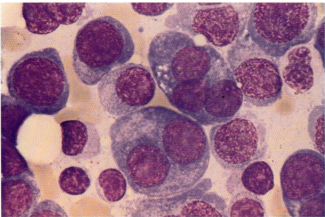

Fig. 162 e – f

e Many multinucleated forms in immature plasmacytoma

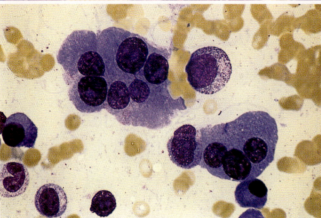

f Giant plasma cells (multinucleated)

Fig. 163 a – g. Multiple myeloma (plasmacytoma)

a, b Immature plasma cells with pleomorphic nuclei in multiple myeloma

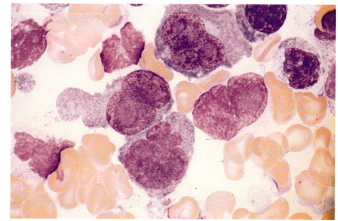

b

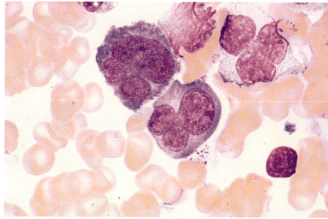

c – e Multiple myeloma with granular plasma cells. Some of the plasma cells contain abundant purple granules that are peroxidase-negative but express the myeloid marker CD33 (**e**)

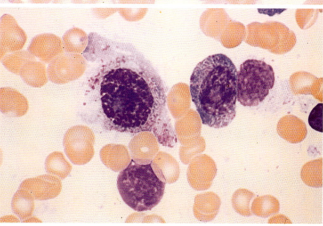

d

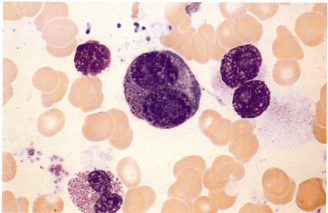

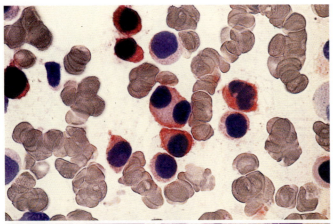

Fig. 163 e–g

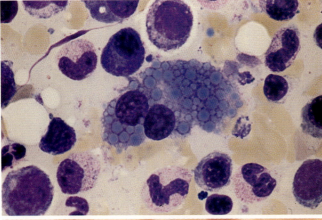

f Binucleated myeloma cell with small Russell bodies in the cytoplasm

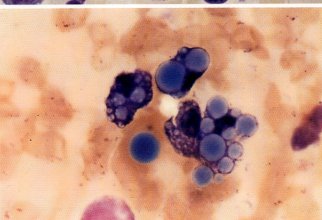

g Large Russell bodies in the cytoplasm of myeloma cells. Some extracellular bodies are also seen

Fig. 164 a – g. Multiple myeloma

a Erythrophagocytosis in myeloma cells

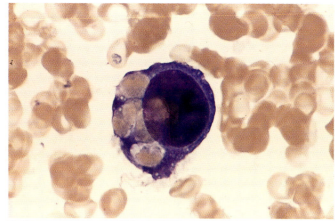

b, c Crystalline inclusions in myeloma cells

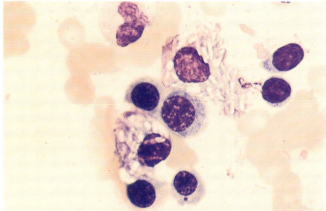

Fig. 164 d – g. Cytochemistry of multiple myeloma

d, e Very strong acid phosphatase activity in myeloma cells

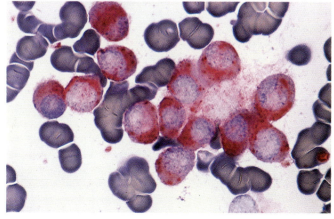

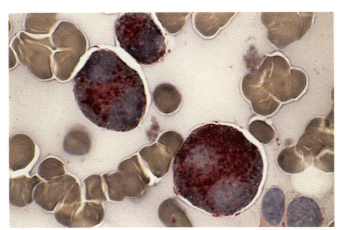

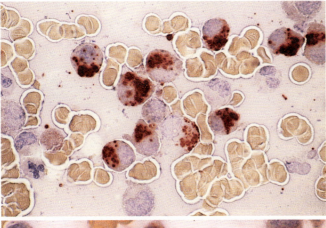

Fig. 164 e–g

f, g Strong ANAE activity in myeloma cells

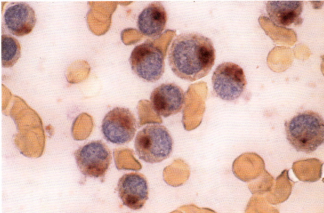

Fig. 165 a – c. Immunocytochemical findings in multiple myeloma

a CD38-positive myeloma cells

b CD56-positive myeloma cells

c As is usually the case, the myeloma cells are CD19-negative

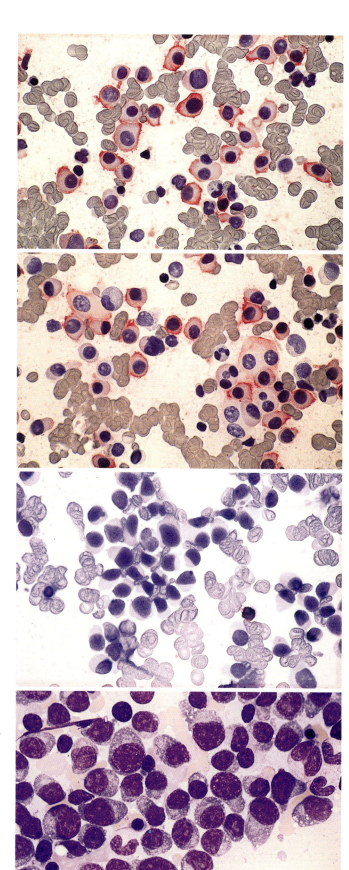

d, e Different case of multiple myeloma before and after therapy

d Bone marrow sample prior to therapy

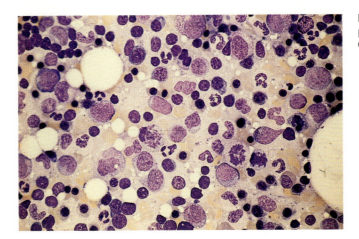

Fig. 165 e. Bone marrow from the same patient 6 months after chemotherapy. Complete remission

Fig. 166 a – d. Histologic section of multiple myeloma (plasmacytoma)

a Giemsa stain. Myeloma cells with intensely basophilic cytoplasm

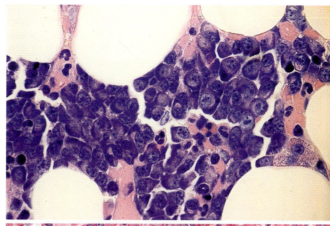

b Immunohistochemical detection of monoclonal kappa chains

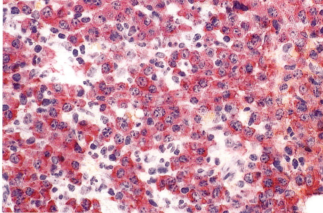

c Higher-power view of the same sample

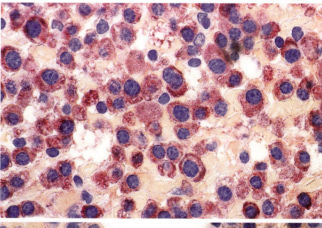

d Section from the patient in **a–c**, λ-chain detection. The myeloma cells are negative, and there are very few interspersed (normal) plasma cells that are λ-chain-positive (*red*)

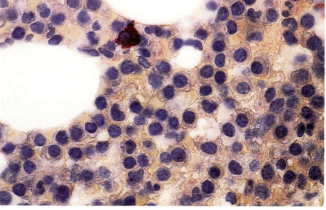

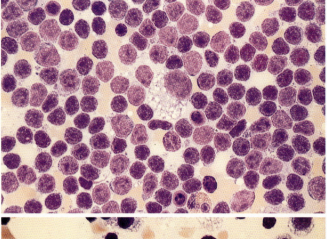

Fig. 167 a–e. Coexistence of lymphocytic lymphoma and multiple myeloma

a Lymphocytes intermingled with large plasma cells with foamy cytoplasm

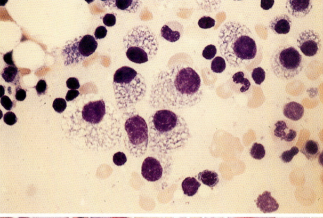

b Different site in the same sample consists almost entirely of foamy plasma cells

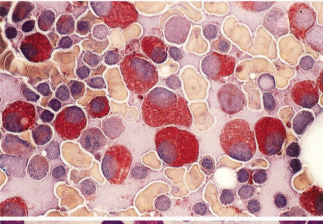

c Acid phosphatase reaction of plasma cells in the same case

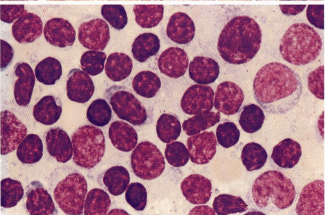

d, e Two different monoclonal proteins – IgA and IgM – in a different patient

d Bone marrow region showing pure lymphatic infiltration

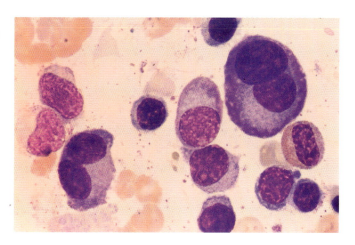

e Different site in the same sample, showing an area of plasma cell infiltration

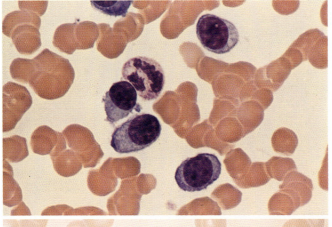

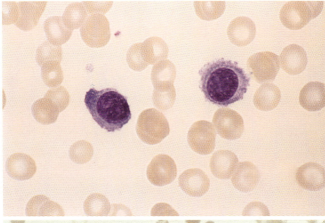

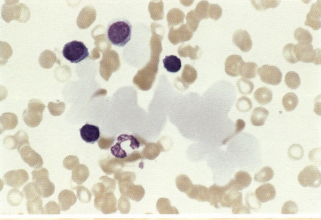

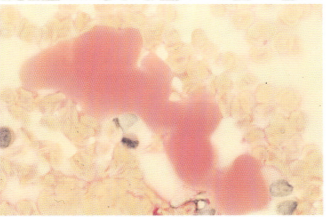

Fig. 168 a – d. Plasma cell leukemia

a Small plasma cells in the peripheral blood

b Small plasma cells in a different case of plasma cell leukemia

c Blood smear from the case in **b** shows peculiar, partially confluent protein globules

d Blood smear from the same patient, PAS reaction. The protein masses stain pink, indicating a carbohydrate component in the protein

Fig. 169 a – d. Plasma cell leukemia

a, b Peripheral blood in a different case of plasma cell leukemia

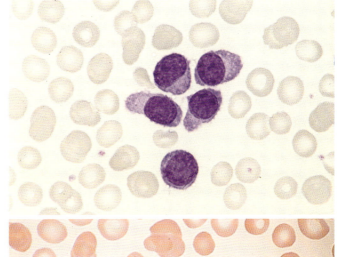

b

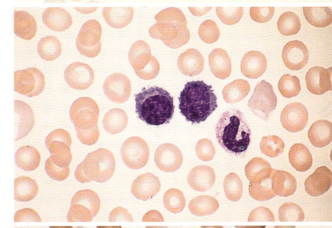

c ANAE in myeloma cells that have entered the peripheral blood

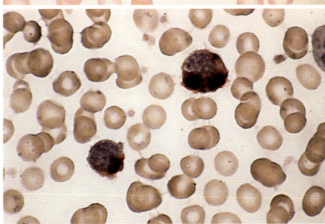

d Bone marrow from the case in b and c

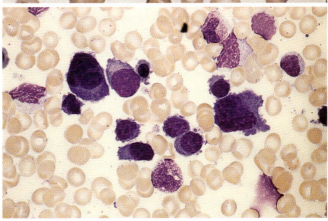

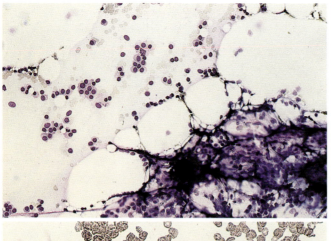

Fig. 169 e, f. Hypoplastic multiple myeloma

e Bone marrow smear from a patient with hypoplastic multiple myeloma shows fatty marrow fragments along with a group of plasma cells

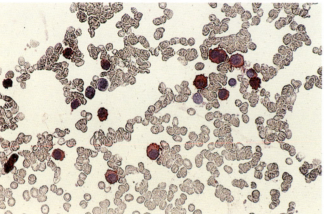

f Higher-power view of the same case with CD56–positive myeloma cells

NK(natural killer)-cell neoplasias

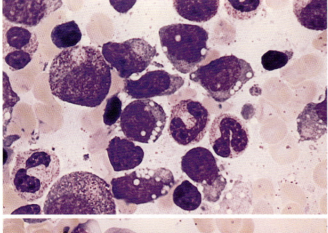

a, b Relatively large blasts with abundant cytoplasm containing distinct reddish granules

b

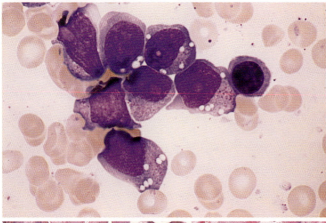

c Intense perinuclear acid phosphatase reaction in a bone marrow smear from the patient in **a, b**

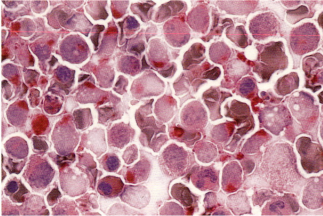

d The blasts are CD56-positive

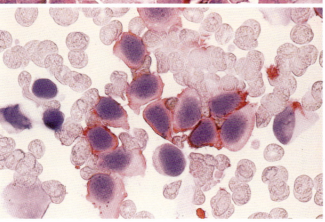

Fig. 170 e–h

e Immunocytochemical analysis also demonstrates CD7 in the blasts. This case is an acute NK-cell leukemia that is very similar morphologically to AML

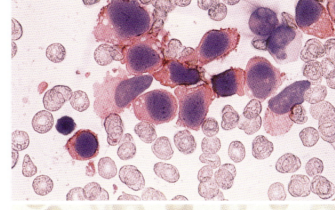

f–h Different case of acute NK-cell leukemia

f–h Similar findings as in **a–e**, with a somewhat narrower cytoplasmic rim. The blasts are also CD56-positive

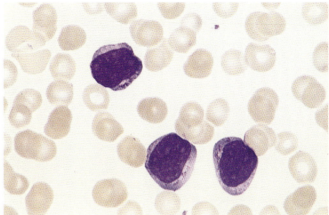

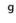
g

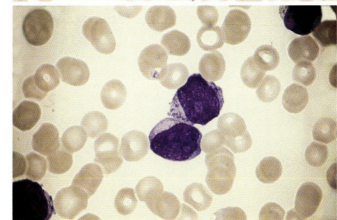

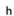
h

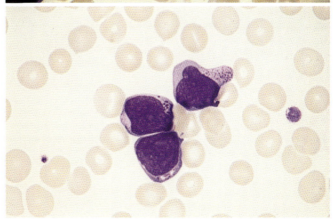

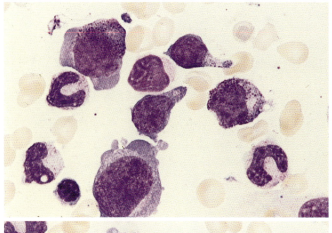

Fig. 171 a–f. NK-cell neoplasia.
Sometimes only isolated granules are found in the abnormal NK cells, and some blasts are devoid of granules

a–c Bone marrow smears in which only isolated blasts with granules are seen

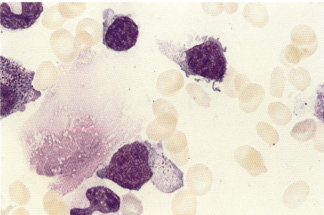

b

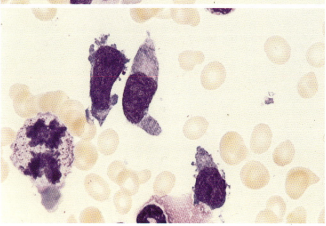

c

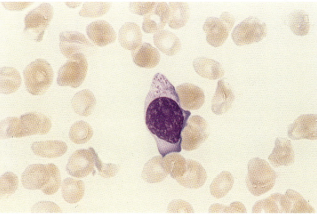

d Peripheral blood smear

Fig. 171 e–f

e Immunocytochemical detection of CD56

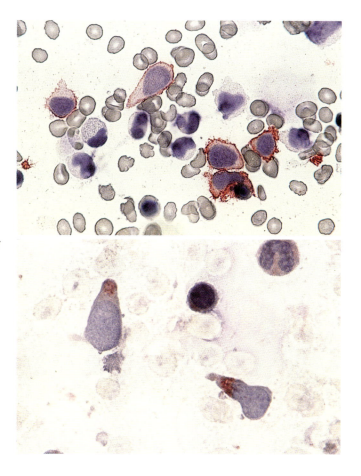

f Detection of acid phosphatase activity

Hodgkin Disease (Lymphogranulomatosis)

At present the diagnosis of Hodgkin disease can be established only by histologic or cytologic examination. All other clinical data, including the blood picture and radiographic findings, provide useful information but cannot verify the diagnosis.

The *cytologic features* of the disease, seen most clearly in lymph node aspirate or touch preparations, are highly diverse but easily recognized. Its distinctive features are the *mononuclear granuloma cells* or *Hodgkin cells* (**Figs. 172–174**) and *multinucleated Reed-Sternberg cells* (**Figs. 172–174**). Both cell types are characterized by a coarse reticular chromatin pattern and especially by very large, often irregularly shaped nucleoli, which usually stain a deep blue. The cytoplasm may be well marginated, but usually it is not clearly demarcated from its surroundings. It stains a pale to dark blue. Mitoses are rare in these cells. In addition, it is usual to find increased numbers of *plasma cells, neutrophils,* and even *eosinophils.* The latter have been described as highly characteristic but in fact do not afford proof of the diagnosis, any more than their absence would exclude Hodgkin disease.

Four subtypes of Hodgkin disease are recognized based on the criteria established by the Rye Conference. They can be accurately classified only by the histologic examination of a biopsied lymph node.

1. Lymphocyte predominance type (LP)
   a) Nodular paragranuloma
   b) Diffuse paragranuloma
2. Nodular sclerosing type (NS)
3. Mixed cellular type (MC)
4. Lymphocyte depletion type (LD)

Recently the WHO recommended the following classification along with the renaming of Hodgkin disease as Hodgkin lymphoma:[1]

Nodular lymphocyte predominance Hodgkin lymphoma
Classical Hodgkin lymphoma
Nodular sclerosis (grades I and II)
Mixed cellularity
Lymphocyte depletion, which includes several forms of "Hodgkin-like ALCL"[1, 2] (anaplastic large cell lymphoma)

The histologic subtype of Hodgkin lymphoma is not considered to have a bearing on prognosis. According to Lennert, the LP type can be further subdivided into nodular paragranuloma (possibly a B-cell type of non-Hodgkin lymphoma), diffuse paragranuloma, and lymphocyte-predominant Hodgkin lymphoma. The LD type corresponds largely to the *Hodgkin sarcoma* of the same authors, while the NS and MC types correspond to *Hodgkin granuloma*. LP and LD can be identified with reasonable accuracy in cytologic smears. NS and MC require histologic differentiation, especially since the "lacunar cells" thought to characterize nodular sclerosis can be recognized only in histologic sections.

---

[1] ALCL = Anaplastic large cell lymphoma
[2] E.S. Jaffe, N.L. Harris. J. Diebold, H.K. Müller-Hermelink: World Health Organization Classification of lymphomas: A work in progress. Ann. Oncol. 9 (Suppl. 5): 25–30 (1998)

Fig. 172 a–e. Bone marrow infiltration in Hodgkin disease

a–c Mononucleated Hodgkin cells with characteristic giant nucleoli

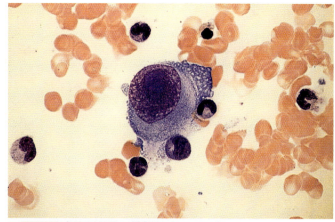

b

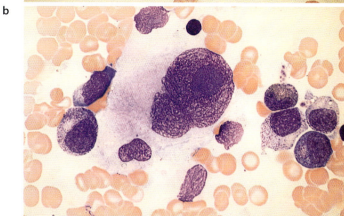

c

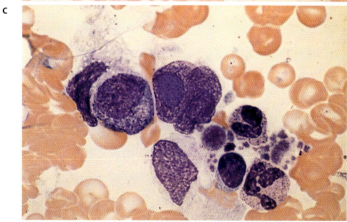

d Constricted, elongated nucleus of a Hodgkin cell with a large nucleolus

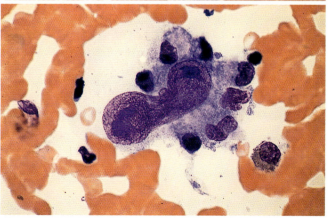

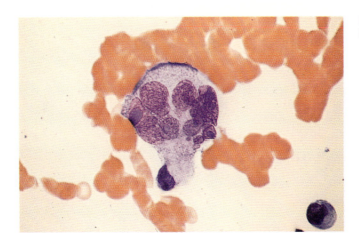

Fig. 172 e. Multinucleated Sternberg-Reed cell

C Lymph Nodes and Spleen

Fig. 173 a–c. Hodgkin disease (lymphogranulomatosis)

a Lymph node. At *center* is a multinucleated Sternberg-Reed giant cell. The large, dark nucleoli are typical

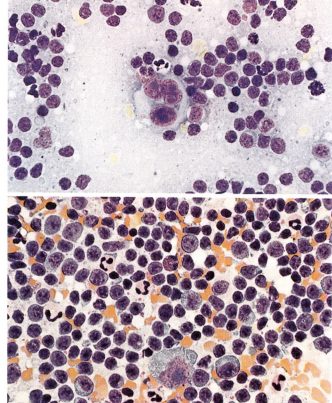

b Spleen. At *bottom center* are a mononuclear Hodgkin cell and several stimulated immunoblasts. At *left* a plasmablast and numerous neutrophils

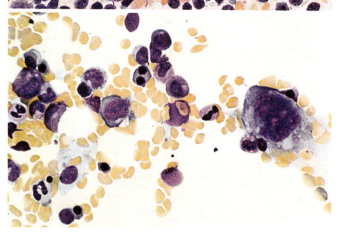

c Bone marrow. At *right* a multinucleated Sternberg-Reed giant cell and several erythropoietic and granulocytopoietic cells

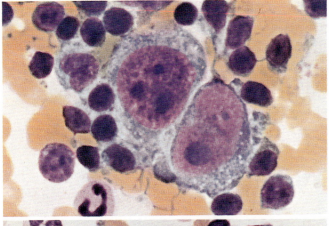

Fig. 174 a – d. Hodgkin disease (lymphogranulomatosis)

a Two adjacent mononuclear Hodgkin cells

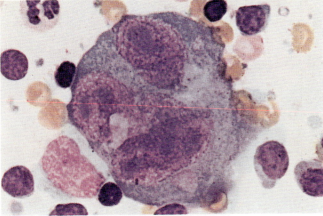

b Multinucleated Sternberg-Reed giant cell

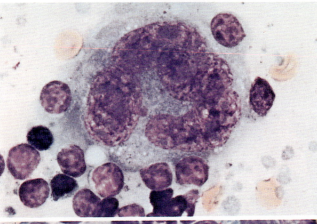

c Multinucleated Sternberg-Reed giant cell

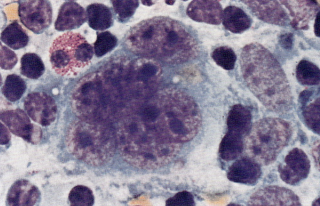

d Multinucleated Sternberg-Reed giant cell. Above it is an eosinophilic granulocyte

D. Tumor Aspirates from Bone Marrow Involved by Metastatic Disease

A number of nonhematologic malignancies can metastasize to the bone and bone marrow. For the staging of these cases, it is important to determine whether bone marrow involvement is present. Not infrequently, however, bone marrow invasion by tumor cells is detected incidentally in patients who are examined for unexplained symptoms or suspicion of leukemia. It can be very difficult to distinguish morphologically undifferentiated tumor cells from the cells of acute leukemia or malignant lymphoma based on morphologic criteria alone.

An accurate classification requires the use of immunologic methods, which also help to assign the neoplastic cells to a specific primary tumor. These methods employ antibodies against components of the cytoskeleton (cytokeratin, vimentin, desmin, etc.), a number of tumor markers, and organ-specific antibodies. Since new antibodies are constantly being offered by various firms, we refer the reader to the monograph by Hastka[1]

---

[1] Hastka J (1997) Immunocytology. Schattauer, Stuttgart

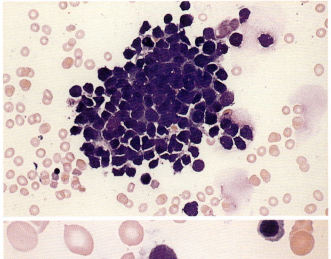

Fig. 175 a–d. Tumor cells from a small-cell bronchial carcinoma in the bone marrow

a Cluster of tumor cells in a bone marrow smear

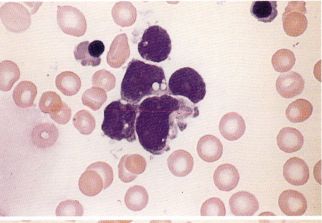

b Same smear at high magnification

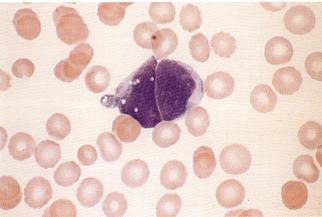

c Two tumor cells in a blood smear from the same patient. (It is unusual to find tumor cells in the peripheral blood unless the sample has been specially concentrated.)

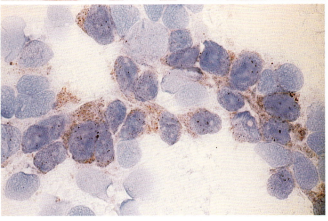

d Neuron-specific enolase (NSE) is a useful immunologic marker for small-cell bronchial carcinoma. Positive detection in a bone marrow smear

Fig. 176 a – e. Cells from breast
carcinoma in the bone marrow

a Pappenheim stain

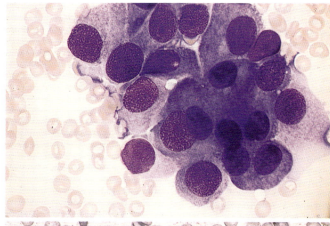

b Immunocytochemical detection
of cytokeratin

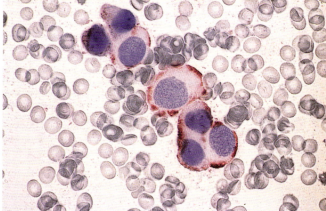

c Histologic examination of a core biopsy
in breast carcinoma. HE stain

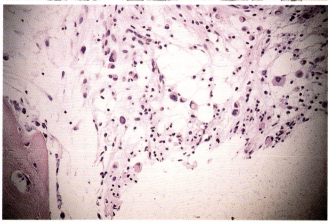

d Histologic detection of cytokeratin in a
bone marrow smear with metastatic
breast carcinoma

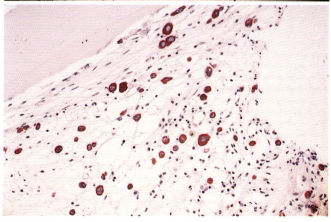

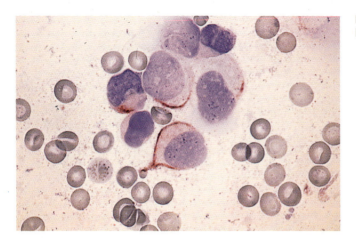

Fig. 176 e. Detection of cytokeratin in a bone marrow smear in breast carcinoma

Fig. 177 a–e. Detection of tumor cells in the bone marrow

a Cells of metastatic gastric carcinoma in a bone marrow smear

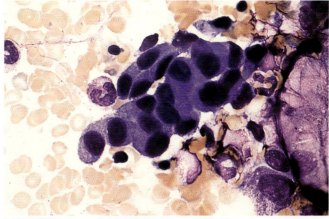

b Detection of cytokeratin in the tumor cells of the same case

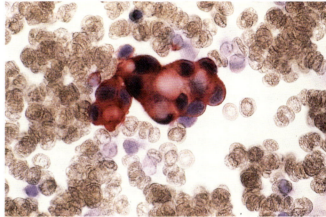

c Osteoclasts along with tumor cells from prostatic carcinoma in a bone marrow smear

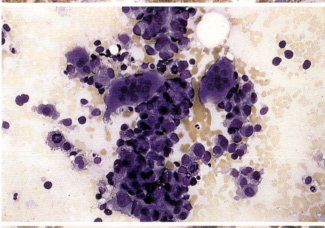

d Tumor cell infiltration in a bone marrow smear

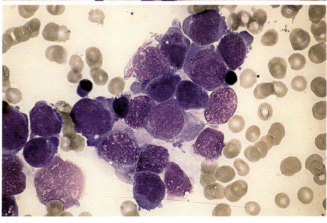

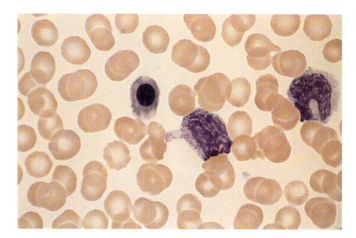

Fig. 177 e. Leukoerythroblastic reaction in peripheral blood from the same patient. A normoblast and myelocyte are seen

| D Tumor Aspirates from Bone Marrow Involved by Metastatic Disease

Fig. 178 a – c. Detection of tumor cells in the bone marrow

a Nest of tumor cells in a patient with prostatic carcinoma

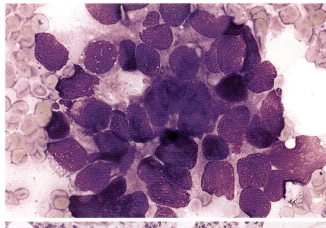

b Histologic examination of a core biopsy in prostatic carcinoma. Adenoid structures can be seen

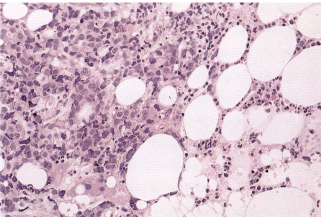

c Vessel-like mass of angiosarcoma cells in a bone marrow smear

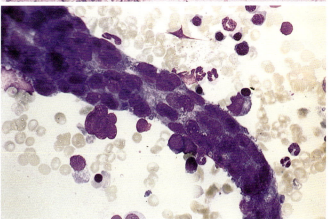

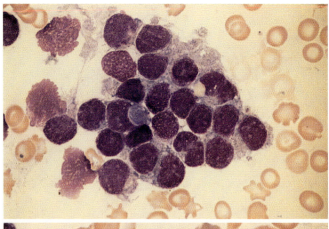

Fig. 179 a – e. Detection of neurologic tumor cells in pediatric patients

a Bone marrow involvement by medulloblastoma. Small, round cells with pale chromatin

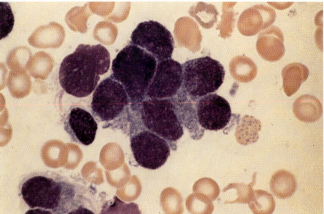

b Higher-power view of the same case

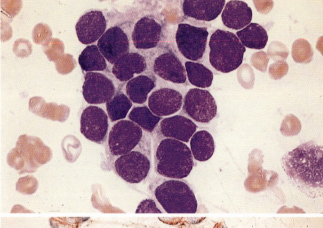

c Cells of neuroblastoma, very similar in appearance to **a** and **b**

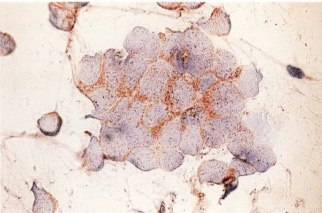

d NSE reaction in a bone marrow smear from the case in **c**

e "Rosette" arrangement of tumor cells in sympathicoblastoma

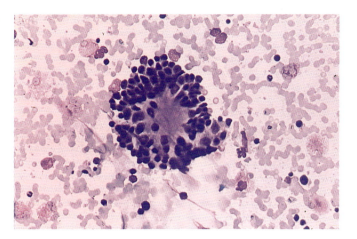

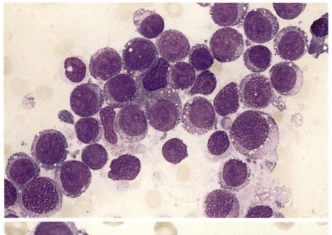

Fig. 180 a – g. Metastatic rhabdomyosarcoma in the bone marrow. Rhabdomyosarcoma can metastasize to the
bone marrow in children and in young
adults. Not infrequently, the cells are
mistaken for those of an acute leukemia

a Rhabdomyosarcoma cells in a bone
marrow smear. These cells are easily
confused with the cells of acute leukemia

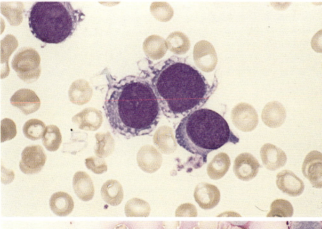

b Higher-power view of the same case

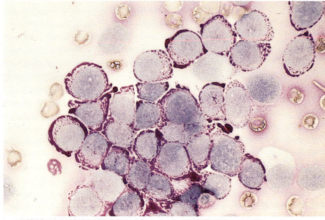

c PAS reaction in the same case. The
degree of the PAS reaction is highly
variable and sometimes is very intense

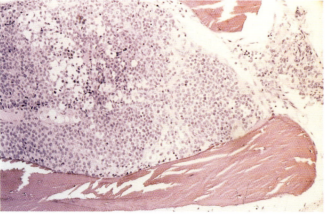

d Metastatic rhabdomyosarcoma in a
histologic marrow section. Note the
relatively pale nuclei

Fig. 180 e – g

e Different case of rhabdomyosarcoma with bone marrow involvement

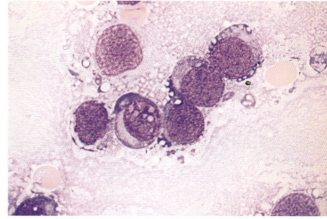

f PAS reaction in the same case

g Same case, showing the detection of desmin in the tumor cells

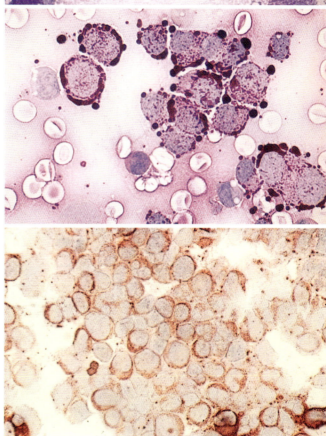

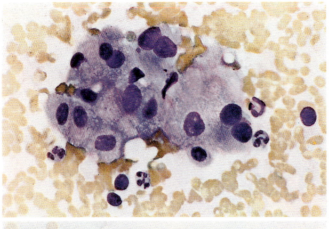

Fig. 181 a, b. Detection of tumor cells in lymph nodes

a Hypernephroma. Cluster of tumor cells

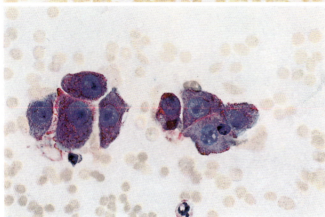

b Hypernephroma. PAS reaction

E. Blood Parasites
Principal Causative Organisms of Tropical Diseases[1]

Malaria

The causative *Plasmodium* organisms are transmitted to man as sporozoites in the saliva of the feeding anopheles mosquito. The organisms travel in the bloodstream from the capillaries to the liver, where they undergo further development. They enter the liver cells (primary tissue forms) in the "pre-erythrocytic phase" of their life cycle, and after a variable period they are released into the peripheral blood as merozoites. There they invade the erythrocytes, inciting a paroxysm of fever. Inside the red cells the plasmodia (merozoites) mature through several stages, culminating in the discharge of merozoites from the remains of the erythrocyte; these then proceed to infect fresh erythrocytes. This process takes about 48 h for the parasite of *tertian malaria (Plasmodium vivax* and *Plasmodium ovale)* and *malignant tertian malaria (Plasmodium falciparum)* and 72 h for the parasite of *quartan malaria (Plasmodium malariae).* The different stages can be recognized in the blood, depending on the time at which the sample is drawn (see **Figs. 182–186**). Besides asexual reproduction through division, the organisms are capable of sexual reproduction in their male and female gametocyte forms. The gametocytes unite *only* in the mosquito, forming oocysts. Sporozoites soon emerge from the cysts and make their way to the insect's salivary glands, to enter the capillaries and bloodstream of the next person on whom the mosquito feeds. Gametocytes that do not enter a mosquito can survive no more than about 40 days in the human body, after which time they can no longer harm their human host.

Cycle in the Tissue

Infected mosquito bites a host
↓
Inoculation of sporozoites
↓
1 Parenchymal cells of the liver (tissue schizont)
↓
2 Strong asexual proliferation (hepatic phase)
↓
3 After several generations, release of merozoites from the schizonts
↓
4 Entry into the blood (erythrocytic phase)

Entry of the Parasite into the Erythrocyte

1. Merozoite recognizes the host erythrocyte.
2. Attaches to the surface of the cell.
3. Must reorient so that its apical end touches the surface of the cell.
4. Invagination develops at the attachment site, and the parasite enters the cell.
5. Erythrocyte reseals, enclosing the merozoite within a vacuole.

Development in the Erythrocyte

1. Ring form with a peripheral nucleus and central vacuole.
2. Trophozoites.
3. Repeated nuclear division.
4. Erythrocyte becomes completely filled with merozoites.
5. Erythrocyte rupture, discharging the merozoites (8–12 *P. malariae*, 18–24 *P. vivax*).
6. Invasion of fresh erythrocytes.

---

[1] Revised by Prof. R. Disko, Munich.

Tertian Malaria (Plasmodium vivax and Plasmodium ovale)

The clinical pattern of paroxysmal fever, splenomegaly, and hepatomegaly is characteristic. The fever usually begins with chills, followed 8–10 h later by sweating and defervescence. The *diagnosis* is established by examination of the blood, i.e., by detecting the parasites in a thick or thin smear. *Serologic tests* using indirect immunofluorescence are not positive until 14–18 days after the parasites gain access to the blood. The course of infection with *Plasmodium ovale* is largely identical to that of *Plasmodium vivax* malaria. Both forms can incite a double tertian fever pattern with daily attacks caused by two nonsynchronous plasmodium populations, each of which has a schizogenic peak on the following day. A maximum of 2 % of erythrocytes are parasitized in both infections. *P. vivax* and *P. ovale* are the only malaria organisms that cause enlargement of the affected erythrocytes with the appearance of "Schüffner dots" in the cells.

Quartan Malaria (Plasmodium malariae)

The fever attacks of quartan malaria occur at 72-h intervals, or every fourth day. In some cases a double quartan pattern is observed. Enlargement of the spleen and liver is not so pronounced as in tertian malaria. Because the parasite burden is only 10,000/mL, more time is required for anemia to develop. The development of a quartan malaria duplicata is possible. Late recrudescence of quartan malaria is known to occur decades after the primary infection has subsided. Relapse is confirmed by identifying the parasites in the blood.

Malignant Tertian Malaria (Plasmodium falciparum)

Malignant tertian malaria (falciparum malaria) is the *most severe, life-threatening* form of the disease. The fever pattern is nonspecific and may resemble that of tertian malaria or may consist of daily attacks mimicking a double tertian pattern. In other cases the fever may be constant or may occur in irregular episodes. Splenomegaly and hepatomegaly are slowly progressive over the course of the disease. The parasite burden is virtually endless due to the "chain reaction" mode of proliferation. Because all parasitized cells are destroyed, the erythrocyte count falls precipitously along with the hemoglobin and serum iron. Untreated, this disease can terminate fatally or cause permanent disability in nonimmune individuals.

The gametes of malignant tertian malaria are crescent-shaped. Some rupture the erythrocyte membrane and consequently are found outside the red cells in smears.

Erythrocytes infected by *Plasmodium falciparum* frequently contain "Maurer spots," which are coarser than Schüffner dots.

Relapse can occur in any type of malarial infection, but a true *recurrence* is seen only in tertian malaria (*P. vivax* and *P. ovale*). Recurrences develop from the persistence of sporozoites in the liver cells (called hypnozoites). These dormant stages may develop into tissue schizonts over a period of time ranging from a few months to five years, and the schizonts provide a source of new merozoites that can reinvade the red cells. The hypnozoites are also responsible for the long incubation periods (up to 1 year) of tertian malaria.

P. falciparum and *P. malariae* do not form hypnozoites, but they may *recrudesce* (for up to 1 year in the case of *P. falciparum*, decades in the case of *P. malariae*). This recrudesence always arises from a nonimmunologic or pharmacologically cured involvement of the blood, and it may occur in tertian malaria as well.

Some cases manifest a *long latent period* in which an infection contracted in the fall, for example, does not produce initial symptoms until the following spring, 7–9 months later. This phenomenon is seen mainly with vivax malaria and is less common in the ovale form.

Fig. 182 a – d. Tertian malaria (*Plasmodium vivax*), Giemsa stain.

Thick smear

a *Left*: erythrocytes are destroyed, and all that remain of the leukocytes (*l*) are nuclei. Parasites (*p*) with a red nucleus (*k*) and blue protoplasm. Typical ring forms (*r*) are scarce in the thick smear

b *Left*: older ring form (*r*) with increased protoplasm and initial deposition of pigment (*pi*)

c *Left*: semiadult schizonts (*h*) with divided nuclei, more abundant protoplasm, and pigment deposits

d *Left*: macrogametocyte (*w*, female gametocyte) with round nucleus, larger than an erythrocyte. Microgametocyte (*m*, male gametocyte) with a bandlike nucleus, roughly the size of an erythrocyte. Pigment is distributed throughout the parasite. Young schizont (*t*), mature schizont (t_1) with 24 – 26 merozoites (*me*)

Thin smear

a *Right*: young ring forms (*r*) with a red nucleus and blue protoplasm surrounding the vacuole. Note that the erythrocytes are not yet enlarged

b *Right*: older rings (*r*). Parasite (r_1) with increased amounts of protoplasm and pigment

c *Right*: semiadults (*h*) with brownish pigment spots in erythrocytes, now enlarged and speckled with Schüffner dots (*s*)

d *Right*: macrogametocyte (*w*), microgametocyte (*m*), young schizont (*t*), mature schizont (t_1), also morula or daisy form with 18 – 24 merozoites. In infections with *Plasmodium ovale*, the affected erythrocytes are slightly enlarged and are distorted into oval shapes. The schizonts contain only 8 – 12 merozoites (**Fig. 185**)

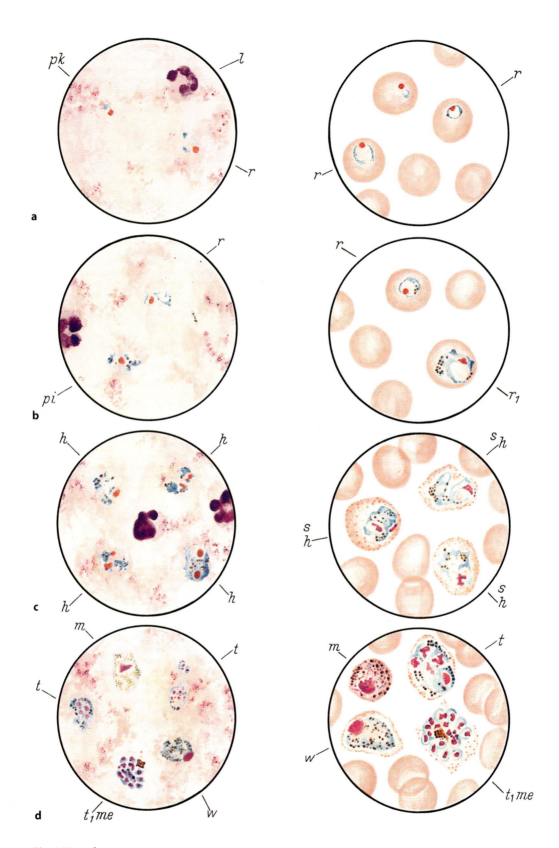

Fig. 182 a–d

Fig. 183 a–d. Quartan malaria (*Plasmodium malariae*), Giemsa stain.

Thick smear

a. *Left*: ring forms (*r*) are more compact than falciparum rings, have red nuclei and blue protoplasm. Leukocyte nucleus (*l*)

b *Left*: band forms (*b*) (a semiadult) and older ring forms (*r*), more compact than in the vivax forms

c *Left*: schizonts (*t*) usually contain 8–12 merozoites (*me*); 16 merozoites are rare

d *Left*: macrogametocyte (*w*, female gametocyte) completely occupies the normal-size erythrocyte; the microgametocyte (*m*, male gametocyte) is smaller than the erythrocyte. Both are smaller than the vivax gametocyte

Thin smear

a *Right*: ring form (*r*) in an unenlarged erythrocyte

b *Right*: band form (*b*) and young schizont (*t*) with pigment and a divided nucleus. No Schüffner dots

c *Right*: schizont (*t*) with 8 merozoites (*me*) and central pigment in an unenlarged erythrocyte

d *Right*: macrogametocyte (*w*) and microgametocyte (*m*). The parasite burden in quartan malaria is the lowest of all the malarias (0.5 % to 1 % of affected erythrocytes)

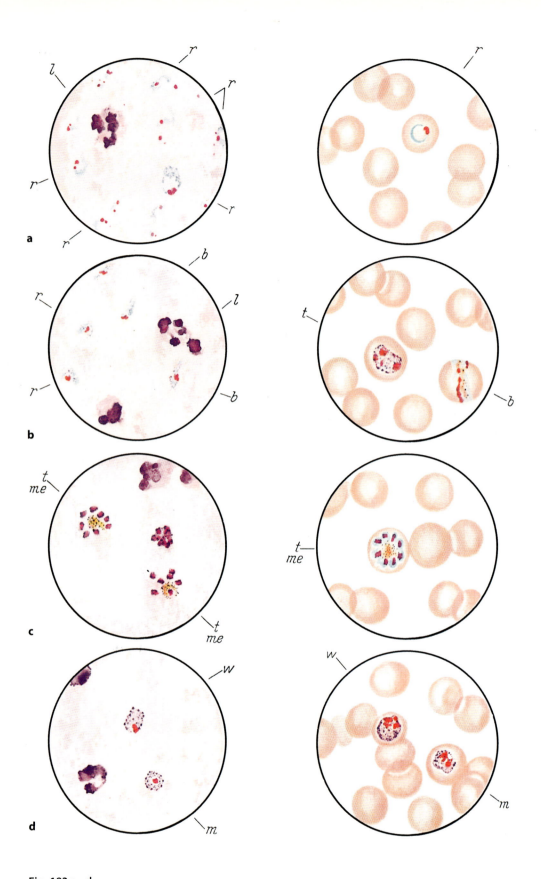

Fig. 183 a – d

Fig. 184 a–d. Malignant tertian malaria (*Plasmodium falciparum* or *P. immaculatum*), Giemsa stain.

Thick smear

a *Left*: numerous ring forms (*r*) with a red nucleus and an adjacent spot of blue protoplasm. The band and segmented neutrophils (*l*) have been distorted by the staining process.

b *Left*: many larger falciparum rings (*r*), some with two nuclei. The parasite burden is highest in malignant tertian malaria (may equal more than 50 % of affected erythrocytes). Remnants of two segmented neutrophils (*l*) are visible in the field.

c *Left*: schizont (*t*) with 8–24 merozoites (*me*), platelets (*thr*), segmented neutrophil (*l*), and lymphocyte remnant (*ly*).

d *Left*: macrogametocyte (*w*) and microgametocyte (*m*), also called crescents, segmented neutrophil (*l*), lymphocyte (*ly*), and cellular debris.

Thin smear

a *Right*: ring forms (*r*) in unenlarged erythrocytes. Infection of one erythrocyte by 2–4 parasites (*r2*) is common. These rings are indistinguishable from young vivax forms!

b *Right*: larger falciparum rings (*r*) in unenlarged erythrocytes, no Schüffner dots.

c *Right*: young schizont (t_1) and mature schizont (t_2) with 24 merozoites.

d *Right*: microgametocyte (*w*) and macrogametocyte (*m*). Remnants of the erythrocyte are still visible around the macrogametocyte, which tends to be longer than the host cell.

The erythrocytes are not enlarged in falciparum malaria, whose early stage is indistinguishable from the three other types of malaria. Therefore the blood examination should be repeated every 12 to 24 h. Falciparum affects all erythrocyte stages, not just the early ones as in vivax malaria

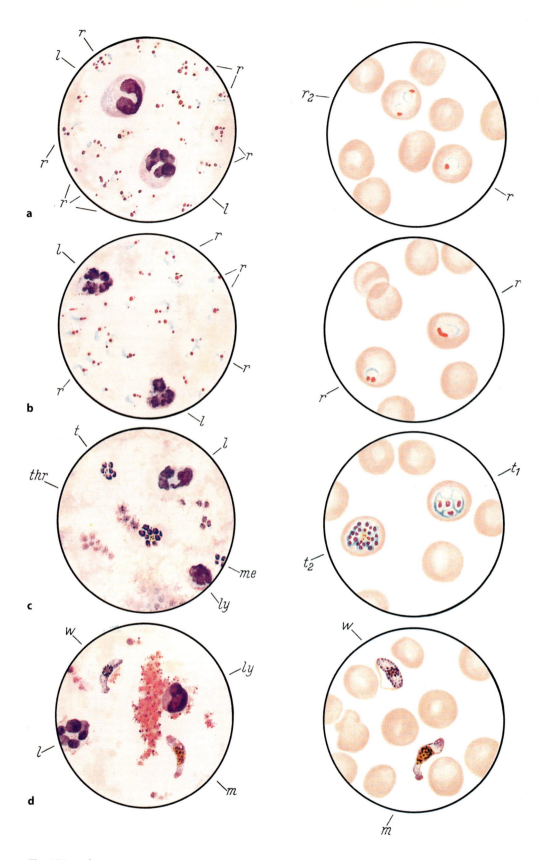

Fig. 184 a–d

Fig. 185 a – d. Malaria

a *Left*: *Plasmodium vivax*: ring form in a slightly enlarged erythrocyte stippled with Schüffner dots

Right: schizont of *P. vivax* in an enlarged erythrocyte

b *Left*: tertian malaria (*P. vivax*): thick smear with large ring forms, segmented neutrophil at *upper left*

Right: young vivax schizonts and several ring forms in a thick smear

c *Left*: *Plasmodium ovale*; ring form in enlarged erythrocytes, which show elliptical distortion and Schüffner stippling

Center and *right*: young schizonts in enlarged, elliptically distorted erythrocytes with conspicuous Schüffner dots

d *Left*: quartan malaria (*Plasmodium malariae*); ring forms in a thick smear (erythrocytes are clumped, not disintegrated!)

Right: thin smear with ring forms and young schizonts in unenlarged erythrocytes

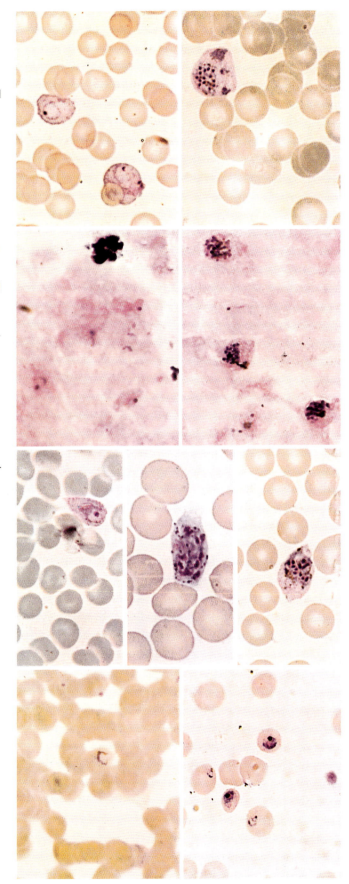

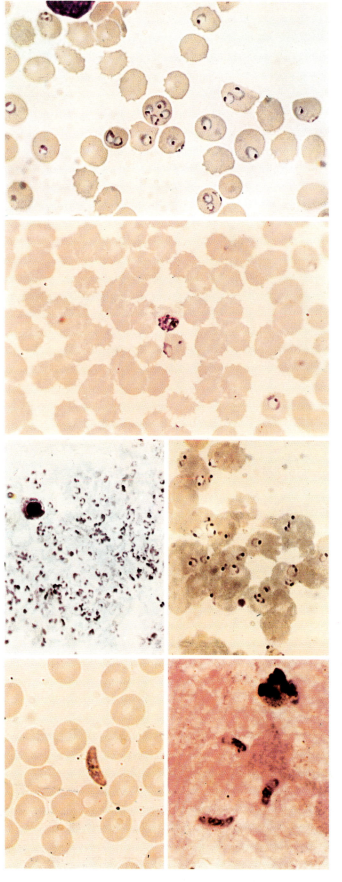

Fig. 186 a – d. Malignant tertian malaria (Plasmodium falciparum)

a Thin smear with numerous rings; some erythrocytes contain 2, 3, or 4 parasites

b Young schizont and ring form in unenlarged erythrocytes

c *Left*: thick smear in falciparum malaria with an extremely heavy parasite burden. Beside the lymphocyte at *upper left*, the field consists entirely of falciparum parasites

Right: thick smear in falciparum malaria

d *Left*: gametocyte in a thin smear

Right: gametocytes in a thick smear

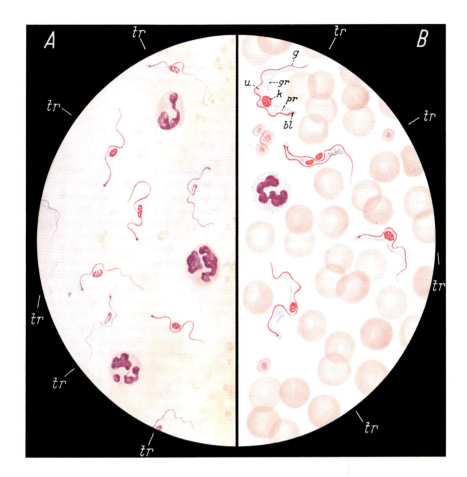

African Trypanosomiasis (Sleeping Sickness)

This is a trypanosomiasis caused by two subspecies of the same species (*Trypanosoma brucei*), which differ in their virulence: *Trypanosoma gambiense*, which occurs chiefly in western Africa and causes protracted illness, and *Trypanosoma rhodesiense*, which is prevalent in eastern Africa and takes a more fulminating course.

The organism is introduced through the bite of the *tsetse fly*. Often a primary focus *(trypanosomal chancre)* develops at the site of inoculation (e.g., on the shoulder, upper arm, or neck), producing central swelling and erythema over an area up to several inches in diameter. The trypanosomes can be detected in aspirates from this area and from the associated regional lymph node.

The second, lymphoglandular phase of the disease is characterized by fever, severe headache, and slight enlargement of the liver and spleen. At this stage the parasites can be detected in *thick and thin blood smears*.

In the final, encephalitic stage of the disease, the trypanosomes invade the central nervous system and can be detected in the *cerebrospinal fluid*.

Fig. 187 a – b. Sleeping sickness (Trypanosoma gambiense), Giemsa stain

A *Thick smear*

Trypanosomes (*tr*) with a red nucleus, which usually is centered red kinetoplasts, and blue protoplasm. The posterior end is usually rounded and contains the micronucleus, which gives rise to the red, whiplike flagellum. The trypanosomes are approximately 13 – 42 µm in length, averaging 20 – 29 µm. They are longer than the erythrocytes. Their shape is pleomorphic, and dividing forms are occasionally seen

B *Thin smear*

Nucleus (k), kinetoplast (bl), flagellum (g), undulating membrane (u), protoplasmic body (pr), dark stained granular inclusions (gr). The kinetoplast is usually rounded or oval

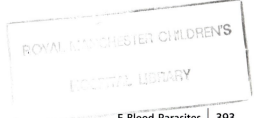

South American Trypanosomiasis (Chagas Disease)

A primary lesion called a *chagoma* forms at the site of inoculation by the *reduviid bug* (triatome). The parasite, *Trypanosoma cruzi*, is introduced not through the bite of the bug but through its infected feces, which are rubbed into the conjunctiva or a break in the skin. The infection spreads rapidly through lymphatic pathways, causing enlargement of the regional nodes. This *oculoglandular syndrome* (Romaña's sign) becomes evident from 4 days to 3 weeks after the infection is acquired.

The disease is particularly life-threatening in infants and small children, as it can progress to a meningoencephalitic form.

The flagellated parasites (Trypanosoma cruzi) can be detected in the blood stream only during the acute febrile phase. Later they are detectable only by animal inoculation and xenodiagnosis (using laboratory-cultivated triatomes). The organisms multiply in an intracellular, nonflagellated form (amastigotic or "leishmanial" form) within the tissue (e.g., the myocardium).

Today serologic methods are also available for the diagnosis of late cases and chronic stages and for identifying *Chagas cardiopathy*. Severe myocardial damage and organ enlargement are late sequelae whose etiology can be established only by serologic procedures.

**Fig. 188. Chagas disease
(Trypanosoma cruzi)**

Blood smear showing *T. cruzi* in the peripheral blood (Giemsa stain). The body of the parasite is stubbier than that of *T. gambiense,* but otherwise its dimensions are much the same: length approximately 20 μm, width 2–3 μm. Typical features are the large nucleus, the large terminal kinetoplast, and the long, usually C-shaped flagellum

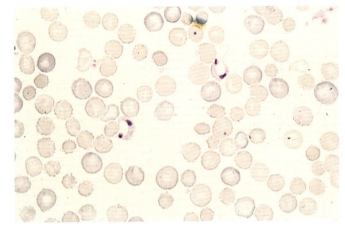

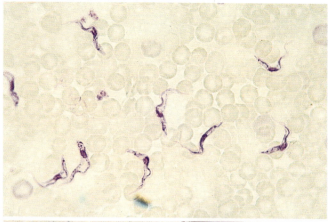

Fig. 189 a, b. Trypanosomes

a *Trypanosoma rhodiense* in a thin blood smear displays a dark red nucleus, blue protoplasm containing darker granules, an undulating membrane, and a flagellum

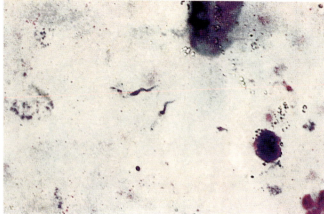

b Thick smear with two parasites at *center*. The general form of the parasite is recognizable, but the fine features of the trypanosome body are not appreciated as clearly as in the thin smear

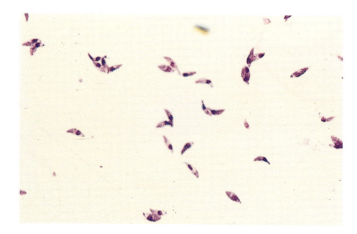

Fig. 190. Toxoplasmosis

Thin smear from the peritoneal exudate of a mouse infected intraperitoneally with *Toxoplasma gondii* shows numerous free organisms shaped like crescents or orange slices with a dark blue nucleus and bluish cytoplasm

Toxoplasmosis

Causative organism: *Toxoplasma gondii*

Infection is usually contracted orally by the ingestion or handling of contaminated food, such as raw meat, or by touching the feces of acutely infected cats, which shed oocytes in the stool. These oocytes are highly resistant and can remain infective for long periods in a moist environment, such as wet soil. The Sabin-Feldman dye test (SFT), indirect immunofluorescence (IIF), and indirect hemagglutination (IHA) test become positive within 6 – 8 days of infection, and the complement fixation text (CFT) becomes positive within 2 – 3 weeks. Recently the enzyme immune test or ELISA assay has been employed to detect toxoplasma infection.

While the CFT becomes negative after a time, the SFT, IHA, and IIF usually remain positive with low titers for the rest of the patient's life, signifying that the infection has entered its latent stage.

Infection must be massive before there is significant lymphadenitis with clinical manifestations such as headache, low-grade fever, and single or multiple lymph node enlargement, particularly in the neck. Involvement of the liver (hepatitis) is occasionally reported.

Severe, generalized forms of the disease are uncommon. Generalized cases with central neurologic involvement and a fatal outcome have recently been observed in patients with AIDS.

The parasite can be detected in the acute stage by animal inoculation or PCR, but the diagnosis is best established by serologic examination of the blood. The histologic examination of an excised lymph node or lymph node aspirate also may be considered.

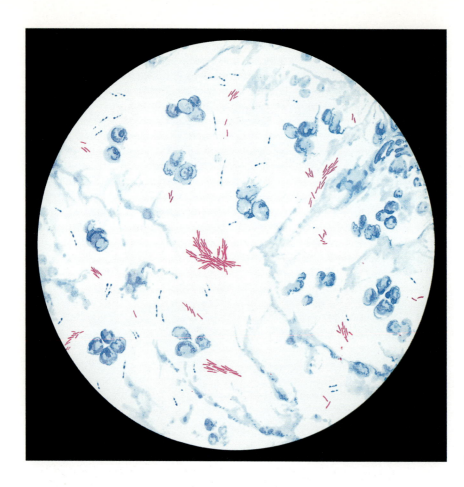

Leprosy

Causative Organism: *Mycobacterium leprae* (Hansen's Bacillus)

The infection is transmitted from person to person and requires prolonged, intimate contact due to the low infectivity of the bacilli. The incubation period is very long (months to years).

The onset of leprosy is insidious. Several forms are recognized:

I. The tuberculoid form develops when resistance to infection is intact. The lepromin test is positive and few bacteria are found.

II. The lepromatous form develops when resistance to infection is impaired (anergic phase). The lepromin test is negative, and bacteria are abundant.

III. The indeterminate form can develop in either direction, i.e., the lepromin test and bacterial count are variable.

IV. The borderline form, in which the lepromin test is usually negative and the bacterial count is usually high.

The natural history of leprosy is marked by periods of activation ("reactions") that commence with chills, fever, and severe malaise. In the wake of this "reaction," new lesions appear due to the dissemination of leprosy bacilli via the blood stream or lymphatic pathways.

Fig. 191. Leprosy (Mycobacterium leprae), Ziehl-Neelsen stain

The leprosy bacillus can be demonstrated in nasal smears or skin biopsies (e.g., from the auricle). Because *M. leprae* is an acid-fast organism, it stains red with Ziehl-Neelsen stain. The bacilli may occur singly or may be grouped into heaps or cigar-shaped clusters. The organisms are 3–4 μm long and 0.4 μm thick.

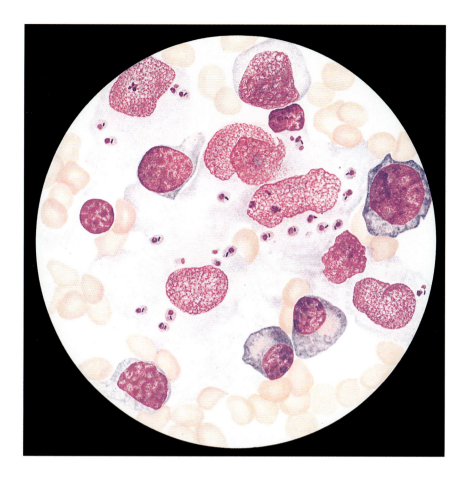

Kala Azar or Visceral Leishmaniasis

Causative Organism: *Leishmania donovani*

The disease is transmitted to humans by blood-sucking sandflies of the genus *Phlebotomus*, with dogs and humans serving as the principal reservoir. The incubation period is highly variable, ranging from days to many months or even years. A nonspecific prodromal stage marked by lethargy and body ache is followed by episodes of fever, often accompanied by chills. In the acute stage, measurements taken at 1 – to 2-h intervals will very often show two fever spikes in a 24-h period.

A very large, hard spleen, a large firm liver, leukocytopenia, thrombocytopenia, and anemia are characteristic. There may also be cardiovascular abnormalities and, without prompt initiation of treatment, permanent myocardial injury. There is reversal of the serum protein ratio with hypergammaglobulinemia, hypoal buminemia.

Fig. 192. Kala azar (Leishmania donovani).

Splenic aspirate contains numerous leishmaniae, most intracellular, with a dark nucleus and rod-shaped kinetoplasts in a pale bluish-red cytoplasm. Some of the organisms are pear-shaped

Fig. 193 a – d. Leishmaniae

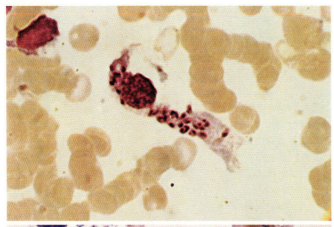

a *Leishmania donovani* in a sternal marrow smear. The numerous parasites are all intracellular

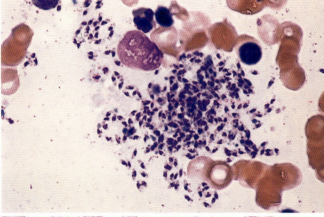

b Sternal marrow smear with extracellular leishmaniae, probably expelled from an infected monocytoid cell that ruptured when the smear was prepared

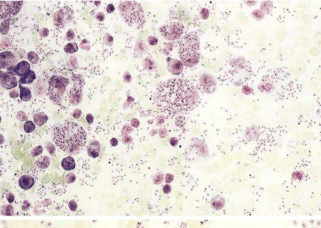

c *L. donovani* in a splenic touch preparation (golden hamster). Macrophages have engulfed massive numbers of the parasites

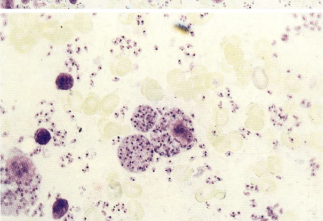

d Free forms in a splenic touch preparation (golden hamster)

Cutaneous Leishmaniasis (Oriental Sore)

Causative Organism: *Leishmania tropica, Leishmania maior*

The disease is transmitted by the bite of the phlebotomus sandfly on unprotected skin. The principal reservoirs are humans (*L. tropica*) and small rodents (*L. maior*). The incubation period ranges from several days to weeks or even months.

Small, red, pruritic papules appear at the site of inoculation and develop into firm nodules. The lesions are most commonly seen on exposed areas of the face (nose, ocular canthi, cheeks, ears) and on unclothed portions of the trunk and limbs. Ulcerating lesions may coexist with nonulcerative lesions that spread to involve adjacent skin areas (*L. recidivans*).

In Central and South America, the causative organisms of cutaneous leishmaniasis are transmitted by flies of the genus *Lutzomyia*. A distinction is drawn between the *L. mexicana* and *L. braziliensis* complexes. Espundia (mucocutaneous leishmaniasis), a malignant form caused by *L. braziliensis*, causes destruction of skin, mucous membranes, and cartilage in the nasopharyngeal region. "Uta," caused by *L. peruviana*, is benign but leads to scarring, especially in the face.

Relapsing Fever

Causative Organisms: *Borrelia recurrentis* (Louse-Borne Relapsing Fever) and *Borrelia duttoni* (Sporadic Tick-Borne Relapsing Fever)

The disease is transmitted by *lice* (*Borrelia recurrentis*, epidemic in Ethiopia central and South America and other countries) or by *ticks* of the genus *Ornithodorus*, for example (endemic in Africa). Following an *incubation period* of 5 to 8 days, the disease begins abruptly with fever up to 40 °C, often accompanied by chills. The fever lasts 3–7 days and is followed by an afebrile period of 2–20 days. The number of relapses is variable. The spleen and liver are enlarged, and there is a propensity for bleeding from the skin and mucosae. The ESR and transaminases are elevated, mild anemia is present, and the leukocyte count is normal.

Fig. 194 a, b. Relapsing fever (Borrelia recurrentis), Giemsa stain.

A Thick smear: *Borrelia* spirochetes (s), leukocyte nucleus (l), cellular debris (z). The spirochetes are appreciably longer than the red cells. Length 15–30 μm with 6–8 turns and pointed ends

B *Borrelia* spirochetes (s) in a thin smear. The sizes of the red cells and spirochetes are easier to compare in this type of preparation

Bartonellosis (Oroya Fever)

Causative Organism: *Bartonella bacilliformis*

This disease is transmitted by female flies of the genus *Lutzomyia*. An animal reservoir has not yet been identified. The flies pick up *B. bacilliformis* when they bite an infected individual and transmit them when they feed again. Bartonella infections occur in the high mountain valleys of the Andes (Ecuador, Peru, and Bolivia). The *incubation period* is from 15 to 100 days.

A clinically nonspecific prodromal stage with remitting or intermittent fever is followed by the development of a severe hypochromic, macrocytic, hemolytic anemia. During this acute stage, which lasts 2–3 weeks, organisms can be detected in the erythrocytes of the peripheral blood. Within several weeks granulomatous skin lesions appear, mainly in exposed areas (verruga peruana). Very massive infections terminate fatally within 10 days.

Fig. 195. Oroya fever (Bartonella bacilliformis), Giemsa stain

Thin blood smear: the bacteria are pleomorphic and stain a bright red in the unenlarged erythrocytes. Most of the organisms are spherical, a few are rod-shaped, and some unite to form small chains. It is typical for several bartonellae to infect one red cell

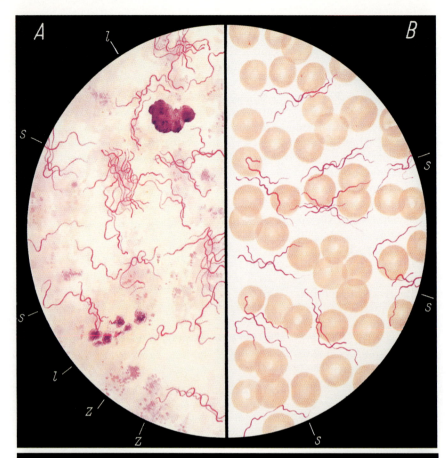

Fig. 194 a, b

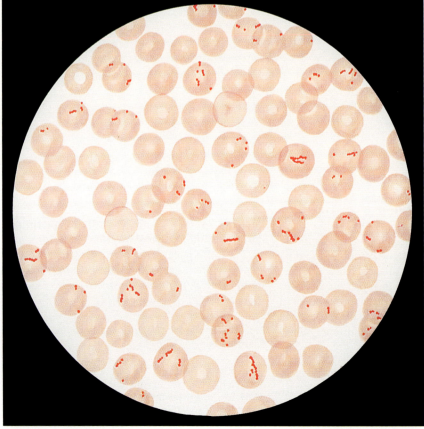

Fig. 195

Mansonella (Dipetalonema) Perstans

Transmission: By biting flies of the genus Culicoides.

Distribution: Western and central Africa and Central America.

This nematode commonly occurs in association with *Loa loa* (**Figs. 197, 199 b, c**) and *Wuchereria bancrofti* (**Figs. 198, 199 d**). The infection is usually innocuous, causing no more than pruritus and transient skin swelling.

Fig. 196. Mansonella perstans, hematoxylin stain.

Thick smears are best for the detection and differential diagnosis of the various microfilariae that occur in the blood (see method on p 19). *M. perstans* microfilariae are 165 – 216 μm long (shorter than the others), slender, and unsheathed. The rows of nuclei extend to the tip of the relatively blunt tail

Filaria Loa Loa

Transmission: By flies of the genus Chrysops. A period ranging from 5 – 6 days to several months passes after inoculation before microfilariae are detectable in the peripheral blood.

Occurrence: Exclusively in the rain forest regions of western and central Africa.

Clinically, severe itching is an early sign and is often accompanied by *Calabar swellings:* tense, circumscribed edematous swellings 1 – 10 cm in diameter with erythema, heat, and moderate pain. The swellings appear on the forearm, face, and occasionally on the trunk and legs. Itching is caused by the migration of the filariae beneath the skin. Migrating filariae can be seen beneath the conjunctiva, where they cause lacrimation and conjunctival irritation. Psychoneurotic

sequelae and severe encephalitic syndromes with microfilariae in the CSF are occasionally observed.

Early diagnosis: The serologic reactions can detect many cases 12 – 18 months before microfilariae appear in the peripheral blood.

Fig. 197. Loa loa, hematoxylin stain.

The *Loa loa* microfilaria is 250 – 300 μm long, larger and thicker than *Mansonella perstans,* with which it often coexists in the blood. Its delicate sheath (*h*) extends past the extremities of the head and tail. The nuclei of the somatic cells are densely arranged and extend to the tip of the tail. This microfilaria occurs in the peripheral blood only in the daytime (hence the old name, *Microfilaria diurna*)

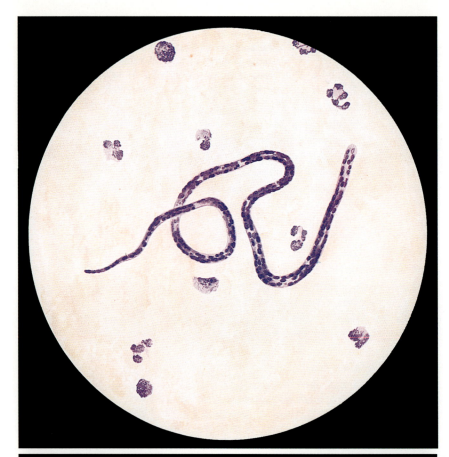

Fig. 196

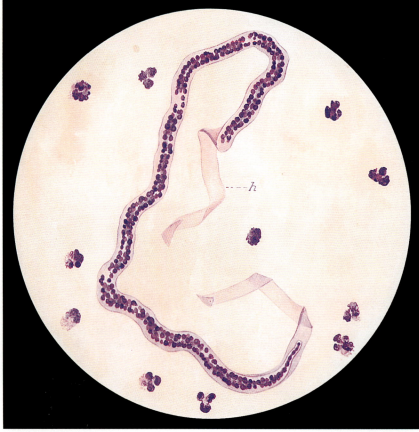

h

Fig. 197

Infections with Wuchereria bancrofti and Brugia malayi

Wuchereria bancrofti and *Brugia malayi* microfilariae are nocturnally active, reaching a peak in the peripheral blood around midnight. A Pacific island subspecies of *W. bancrofti* (var. *pacifica*) does not show this nocturnal periodicity.

Geographic distribution of *W. bancrofti*: Western, central, and eastern Africa, Egypt, Madagascar, Comoro Islands, Central and South America, India, Southeast Asia, Sri Lanka, China, Korea, New Guinea, and the South Sea Islands. *B. malayi is* found in India, Sri Lanka, and Southeast Asia. Both parasites have many features in common. They are found in the lymphatic vessels and in the sinuses of the lymph nodes.

Transmission: By *Anopheles, Culux* and *Aedes* species of mosquitoes.

Initial symptoms appear 3 to 16 months after the infection is acquired and include deafness, limb weakness, and itching in the axilla and groin. Periodic pain in the extremities and testes also occur. Pea- to walnut-sized lymph nodes develop at the base of the thigh, in the axilla, and at the elbow, and lymphangitis develops in the genital region and extremities. A syndromic condition may arise that has been described as "tropical eosinophilia," i.e., a pulmonary filariasis with no detectable microfilariae in the peripheral blood. This form occurs predominantly in Asia.

Late Sequelae: Lymph scrotum, chyluria, and elephantiasis

Very often, serologic reactions become positive approximately 4 to 8 weeks after the infection is acquired. Considerable time passes before microfilariae can be detected in the peripheral blood.

Fig. 198. Wuchereria bancrofti, hematoxylin stain.

The microfilaria of this species is 224 – 296 µm long and sheathed (*h*). The nuclei (*k*) of the somatic cells are loosely arranged and do not extend to the tip of the tail (*s*). The parasites tend to form large, smooth coils in thick smears

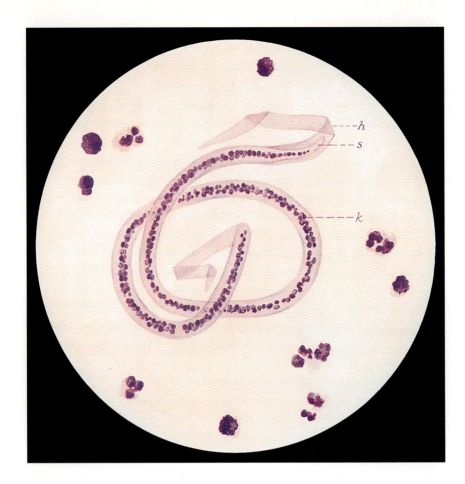

Fig. 198

Fig. 199 a – d. Filariasis

a Microfilaria of *Mansonella perstans*, see also **Fig. 195**

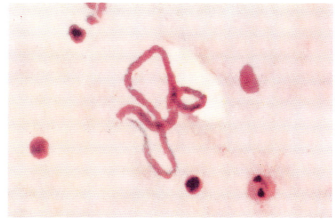

b High-power view of a *Loa loa* microfilaria with granules in the cell body and conspicuous protoplasm (see also **Fig. 197**)

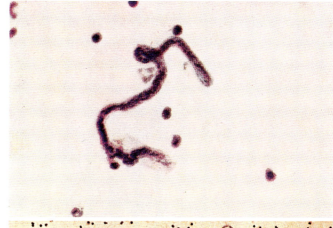

c Low-power view of numerous *Loa loa* microfilariae in a thick smear

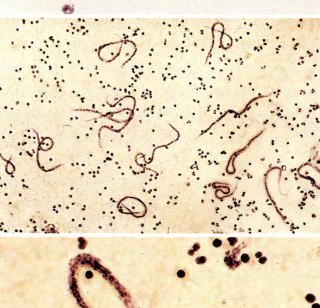

d *Wuchereria bancrofti*, see also **Fig. 198**

Subject Index

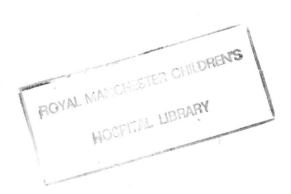

Printing and binding: Druckerei Triltsch, Würzburg

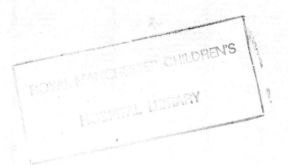